献 辞

谨以此书献给我所有的师长，包括我的父母和弟兄，

尤其是室利 · 室利摩德 · A.C. 巴克提韦丹塔 · 斯瓦米 · 帕布帕德，

是他将印度巴克提瑜伽哲学带给当代世界；

亦献给所有寻求理解此哲学的学人。

Dedication

This book is dedicated to all my teachers (parents and brothers included)

most especially Srī·Srīmad ·A.C. Bhaktivedānta Swami Prabhupāda ,

who has brought Indian philosophy of Bhakti Yoga to the modern world ;

and to all who seek to study this philosophy.

瑜伽哲学经典

Classic of Yoga Philosophy

服务克里希纳

KRISHNA-SEVA

——巴克提瑜伽实践中的传统仪礼

——Traditional Ritual in the Practice of Bhakti Yoga

【美】肯尼斯·R.华培 Kenneth R.Valpey 著

李丹阳 李玉伟 译

云南大学出版社

YUNNAN UNIVERSITY PRESS

【美】肯尼斯·R.华培

Kenneth R.Valpey 著

李丹阳 李玉伟 译

服务克里希纳

KRISHNA-SEVA

——巴克提瑜伽实践中的传统仪礼

——Traditional Ritual in the Practice of Bhakti Yoga

图书在版编目（CIP）数据

服务克里希纳：巴克提瑜伽实践中的传统仪礼 / (美) 肯尼斯·R.华培 (Kenneth R.Valpey) 著；李丹阳，李玉伟译. -- 昆明：云南大学出版社，2018

书名原文：KRISHNA-SEVA:Traditional Ritual in the Practice of Bhakti Yoga

ISBN 978-7-5482-3289-6

Ⅰ.①服… Ⅱ.①肯… ②李… ③李… Ⅲ.①瑜伽—文化—研究 Ⅳ.①R793.51

中国版本图书馆CIP数据核字(2018)第058242号

策划编辑： 万　斌
责任编辑： 万　斌
封面设计： 王婳一
图片摄影： 帕罗姆·托玛内（Param Tomanec）

出版发行： 云南大学出版社
印　　装： 廊坊市海涛印刷有限公司
开　　本： 787mm×1092mm　1/16
印　　张： 18
字　　数： 314千
版　　次： 2018年12月第1版
印　　次： 2018年12月第1次印刷
书　　号： 978-7-5482-3289-6
定　　价： 68.00元

社　　址： 昆明市一二一大街182号
（云南大学东陆校区英华园内）
邮　　编： 650091
电　　话：（0871）65033244　65031071
E-mail： market@ynup.com

若发现本书有印装质量问题，请与印刷厂联系调换，
联系电话：0316-2507000。

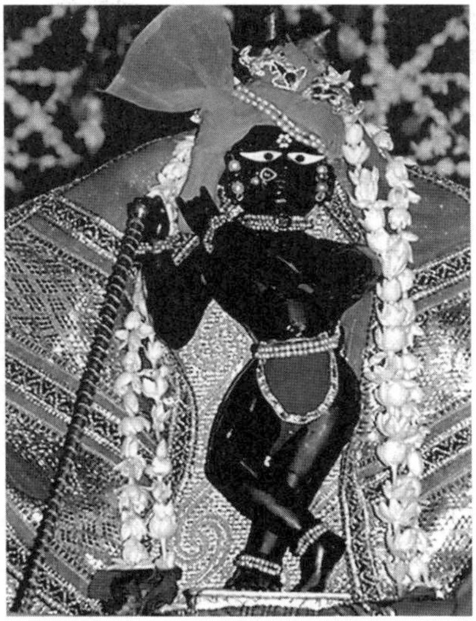

图 1　茹阿达罗曼

克里希纳神像。身着轻薄夏装，佩戴少量装饰品。据说这是一尊“自显的”神像，16 世纪末示现于温达文。

Fig. 1. Rādhāramaṇa—an image of Krishna in minimal summer dress and ornaments. The image is said to be “self-manifest，” having appeared in Vrindavan in the late 16th century.

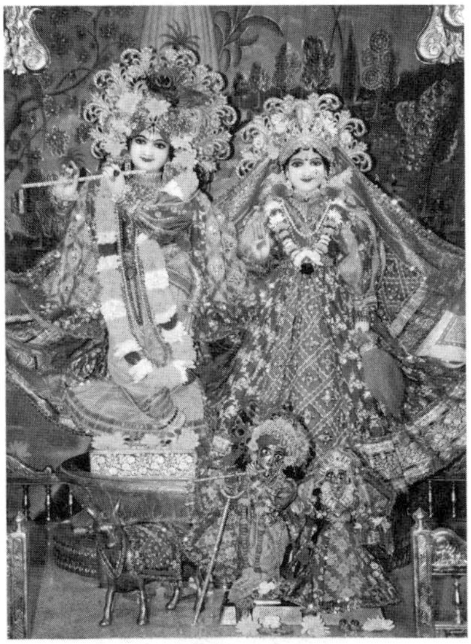

图 2　茹阿达 – 哥库拉南达

茹阿达 – 克里希纳神像。1973 年安设于伦敦附近的巴克提韦丹塔庄园。

Fig. 2. Rādhā-Gokulananda—images of Rādhā and Krishna, established in 1973, at Bhaktivedanta Manor, near London.

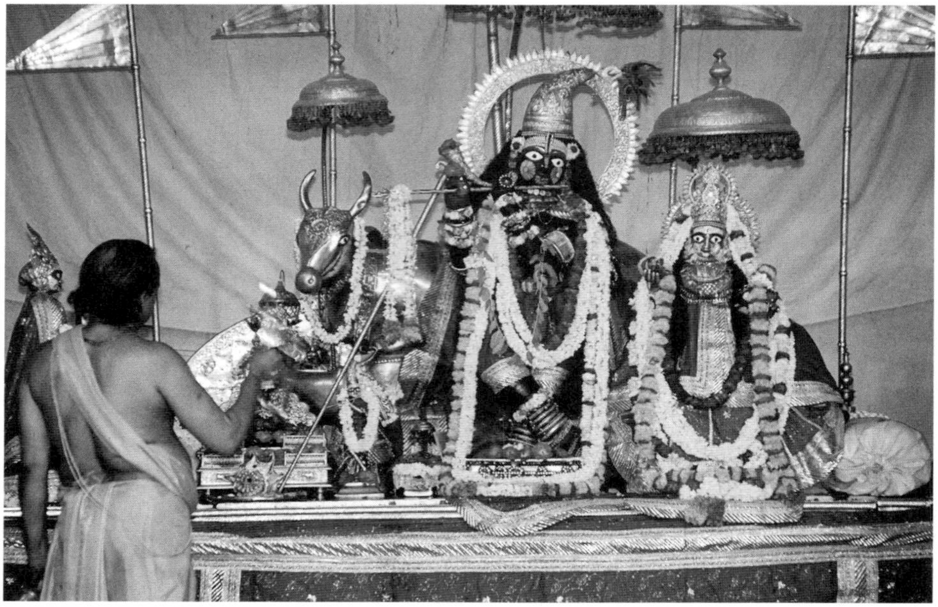

图 3　茹阿达 • 哥文达提婆

茹阿达和克里希纳神像。位于印度拉贾斯坦邦的斋浦尔（皇宫神庙）。如图所示，一位祭司正在做吉祥灯仪（阿尔提）。

Fig. 3. Rādhā-Govindadeva—Images of Rādhā and Krishna in Jaipur（palace temple），Rajasthan，India，with priest offering ārati.

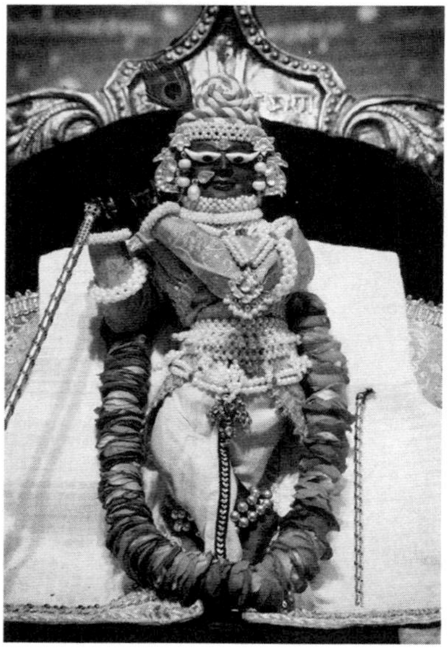

图4　茹阿达罗曼

与图 1 是同一尊神像，不过穿上了冬装，佩戴的饰物也较多。

Fig. 4. Rādhāramaṇa—same as Fig. 1, but wearing winter dress and ornaments.

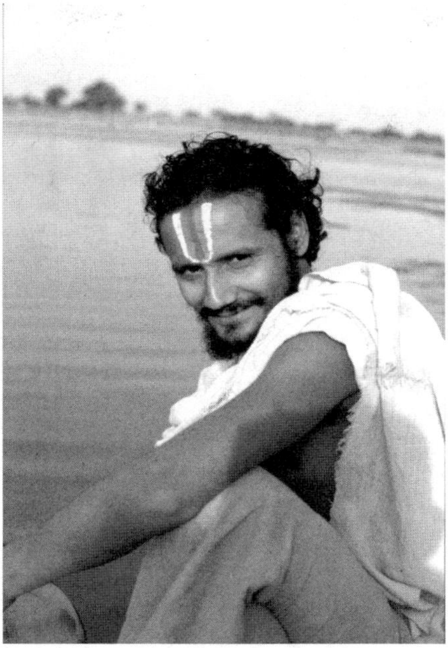

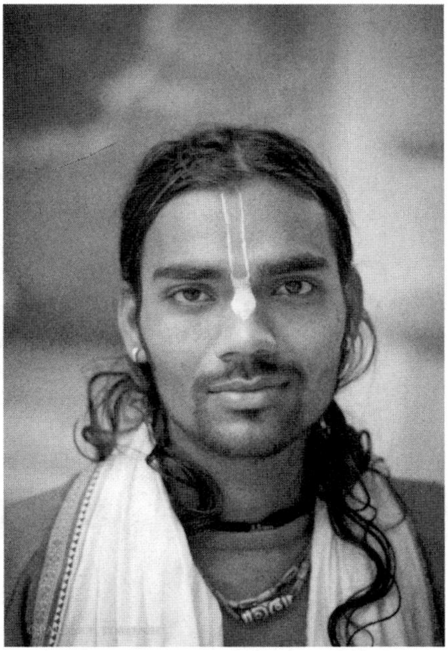

图 5 和图 6　外士那瓦圣人

服务毗湿奴 / 克里希纳的苦行者。额头上的“提拉克”标志，表明他们各自属于两个不同的外士那瓦传统。

Fig. 5. & 6. Vaishnava sādhus (ascetic practitioners of Vishnu/Krishna sevā), wearing “tilak” markings that indicate their affiliation to two different Vaishnava traditions.

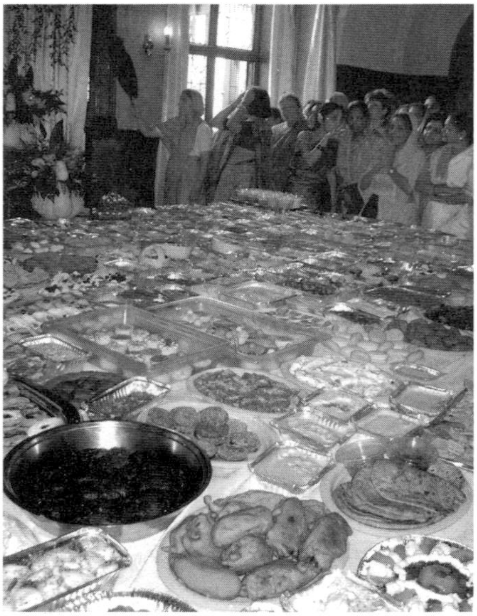

图 7　盛筵供奉

在克里希纳圣诞日（詹玛斯塔米），为供奉仪式烹调大量素食，准备献给克里希纳。

Fig. 7. Vegetarian food preparations, prepared for ritual offering to Krishna, on the occasion of Krishna's birthday celebration (Janmāṣṭami).

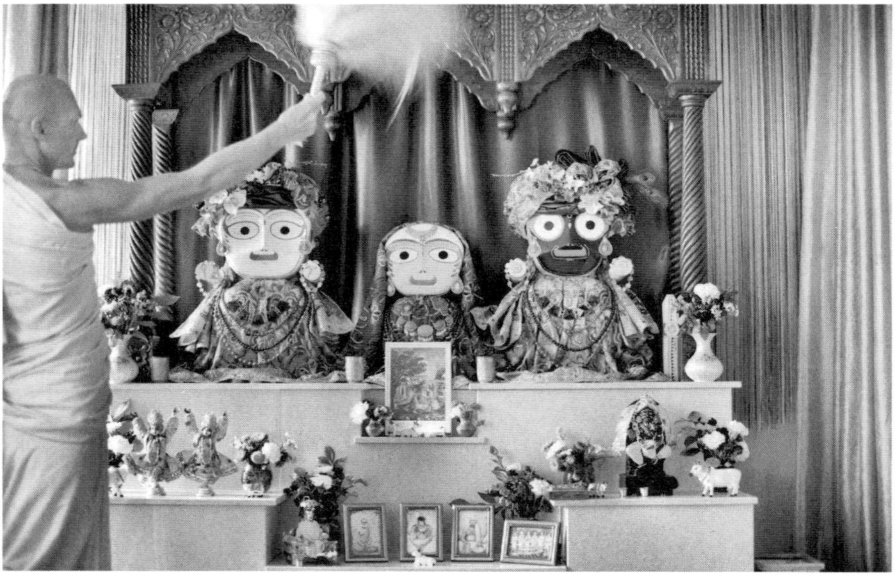

图 8　手持拂尘的祭司

欧洲，克罗地亚。一位祭司正手持拂尘侍奉佳甘纳特（右）、苏巴朵（中）和巴拉提婆（左）。

Fig. 8. Priest waves a fly whisk (chamara) to images of Jagannātha (right), Subhadrā (middle) and Baladeva (left), in Croatia, Europe.

原英文版致谢

本书最初是我在美国加利福尼亚大学伯克利分校联合神学研究院的文科硕士学位论文。所以，我首先要对论文委员会成员表达感激之情，这一课题整个研究与论文的写作过程得到了他们的指导和帮助。我的导师，多明我会的约翰·希拉里·马丁教授，不但帮助我对治学的彻底精神和力求精准的态度有了几分认知；而且他就我的论文本身，耐心地给予了有益的指导，使之呈现“可以见人”的得体模样。德伍德·福斯特教授，出于纯粹的友善和良好的祝愿，同意作为委员会成员参加论文答辩会，可以看出他决心不让退休妨碍自己积极而持续的学术生命。理查德·佩恩教授向我提供了富有真知灼见和启发性的建议，一向是我的鼓励者和支持者。同时，我也非常感谢耶稣会的弗朗西斯·X. 克卢尼教授，在比较神学研究之路上，他给了我颇有价值的指导和鼓励。

我还要由衷感谢鼓励我在神学院从事学习和研究的外士那瓦（毗湿奴派）研究所的诸位学者，特别是霍华德·雷斯尼克博士（H. D. 哥斯瓦米）、威廉·沃尔博士以及罗伯特·科恩。同时，对伯克利新佳甘纳特·普瑞神庙的社区居民，我也要表达感谢之情，因为他们对我表示欢迎，并宽容我为学期间的很少露面。此外，我还要特别感谢我的学生们，他们一直协助我，还为我精心烹饪。这一研究项目要是没有众多外士那瓦社团成员，尤其是欧洲外士那瓦的支持，是不可能完成的。对于他们中的每一个人，我永远表示感谢。

Original Acknowledgements for English Version

As I wrote this originally as a dissertation for the degree of Master of Arts at Graduate Theological Union（Berkeley, California，U. S. A. ）I first want to express my gratitude to the members of my Thesis Committee for their help in guiding me through the process of completing this project. My Advisor, Professor John Hilary Martin，O. P. ，has helped me gain some understanding of thoroughness and precision in scholarship，and he has patiently rendered helpful guidance to bring this work into presentable form. Professor Durwood Foster，out of pure kindness and well-wishing spirit，has agreed to be on this committee as part of his determination not to let retirement stand in the way of continued active academic life. Professor Richard Payne has provided helpful insights and suggestions and has been a source of encouragement and support. I am also very grateful to Professor Francis X. Clooney, S. J. ，who has given me valuable guidance and encouragement on the path of comparative theology.

I wish to sincerely thank the members of the Institute of Vaiṣṇava Studies for encouraging me to take up study at the Graduate Theological

Union, especially Dr. Howard Resnick (H. D. Goswami), Dr. William Wall and Robert Cohen. I am also grateful to the residents of the New Jagannatha Puri Temple community in Berkeley for extending their welcome and tolerating my minimal participatory presence during my studies. I have to especially thank my own students for their constant assistance and excellent cooking. This project would not have been possible for me to execute without the generous financial assistants of numerous members of the Vaiṣṇava community, especially in Europe, to each of whom I am ever grateful.

中文版序

我第一次访问中国是在 25 年以前。记得当时广州的大街小巷有无数人在骑自行车。如今，多年过去了，自行车已然被汽车取代。我们现代的世界，变化何其迅速！何止广州！何止中国！放眼看去，整个亚洲正经历着巨大的变化，其步伐之快或许足以使我们忘却了层层文化和文明的历史积淀。而正是在那层层积淀之上，我们如今所见闻和所经历的一切才得以建树。自 1978 年以来，我一直定期拜访印度，那里也发生着同样的事。中国和印度都有着世界上主要的古老文明。然而，两国各自经历的“变化”之强风令其博大精深、辉煌荣耀的文化以及几千年来生生不息的文明变得面目模糊、难以辨认。

当我花费大量时间在印度探索那块土地上的智慧传统时，这些传统当中的一个方面渐渐浮出水面，令我特别感兴趣，恰恰就是因为在当今的印度依然能够强烈感受到它的存在。然而，尽管今天这传统还清晰可见，但很多人，甚至连印度本土人都对他们自己的这部分传统不甚理解。鉴于此，我把自己的研究成果写成《服务克里希纳：巴克提瑜伽实践中的传统仪礼》一书，作为一个小小的尝试，希望藉此“打开”这个人们知之甚少却又颇为重要的文化实践之包裹，以飨那些对印度人生活和思想方式完全陌生的读者。

我在中国的许多朋友鼓励我将这本书以中文出版。他们说，这样不仅有助于理解和欣赏这一古老的印度传统，而且可以间接激发中文读者，增益对其自身仪礼传统的欣赏和珍视。中国传统仪礼文化或许在某些方面与印度传统存在共鸣的因素。中国和印度是邻居，有着重要的文化联系。我希望拙著在增进两国跨文化理解与欣赏方面贡献绵薄之力。我们决定将这本书做成英汉双语学术读物，以鼓励那些懂英语、想要读原文的读者，或许可以借此机会丰富他们的英语知识，同时，也可了解某些具有一定难度的概念是如何译成中文的。

非常感谢所有在本书翻译、出版过程中给予帮助的朋友们，尤其要感谢云南大学出版社的全体员工，是他们的辛勤工作才促成了本书的出版问世。

——肯尼斯·R. 华培，英国牛津大学印度学、动物伦理学研究中心

Preface for Chinese Version

The first time I visited China was more than twenty-five years ago. I remember seeing the streets of Guangzhou filled with countless bicyclers. Now, a few years later, the bicycles have been replaced by automobiles. How quickly our modern world is changing! And all this is happening throughout Asia, at a pace that might lead us to forget the many layers of culture and civilization upon which what we see and experience today has been built. The same is true in India, where I have been regularly visiting since 1978. Both China and India are major ancient cultures of the world, and in both countries the strong winds of change have made it difficult to discern the great and glorious depths of the cultures that have carried these civilizations through the ages.

As I have spent much time in India exploring the wisdom traditions of that land, one aspect of these traditions emerged as of particular interest to me, precisely because its presence is strongly felt in present-day India. Yet although it is a very visible tradition today, still, many people even within India have lost their understanding of this aspect of their own tradition. *KRISHNA-SEVA*: *Traditional Ritual in the Practice of Bhakti Yoga* is a small attempt to "unpack" this little understood yet important cultural practice for people completely unfamiliar with Indian ways of life and thought.

Many friends in China have encouraged me to bring out this study in Chinese, as they say it can serve to gain an appreciation not only of this aspect of ancient Indian tradition, but also indirectly it can inspire Chinese readers to have greater appreciation of their own traditions of ritual, some of which may resonate with aspects of the Indian tradition. As China and India are neighbors with important cultural connections, my hope is that this book may serve as one small contribution toward an increase of cross-cultural understanding and appreciation. We decided to make this a dual-language book–English/Chinese–to encourage those Chinese readers who know English and would like to see the original (possibly to improve their English knowledge, or to see how certain fairly difficult concepts have been translated).

I am most grateful to all my friends who have helped in the translation and production of this publication, and I am especially grateful to the staff of Yunnan University Press for facilitating its publication.

——Kenneth R. Valpey, Oxford Centre for Hindu Studies and Animal Ethics, Oxford University, U. K.

梵语发音指南

针对书中提到的一些梵文词汇，给出些许发音上的指导，可能会对读者有帮助。本书梵文和孟加拉文的拉丁转写方法，采用的是学术性出版物的标准体系。大体上，元音字母发音通常和意大利语中的元音字母发音类似，上面带一横线的，表明其音长是不带横线的元音的两倍（如“ā”的发音是“a”的两倍长）。字母“c”的发音通常与英文中的“ch”相同。“ś”的发音和德语单词 *sprechen* 中的“s”一致。“ṣ”按照英语单词 *shine* 中的第一个辅音音素（[ʃ]）来发音。*visargaḥ* 中的 ḥ，表示需稍微重复一下它前面的元音，因此 *visargaḥ* 读作“visargaha”。*anusvāraṁ*（*ṅ*）中的 ṁ 或 ṅ，表示发完它们前面的元音之后是一个鼻音，就像英语中的“ng”，都是用鼻腔发音。送气辅音“th”，与英语单词“ho*th*ouse”中的双辅音“th”发音相同。其他送气辅音按照英语中相应的双辅音发音即可。

Pronunciation Guide

This book makes reference to several terms in Sanskrit, for which a minimal guideline on pronunciation may be helpful. The system of transliteration of Sanskrit and Bengali used in this work is a standard system in scholarly publication. Briefly (and roughly), the vowels generally are pronounced as in Italian, with a line over the vowel indicating twice the length of pronunciation of those without ("ā" =aa). The letter "c" is always pronounced as "ch" in English; "ś" is as in the German word *sprechen*, "ṣ" is as in the English word *shine*. The *visarga* (ḥ) indicates a slight repetition of the vowel immediately before it. Thus *visargaḥ* would be pronounced "visargaha." The *anusvāra* (ṁ or ṅ), indicates a nasalization of the vowel before it, roughly equivalent to the English "ng". The aspirate consonant "th" is pronounced as in the double consonant in "ho*th*ouse". Other aspirated consonants follow the same principle.

目　录
Contents

导　言

起源于印度的种种瑜伽传统，构成了一幅辽阔的图景，其中最为显著、突出的是巴克提（虔爱）瑜伽。公元 16 世纪，这种瑜伽形式在一位颇富感召力的年轻圣哲室利·柴坦尼亚的推广下发扬光大。他在印度各地游历，凡其所见之人，不论学者白丁，不论富者贫者，都勉励他们练习一种简单的“哈瑞克里希纳－摩诃曼陀罗”①冥想。近年来，巴克提瑜伽更为广泛地在社会上普及起来，乃至流行音乐家们以百老汇音乐剧《长发》为开端，录制了数场瑜伽唱诵音乐专辑。②与这种曼陀罗冥想形式相比，不为人熟知且不为大多数人所理解的是，各冥想中心在进行同样的吟唱时，还伴有每日精心服务神像的复杂程序，作为巴克提瑜伽——灵性奉爱的规范修习（*vaidhi-bhakti-sādhana*，外迪－巴克提－萨达纳）中不可或缺的一个要素。这一程序亦称为外士那瓦宗的毗湿奴崇拜（Vaiṣṇavism），即参与到和“毗湿奴”这一名字密切关联的终极宇宙秩序的文化体系中。为了有助于理解巴克提的灵性原则，本书尝试呈现高迪亚－外士那瓦（Gauḍīya Vaiṣṇava）的神学理论与见地，③因为这与巴克提瑜伽实践中的传统仪礼——“服务神像”直接相关。“服务神圣形象”，是通过看得见的形体、相貌来理解神圣性的一种途径。对于神圣的听觉形式——圣名“哈瑞纳玛”（*harināma*），神像以视

---

① 参见《梵文和孟加拉文转写发音指南》，第 4 页。

② 盖伊·L. 贝克：《搅拌寰球甘露之洋：圣帕布帕德的奉爱音乐》，《毗湿奴派研究期刊》第 6 卷，1998 年春，第 2 期，第 133~135 页。此音乐剧于 1968 年 4 月在美国纽约百老汇首演。

③ 或许引用理查德·戴维斯的表述更精确一些，他说：“命题的矩阵，构成了外士那瓦对仪式进行概念化并将其付诸实践的世界。”理查德·H. 戴维斯：《振荡宇宙内的仪式：中世纪印度的湿婆崇拜》，新泽西，普林斯顿：普林斯顿大学出版社，1991 年，第 22 页。

觉形式给予补充，使之完美无缺。这一点尤为起源于印度东北孟加拉的毗湿奴派所认可。

关于高迪亚（孟加拉）外士那瓦宗[①]的历史，已有相当数量的英文论著出版问世，研究的主题也涉及若干方面。[②]然而，就高迪亚传统中服务神像的理论体系，在以往研究中却鲜有涉猎。而且，也未发现以比较神学为视角作出的有意义的尝试——将高迪亚－外士那瓦神像崇拜理论与可能存在的反对或质疑，特别是犹太－基督教传统所表述的观点，进行比较性研究。在庙宇和居士家中服务克里希纳神像，正日益成为世界各地的冥想和瑜伽景观中的一部分。但由于很多人士对这一传统并不熟悉，自然会认为它是陌生的、怪异的，甚至是危险的、邪恶的。因此，有必要对服务神像（*mūrti-sevā*）的神学理论予以关注和研究，以便理解和鉴赏这一宗教现象。尤其是印度人越来越多地移居世界各地，这一传统也随之不断流传到世界各个角落，故而需要对服务神像传统进行更深层次的解读。基于此，本书将主要探讨以下神学核心议题：根据高迪亚－外士那瓦神学理论，一个显然毫无生气的物质形体，在何种意义上被视为神圣并因而受到尊崇？这种正式的神像崇拜（*arcanam*）[③]实践，在哪些方面被认为是解决了接近至尊者或为至尊者所接近的问题？上述问题的答案在于化身（*avatāra*，神圣降临）理论与奉爱实践之间的相互关联性。其中，最为关键的是，吠檀多毗湿奴教派柴坦尼亚支派

---

① 要理解“外士那瓦宗（Vaiṣṇavism）”这一术语，首先需了解 Vaiṣṇava 的由来。“Vaiṣṇava（音译外士那瓦，意译毗湿奴派。文中根据行文需要采取这两种译法——译者注）”从“Viṣṇu（毗湿奴）”衍生而来。“毗湿奴”，是“薄伽梵”，即“神”的主要名字。一般而言，毗湿奴派与湿婆派，即将湿婆视为至尊的崇拜者，形成对比。尽管高迪亚－外士那瓦们（Gauḍīya Vaiṣṇavas）崇拜毗湿奴，但他们清楚毗湿奴不过是克里希纳的一个扩展。故在其传统中，占中心地位的是克里希纳，而非毗湿奴。高迪亚－外士那瓦（Gauḍīya Vaiṣṇava）亦称为：毗湿奴派孟加拉支派，或毗湿奴派柴坦尼亚支派（文中一般采取音译，即“高迪亚－外士那瓦”——译者注）。

② 关于在孟加拉的孟加拉语外士那瓦宗的全面研究文献，参见拉胡·彼得·达斯所撰《关于孟加拉语外士那瓦宗的最新论著》，作为其中一章，收录于《孟加拉外士那瓦宗研究论文集》，加尔各答：福尔摩出版公司，1997 年。要了解外士那瓦宗在西方兴起的历史和现状的研究成果，特别是国际克里希纳意识协会，请参见查理斯·R. 布鲁克斯、斯蒂尔森·犹大、金·诺特、伯克·罗齐福特和拉里·希恩及其他学者的著作。

③ *Arcanam* 发音为“阿尔查拿摩”，与意为“秘密”或“神秘知识”的拉丁词汇没有明显的词源关系。

所持的“不可思议即一即异论”（*acintya-bhedābheda-tattva-vāda*）或称“不可思议不一不异论”，即至高无上者与多样性的生物之间不可思议地既同一又有差异的理论。

由于实践是高迪亚－外士那瓦神像崇拜理论的核心，所以我会就每日神像崇拜中某些特定仪式程序给予简要论述，譬如，为神像沐浴、更衣和装扮，供奉食物，在神像前挥动油灯，吟诵曼陀罗等。但是，因为其中诸多细节，呈现出与南亚其他神像崇拜实践的相似之处，故而，直接关注高迪亚－外士那瓦宗化身理论的独特性颇具意义。在檀车节（*Jagannātha-Rathayātrā*）这样一个特定节日的诸多方面，以及记载克里希那的虔爱者所达到的造诣与境界的经典中，这些独特性得到彰显。这里所说的“檀车节”，乃是公众拖动“宇宙之主”的檀车进行巡游的庆典。

本书以我在印度诸多神庙和圣地所从事的长期田野调查为基础，主要运用神学阐释[①]与比较神学的研究方法，力图呈现高迪亚传统中的神像崇拜是由虔爱者（*bhakta*）与克里希纳（**Krishna**）之间的动态关系来维系这一原理，而通过巴克提实践，虔爱者体验到克里希纳临在于神像中。以“功能性”视角来看，神像崇拜实践作为高迪亚－外士那瓦宗正式仪轨的焦点，可被理解为是一种将即时性的直接体验感融入巴克提核心思想的方式。“巴克提”这个词表示一种持久不衰、转化内在的虔信奉爱心态，以对至高神圣者的积极主动的服务为特征。高迪亚－外士那瓦传统认为，这里所说的“至高神圣者”，即是以其最为圆满的品质所示现的克里希纳。巴克提的这种即时性，在“克里希纳－塞瓦”（**Krishna**-*sevā*），即“（直接）服务克里希纳”这一表述中有所揭示。服务克里希纳至关重要的核心理念是，出于持久不变的热情，以指定的崇拜程序为依据，积极主动地服务。对于这样的奉献者，至尊者让自己变得容易接近和触及。而在这一互动中，绵密稳定（持续而不间断）的热情，或许是整个崇拜仪式程序中最为突出的特色。

我使用“功能性”这一词汇，是颇为慎重的。因为它可能会使读者对

---

① 保罗·格里菲思指出，在宗教学领域的学术研究中，“教义的义理研究”呈衰落之势，让位于以社会学、政治学、历史学和哲学语境对教义的分析。格里菲思在其著作《论成佛》一书中提出“旨在使恰如其分的义理研究成为可能”的理论。保罗·J. 格里菲思：《论成佛：佛果的经典教义》，纽约，奥尔巴尼：纽约州立大学出版社，1994 年，第 2 页。我采用的研究方法，并未强求与其方法完全一致，但其“精神”或许类似。

正在讨论的主题抱有一种简化论的观点。而这完全有违我的初衷。更确切地说，本书研究的根本旨趣在于，探讨被认为是克里希纳－巴克提的超验领域，与克里希纳－巴克提实践必然被展示其中的偶然世界间的动态交流。在这一语境中，既然具体有形的形象被实践者理解为，至高者依据“关系”所展现的终极实相，那么，以“神像崇拜”为研究对象再恰当不过了。这里所说的“至高者”，梵文称之为“薄伽梵”（*bhagavān*），是至高无上的人，被认为是最高我（*paramātmā*，赋予万物以生机的本体意义上的“大我”）与梵（*brahman*，被视为非二元性的绝对存在）的绝对源头。公元 16 世纪高迪亚－外士那瓦主要学者之一茹帕·哥斯瓦米（Rūpa Gosvāmī），将“薄伽梵”定义为“至尊人”，即“那个拥有无限灵性关系之甘露（*rasāmṛta*）的特有形象”[①]。梵文术语“茹阿萨”（*rasa*，原意为液体、审美/品味、精华），自古以来，在印度美学话语中占据主导地位，体现了高迪亚－外士那瓦理论的核心关怀。神像崇拜的终极目标是依据某种特定的爱的交流方式，参与到与克里希纳的一种永恒关系当中。可见茹阿萨理论与神像崇拜有关，是以，有必要对这一理论进行简要讨论。此外，与神像崇拜相关联的还有外迪－萨达纳－巴克提（*vaidhi-sādhana-bhakti*）的实践，其特点是以遵守规范原则为主，神秘性较少。这一层面的神像崇拜实践，以不断获取灵性晋阶为导向；通过参照大量被公认为擅长与克里希纳进行情感（*rasa*）交流，并因而被视为处于灵性进程中最高层面的虔爱者（*bhaktas*）崇拜神像的故事，使自身的实践在持续稳定中不断丰富和发展。

本书篇章结构如下：首先简略探讨高迪亚－外士那瓦的认识论。然后，根据吠檀多哲学所构想的“不可思议即一即异论”，简要呈现这一传统的化身理论。接下来阐释巴克提理论的基本原理，以及萨达纳（*sādhana*，规范练习）的概念，并考察声音和形象是如何相互关联，以使有情众生在灵性上获得提升。第三章主要关注的是茹阿萨（*rasa*）理论以及擅长与神像发展关系、品味神圣情感的圣人们的经验。

第四章，“外士那瓦（Vaiṣṇavas，毗湿奴派信徒）是偶像崇拜者吗？”旨在比较神学研究。借这一研究方法，将高迪亚－外士那瓦宗的克里希纳－

---

① 《奉爱甘露之洋》第 1 篇第 1 章第 1 节。

巴克提传统神像崇拜理论，与亚伯拉罕诸教所持的对神像崇拜的异议并列起来，进行比较性研究。关注的焦点再次回到巴克提的本质上。认为巴克提是终极的灵性方法与程序，引向并最终带来普瑞玛——对至尊人克里希纳“从心所欲而不逾矩”的爱。

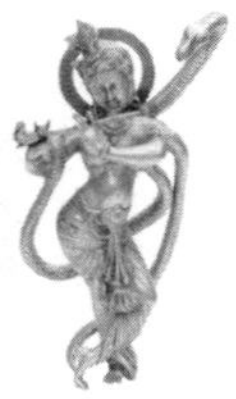

第一章 神圣降临的理论

啊，宇宙之魂！这当然令人困惑：你虽无为，却无不为；你虽是生命力，不经出生就存在，却诞生在这尘世。你本人降生在动物、人类、圣哲和水生物当中。这一切实在让人困惑不已。

——《薄伽梵往世书》1. 8. 30[①]

第一节 知识的源头

要理解任何一个印度传统中的神像崇拜理论体系，而不仅仅限于高迪亚－外士那瓦传统，需要进入浩如烟海的吠陀相关文献。这一系列古老的梵语文本被所有印度传统视为阿袍茹赛亚（apauruṣeya），即并非出自人类之创作，而是天启圣典。无须拘泥于众多注解原初《吠陀经》的复杂的文本，在此，或许读者只需注意，在这些导致迥然相异之结论的哲学或神学著作背后，认识论一向是首要的关注点，尤其在力求系统阐释诸《奥义书》文本所

① 除非特别注明，本书引用的《薄伽梵往世书》《薄伽梵歌》《柴坦尼亚生平甘露》中所有译文，皆出自 A. C. 巴克提韦丹塔·斯瓦米·帕布帕德的译著。他是柴坦尼亚·摩诃帕布以降的高迪亚－外士那瓦师徒传承中的一位导师，梵文学者，20 世纪杰出的外士那瓦（毗湿奴派）巴克提传统的倡导者。我不时会提供某个词或短语的另外一种看起来更贴切或更加忠实于原文的翻译，或在括号内加入某个英文词汇或短语所对应的梵文。此外，我还会在脚注中列出每段译文的梵文拉丁转写。帕布帕德翻译《圣典薄伽瓦谭》（又名《薄伽梵往世书》）所用的版本是克里希纳·桑卡尔·萨斯垂编辑的《室利摩德－巴嘎瓦塔－摩诃普然纳》，印度，艾哈迈达巴德：室利－巴嘎瓦塔－维迪亚琵塔出版社，初版日期不详，现存本为 1968 年版。

构成的吠檀多语境中。[①]

我们所关注的这一脉络的神学传统和反思，在六哥斯瓦米的著作中有详尽阐释。作为室利·柴坦尼亚·摩诃帕布[②]的弟子，他们受其导师委托，汇编整理既有文献中有关灵性奉爱的教导，使之系统化，并基于个人洞见加以详尽注释（而柴坦尼亚·摩诃帕布本人著述不多，只留下了以八个诗节概括其教导的《八训规》）。六哥斯瓦米中的吉瓦·哥斯瓦米[③]经与同游磋商，撰写了高迪亚－外士那瓦最为全面的神学注释《六论》。《真理论》为其第一篇，其中专门探讨了认识论的问题。

吉瓦在开始正文之前，为了确立高迪亚－外士那瓦宗特定文献的核心地位，表达了自己对吠陀天启的信心：

> 人类必然有四种缺陷：易受错觉迷惑；会犯错误；有欺骗的倾向；有着不完美的感官。因此，他们的直接察知及推理等都是有缺陷的。既然上述获取知识的手段并不能帮助他们接近不可思议的灵性实相，那么，对于好奇爱问的我们来说，想要了解超越于万物而又撑持万物——寰宇之中最不可思议和令人称奇的那一位，直接的察知、推理等都不是获取知识的恰当手段。有鉴于此，唯一适合的方法当是吠陀文献——自太初以来就存在的超验文字。作为一切世俗知识与灵性知识的起源，吠陀文献经由师徒体系世代传承下来。[④]

通过这段话，吉瓦·哥斯瓦米告诉读者，不必花费力气确认吠陀文献的

① 《奥义书》是一部哲学典籍汇编。有学者认为其约成书于公元前800年至公元200年之间。霍尔德里奇、芭芭拉·A:《吠陀经与摩西五经：超越经典之文本性》，纽约，奥尔巴尼：纽约州立大学出版社，1996年，第449页脚注。

② “摩诃帕布”是一个尊称，字面意思是“伟大的导师”。

③ 另外五位哥斯瓦米分别是：茹帕、萨纳坦、哥帕拉·巴塔、拉古纳特·巴塔、拉古纳特·达斯。

④ 萨提亚·那罗延·达斯：《圣吉瓦·哥斯瓦米·帕布帕德的〈神圣真理六论〉》，德里：吉瓦毗湿奴派研究学院，1995年，第18、27页。

权威性。与其他的知识来源相比，这是绝对可靠、毫无谬误的真理之源。[①] 然后吉瓦的思路迅速跳离原初《吠陀经》，转而斟酌相关文本——《宇宙古史》。他运用淘汰法，通过核对经文谨慎支撑自己的判断，最后确定一部特别的文献——《薄伽梵往世书》（亦称为《圣典薄伽瓦谭》或《宇宙古史——薄伽梵之部》）[②] 为天启圣典。他认为这部经典是最根本、最清晰易懂、最为恰当[③]、最具权威的。包括非婆罗门在内[④]，人人都可亲近此经典。关于《薄伽梵往世书》的作者等问题，吉瓦·哥斯瓦米经考证认为，

---

① 由吠陀证言所产生的认识论（*pramāṇas*，量），其权威性为中世纪印度六大正统哲学流派（印度六派哲学）所公认，每一流派都接受两种或两种以上的“量”（*pramāṇas*），从属和支持吠陀的地位。吉瓦·哥斯瓦米以及后来的巴拉提婆·维迪亚布善都认可，直接察知（*pratyakṣa*，现量）及由类推得来的知识（*anumāna*，比量），包含所有其他被公认为权威的量，而且，只要能给平凡的生命以启迪，也被视为从属并支持吠陀（*śabda-pramāṇas*，圣言量）。或许有人记得托马斯·阿奎那就知识与信念所作的区分：那不可能自动为人所知的事物属于信仰的领域，属于某种天启的教义信条。而吠陀文献及其推论描述的是超凡之人的体验。18 世纪高迪亚 – 外士那瓦评论家巴拉提婆·维迪亚布善追随所有声名卓著的外士那瓦评论家以及商羯罗，将《吠陀经》（*śruti*——《天启经》，“耳闻得来”）视为直接经验（*pratyakṣa*，现量），由吠陀得出的推论（*smṛti*——《圣传经》，“由记忆得来”，口耳相传的）为间接推理（*anumāna*，比量）。参见苏德什·纳朗《巴拉提婆·维迪亚布善的外士那瓦哲学》，德里：纳格出版社，1984 年，第 30~42 页。盖伊·L. 贝克观察到：“诚然，西方意义上的理智，或称理性思维在印度人思想中占有重要而独特的位置。然而在天启圣典面前，则退居次位了。吠陀乃天启圣典，因而是‘非理性’和超自然的。从某种角度来看，它构成印度人一切真理的基础。”印度思想中理性的运用（即严格意义上的印度哲学），由此限于将人类经验及经验观察与启示圣典相调和的努力上面。参见盖伊·L. 贝克：《声音的神学：印度教与神圣音振》，德里：莫提拉·班那西达斯出版公司，1995 年，第 10~11 页。虽然吉腾德拉·莫汉蒂认为圣言量（启示的证言）优越性理论中存在弱点，但他在就此呈现自己的哲学分析后，还是承认道：“称圣言为一种量（*pramāṇa*，权威），这种声明可能会被我的论证所削弱……不过它仍处于界定印度思想核心要素的基础性地位上。”吉腾德拉·莫汉蒂：《理性与印度思想传统：论印度哲学思想的本质》，牛津：克拉伦登出版社，1992 年，第 259 页。

② 关于《薄伽梵往世书》成书时代，现代学者认为约成书于公元 900 年。该书自述出现于喀历年代初期，即大约 5000 年前。现存修订版或许真的成书于 10 世纪，而口述传统或可上溯至更早的时期。

③ “最为恰当”是指《薄伽梵往世书》尤其适合于当今的年代，也就是喀历年代（*kali-yuga*），灵性的黑暗时代。

④ 婆罗门：按照印度传统社会阶层体系的划分，属知识分子阶层。

该书是室利·毗耶娑[①]本人对《梵经》[②]作出的评注，而他的《六论》实际上是对《薄伽梵往世书》的评注。文中他只是时而参考旧注，而不总是步先前注释者[③]之后尘。与其他《往世书》[④]文本不同，这部《薄伽梵往世书》广泛论及化身（阿凡达，*avatāra*），即“神圣降临”的理论，确认克里希纳（Krishna）为所有化身的源头（*avatārin*）。

为了便于分析《薄伽梵往世书》的内容，高迪亚－外士那瓦学者将其划分为三个范畴。其一，*Sambandha*——“关系”，涉及主宰者即神与世界的关系、主宰者与个我即生命体的关系、生命体与世界的关系；其二，*Abhidheya*——“程序”，是指有情众生在了解上述关系的基础上用以接近神的方法；而接近神，便是理解“关系”与实践“程序”的宗旨和目的，即 *prayojana*，乃第三个范畴。[⑤]

本书第一章探讨化身理论，主要关注第一个范畴“关系”中所包含的原则。第二章阐释巴克提，这是第二个范畴“程序”中的实质性原则；而第三个范畴“目标”，特别是通过茹阿萨（*rasa*，甜美关系之品味）原则致达目标，将是第三章将要探讨的重点，茹阿萨彰显的是虔爱者与神之间的圆满关系中唯美的主动原则。

① 毗耶娑：克里希纳·兑帕亚纳·毗耶娑，传统上被公认为是梵文史诗《摩诃婆罗多》及《宇宙古史》的编纂者。

② 《梵经》：是《奥义书》最重要的评注，高度凝练的格言警句是其成书风格。作为标准典籍，各吠檀多哲学流派都被期望就此作出注释。O. B. L. 卡普尔：《室利·柴坦尼亚的哲学和宗教：哈瑞－克里希纳运动的哲学背景》，德里：曼施罗摩－玛诺哈拉出版社，1977年，第70页。

③ 特别是室利陀罗·斯瓦米、罗摩奴阇以及摩陀婆。

④ 《往世书》是梵语文献，主要以叙事的方式记载全宇宙范围内的神圣历史。有学者认为，其写作时间始于公元3或4世纪，直到15或16世纪。传统上认为其成书年代更为久远，即在现今这个宇宙年代开始不久，大约始于公元前3000年。

⑤ 卡普尔：《室利·柴坦尼亚的哲学和宗教：哈瑞－克里希纳运动的哲学背景》，德里：曼施罗摩－玛诺哈拉出版社，1977年，第74~75页。

第二节 吠檀多毗湿奴派的本体论

一、伊斯瓦尔——主宰者

吠檀多毗湿奴教派五大派系[①]皆强调生物与神在本体论方面存在差别，否认多样性即摩耶（*māyā*，幻象）的一元论主张，从而驳斥了商羯罗及其追随者吠檀多不二一元论的哲学观点。吠檀多的核心问题在于，永恒不变的梵（***brahman***），或称绝对存在，是如何与这个偶然世界相互关联的。摩陀婆（1197—1276）以其二元论哲学强调梵与偶然世界的差别。罗摩奴阇（1050?—1137）不是那么激进的二元论者，可毫无疑问他是摒弃不二一元论的。其限定不二论持“宇宙乃神之身相”一说，以调和神与世界截然对立的二分法。高迪亚－外士那瓦学者（Gauḍīyas）力图以其不可思议即一即异论（***acintya-bhedābheda***），即最高存在与多样性生物之间“不可思议地既同一又有差异的理论”，来调和二者的关系及各自的定位。**O. B. L.** 卡普尔在此学说基础上，陈述问题并提出解决路径，用自己的话为吉瓦·哥斯瓦米的主张作了注解：

> 哲学史表明，无处不在和超验性都不能解决神与世界的关系问题。同一性和差异性这两个概念亦均不足以充分描述存在的本质。只强调其一，实际上会导致对世界的否定，以其为幻象（一元论）；而只强调另一个，又会将实相一分为二，在神与世界之间筑起一道不可逾越的鸿沟。然而，这两个概念似乎同等重要。同一性是理性的必然要求，而差异性则是基于经验的不可否认的事实。同一性与差异性的完美结合必然是为哲学所珍视的目标。然而，这种结合，虽说必要，却是不可能或无法想象的。这是对人类逻辑的最终测试，结果失败了。但是，在人类逻辑败下阵来的地方，那位无限者的逻辑获胜了。在完美者那里，不存在必然性与可能性之间的

① 吠檀多毗湿奴教派五大派系，即罗摩奴阇、摩陀婆、尼跋迦、筏罗婆和柴坦尼亚的追随者们。详查上述每一位吠檀多学者，请参见曼珠·杜贝：《外士那瓦哲学体系中神的概念》，瓦拉纳西：桑杰书籍中心，1984年。

矛盾。在那里，同一性与差异性的必然结合向我们昭示了实相何以成其为实相。[①]

高迪亚－外士那瓦学者提出的方案，承认要解决同一性与差异性相调和的形而上学问题[②]应建立在圣典文本基础上，且应以 *acintya-śakti*，即“神不可思议的能量”这一概念为依据。通过这种能量，相互排斥的概念在“更高结合”的维度上达成完美的统一。这一学说详细阐释了能量转化（*śakti-parināma*）概念，以此来维持梵的永恒不变性。梵，即神，亦即绝对存在，本身不会被转化，或者说，不为多样性所改变；相反，多样性只是神的能量转化，不可能离开神而独立存在。[③]

以不同视角切入，这种解决方案可进一步呈现微妙、细腻的描述。梵（最伟大者）可被构想为另两种同样有效的表述方式，即 *paramātmā*（最高我）和 *bhagavān*（一切富裕的最高拥有者）。尽管以上三种视角在某种意义上有着同等效力，但还是可以依据领悟的提升加以分级。为了证实这一点，吉瓦·哥斯瓦米援引了另一部为外士那瓦推崇的圣典《毗湿奴往世书》：

> 所谓（非人格的）“梵”，即未展示的、不变老的、不可思议的，不经出生就存在，没有任何缩减，无法言说，无形无相，无有手足肢体，无所不能，无处不在，永恒长存，一切物质元素之本源，没有起因，虽遍存万有，然无物处于其中；万物由此而流衍。天神（高度进化的灵魂）将“梵”视为至高的居所；对于那些渴望解脱之人来说，“梵”是其冥思的对象。吠陀祷文描述“梵”为毗湿奴隐而不显的、微妙的灵性光灿和居所。“梵”可以被理解为

① 卡普尔：《室利·柴坦尼亚的哲学和宗教：哈瑞－克里希纳运动的哲学背景》，第 152 页。

② 杜贝：《外士那瓦哲学体系中神的概念》，第 41 页。我们可能会注意到，这实际上是一个形而上学问题，而不仅仅是卡普尔所说的“人类逻辑测试”问题。因为逻辑是人类心智运作模式，而超越逻辑的是有别于人类心智功能的、另一种秩序和规则的形而上学悖论。

③ 将此学说中神的能量概念，与正统基督教教义中神的能量概念相对比会很有意思。后者断言，离神最近的人或许直接见到了神本人，同时也会见到神的能量。

> “薄伽梵”的绝对真理方面，而最高我（*pramātmā*，超灵）则是永恒不朽的至尊人薄伽梵（*bhagavān*）超验形象的局部展示。①

薄伽梵，或神，被定义为“最高存在，无限量地拥有六种富裕（opulence）”②。正是这种将薄伽梵视为一切力量拥有者的界定，赋予其成为至尊人（*puruṣottama*）的资格。而将其称为 *saguna-īśvara*③，意思是说，神作为拥有一切品质的主宰者，优于不具属性的绝对存在梵（*nirguna-brahman*）。我们会看到，正是这位至尊人被认为是所有化身（*avatāras*，来到尘世的神圣降临者）独一无二的源头。

二、吉瓦——生物体

吉瓦·哥斯瓦米再次引用《毗湿奴往世书》，支撑薄伽梵（*bhagavān*，神）通过三方面展示其能量的理论。这三方面分别为：内在能量（*svarūpa-śakti*）、中间能量（*tatastha-śakti*）、外在能量（*bahirāṅga-śakti*）。④ *tatastha-śakti*，亦称为吉瓦－沙克提（*jīva-śakti*），字面意思是“处于边界的能量”，即“生物能量”。*bahirāṅga-śakti* 被视为摩耶－沙克提（*māyā-śakti*，迷幻能量、幻力）。正如曼珠·杜贝所提出的：“吉瓦－沙克提负责个我灵魂的存在，摩耶－沙克提负责世界的创造、维系和毁灭。而最高我作为这一切的撑持者，扮演众灵魂和世界监管者的角色。”⑤

外士那瓦强烈反对一元论所持的世界和众生都没有实质根基的主张，同时也反对泯灭个体性而融入一个有意识的至高存在的观点。他们想要保持神

---

① 这段引文的梵文诗节参见《毗湿奴往世书》第 6 篇第 5 章第 66~69 诗节。参见拙译著《论至尊人格首神》第 3 章第 2 诗节。

② 《毗湿奴往世书》第 6 篇第 5 章第 47 诗节。斯瓦米·帕布帕德所著《觉悟自我的科学》第 1 章中引用此诗节。根据《毗湿奴往世书》，这六种富裕分别是：力量、声望、财富、知识、美丽和弃绝。还有六种与薄伽梵的可接近性相关的富裕或属性，参见第 19 页脚注③。

③ 杜贝：《外士那瓦哲学体系中神的概念》，第 5 页，引自《毗湿奴往世书》第 6 篇第 5 章第 12~14 诗节（版本不详）。

④ 杜贝：《外士那瓦哲学体系中神的概念》，第 44 页。

⑤ 杜贝：《外士那瓦哲学体系中神的概念》，第 44 页。

与生物之间永恒的主仆关系。作为中间能量的产物，生命体是阿努（*anu*）本质上极其微小，而神是维布（*vibhu*），本质上无限大，生命体依存于其与神的关系当中。尽管如此，生命体本应作为永恒解脱的灵魂，与内在能量相契合，按其原本身份行使相应职责。可是，由于愚昧无明，生命体受制于摩耶－沙克提——现象世界正是通过这种幻力被创造、维系和毁灭的，而生命体看似独立的欲望也正是通过这种力量被促成的。

外士那瓦宗与大多数倾向于消减生物与湿婆之间差异的湿婆教派形成对比，后者甚至认为吉瓦（*jīva*，个我）会在一定程度上体悟到可与湿婆本人相媲美的"湿婆性"。[①]而某些湿婆教派和所有的外士那瓦宗都明确肯定每一生物永恒的个体性。在后者看来，个我一向是依靠和从属于薄伽梵的微小部分，从来不是一个独立的存在。正如印度几乎所有的宗教哲学流派所主张的那样，外士那瓦宗确认，个我的根本问题在于被系缚在不断重复的生死轮回中。在外士那瓦看来，导致这种系缚的起因是个我的愚昧无明，在与薄伽梵的关系当中自我的真实身份是什么，他们对此一无所知。而解决问题的出路在于：解脱（*mokṣa* 或 *mukti*）。只有去除"我是不受约束的独立行为者、控制者或主人"这种虚假概念，重建服务关系，"解脱"才会发生。与此同时，为了达成个我的"解脱"，薄伽梵也展示其主动性，作为各类不同的化身降临世界，使受缚的吉瓦更易接近他。不仅如此，作为场域即个我躯体境况的知悉者，作为最高我（*paramātmā*），薄伽梵也在吉瓦（*jīva*，个我）心中采取行动，由内而外，指导其于捆绑中脱身。

三、伽嘎塔——世界

通过薄伽梵的迷幻能量（*māyā-śakti*，摩耶－沙克提，幻力），为个我灵魂（*jīvātmā*）提供完美的适宜其实现愿望的便利条件。而种种便利背后的舞台就叫伽嘎塔（*jagat*），即"那个变易不居者"——充满短暂名相的不确定的偶然世界。每一生命体在外形结构上被配置一套感觉器官，这些器官合起来构成其物质身体，而物质身体易受物质的束缚。

从另一视角来看，是神的迷幻能量（*māyā-śakti*）使这个无生命的世界

① 戴维斯：《振荡宇宙内的仪式：中世纪印度的湿婆崇拜》，第 84、135 页。

产生出来的，神通过幻力展示自身。由于神真实不虚，故而他的能量以及能量的展示亦复如是——这里所说“能量的展示”是指能量的转化，而非充满活力的能量源的转化。作为神的能量的转化，世界并非神受到摩耶影响而示现的身相；世界的存在亦非对其地位的妥协。由此，被系缚其中的生物所经验的种种快乐与痛苦、希望与恐惧（连同对一已行为所应负的道德责任）都不是无足轻重的。世界是由真实起因产生的真实结果，正因为如此，它是神至高无上的品质之一。[①]杜贝在比较五大毗湿奴派神学体系时指出：

> 将物质世界归结为摩耶－沙克提是孟加拉外士那瓦宗的重要理论特征。这种观点强化了终极实在不二一元的理论。“不可思议即一即异论”尝试解决能量与能量拥有者之间同一性和差异性的难题。孟加拉学派并没有将一方视为真实，将另一方视为不真实，而是将二者归于一种超乎逻辑和不可思议的关系中。[②]

世界为生物提供了方便，不过它也为神提供了便利。18世纪高迪亚－外士那瓦评论家巴拉提婆·维迪亚布善引用《薄伽梵往世书》第11篇第9章第21诗节的一个类比，来阐明这一点：

> 正如蜘蛛凭其自身制造了蛛网，游戏一段时间，然后又将其吸入体内。同样，主创造了世界，维系一段时间之后，最终收回。蜘蛛作为一个生命体，它有意识的部分并未转化成蛛网，而是不存在意识的蜘蛛躯体将蛛网编织出来的。[③]

蜘蛛在自己编织的蛛网上占有一席之地；同样，那个永恒不变的、无所

---

① 苏德什·纳朗：《巴拉提婆·维迪亚布善的外士那瓦哲学》，德里：纳格出版社，1984年，第77页。

② 杜贝：《外士那瓦哲学体系中神的概念》，第76页。

③ 苏德什·纳朗：《巴拉提婆·维迪亚布善的外士那瓦哲学》，第82页。

不能的神，为了展现其丽拉（*līlā*），即娱乐活动，由他的内在能量协助[①]，也在他自己的创造之内扮演某一角色。他以各种化身的形象做事，在不同年代以不同形象显现在宇宙之内。

第三节　宇宙论

一、创造、维系和毁灭

高迪亚－外士那瓦对宇宙创造和毁灭的理解，与印度古典数论哲学体系的理解方式大致相同。[②]他们认为，创造是若干元素和原则的展开过程——每一个都自其前一个而来——由此，个我生命的躯体便形成了。固定的天文周期过后，宇宙毁灭，接着创造过程重新展开。有关薄伽梵（*bhagavān*，神）是如何以各种拥有特别权威的不同形象，通过一个设计相当周密的扩展或显现程序参与宇宙演进过程的，[③]高迪亚－外士那瓦基本上接受《往世书》（Purāṇas）和五夜派（Pañcarātra）[④]经典的记载。神，被认为是菩鲁沙（*puruṣa*，原初之人），这些不同的形象被视为神的展示，当他们降临到由自身所创造的世界，便以"原人之化身"见称，梵文称之为 *puruṣa-avatāras*（菩鲁沙－阿凡达）。

---

① 内在能量可进一步分为三种能量，其中一种能量协助神的娱乐活动，使之免于受外在能量污染之危险。

② 苏德什·纳朗:《巴拉提婆·维迪亚布善的外士那瓦哲学》，第 83 页。因此，这也与湿婆圣典派（湿婆悉檀多派）宇宙观颇为相似，像毗湿奴派教义一样，这种宇宙观拒绝接受一元论将摩耶（*māyā*）看作独立存在的实体而非错觉幻象的观点（戴维斯:《振荡宇宙内的仪式：中世纪印度的湿婆崇拜》，第 44 页）。

③ 这一规律也为其他几个印度宗教与哲学体系所认可。在湿婆圣典派宇宙观看来，"释放发散"与"重新收回"构成"宇宙振荡"。就二者对称性以及与此观念相联系的仪式程序，戴维斯给出了详细而有趣的阐述（戴维斯:《振荡宇宙内的仪式：中世纪印度的湿婆崇拜》，第 42~74 页）。

④ 梵语文献学的一个分支广泛探讨了神像崇拜的理论与实践，强调"扩展"的观点，即不同的神像形体皆由一个原初形象而来。有关五夜派的更多讨论，参见 A. K. 马宗达《柴坦尼亚的生平与教导：外士那瓦宗研究》，孟买，焦帕蒂：帕腊提亚－维迪亚－巴万出版社，1969 年，第 296~297 页。该书简要探讨了高迪亚－外士那瓦学说与五夜派文献相关的特殊性。

此外，据《薄伽梵往世书》记载，还有一类化身，即三个属性（三德）化身——梵天（*Brahmā*）、毗湿奴（*Viṣṇu*）、湿婆（*Śiva*），促成第二级创造、维系和毁灭。在这一层级上，三位化身中的两位——梵天和湿婆的概念有些不确定性。而毗湿奴（那个进入者）是薄伽梵的一个“圆满”形象，因而属于毗湿奴范畴，具有毗湿奴真如本性（*viṣṇu-tattva*）。而梵天一般属于受物质世界束缚的个我灵魂范畴（*jīva-tattva*），不过高迪亚－外士那瓦评论家有时亦将其列入毗湿奴范畴。至于湿婆，被外士那瓦宗上师视为自成一类，称为 *śiva-tattva*（这并不奇怪）。《梵天本集》中有段非常重要的诗节，分别将毗湿奴和湿婆比作牛奶和酸奶：牛奶可以制成酸奶，可酸奶不能反过来制成牛奶。两者存在着密切的亲缘关系，然而牛奶因为是酸奶之源，故其地位上被视为高于酸奶。

在这一层级的创造中，当外在能量（*bahirāṅga-śakti*）差异性不断增大，由此带来的些微负面因素会给梵天和湿婆带来影响；而毗湿奴，作为薄伽梵，则完全保持超然，远离物质玷污。由此，正是靠毗湿奴的神力介入，这个物质展示的微妙平衡才得以维系——不论从物质自然角度，还是从道德精神层面而言均是如此。薄伽梵正是以毗湿奴的身份，通过俯瞰监督“因果报应”的法则，即（恰当与不恰当的）行为所支配的无形的精神上层建筑，来履行他被期望的威严①主权。同时，也正是透过毗湿奴，众多逍遥时光化身（*līlā-avatāras*）降临世上，执行三重功能。其一，祝福中正之人；其二，降伏邪恶之人；其三，重建宗教原则（*dharma*，达摩、法）。以上三方面均属逍遥时光化身的神圣娱乐活动（*līlā*，丽拉）。

《薄伽梵往世书》列举了其中较为重要的逍遥时光化身（*līlā-avatāras*）后，对其基本特性作了综述，接着确认了理解这一主题的方法：

> 主的活动永无瑕疵，他是六个感官的主人，是绝对拥有六种富裕的全能者。他创造、维系并毁灭这个展示了的宇宙，而其自身丝毫不受影响。他在每一生命体之内，永远是独立的。因为他像演员演戏一样在娱乐、游戏，知识贫乏的愚者不能够知晓他的形象、名

① 这段说法，我参考的是约翰·B. 卡曼的著作《威严与柔和：上帝概念反差与和谐的比较研究》，密歇根，大溪城：伊尔德曼斯出版公司，1994 年。

字以及活动，也无法凭其推测或言语来描述此类事情。唯有那些一直不断、毫无保留地为手持车轮[①]的主克里希纳的莲花足作出顺意服务的人，才能够洞悉这位宇宙创造者全然的光荣、力量和超然存在。[②]

二、扩展与降临：更易接近

薄伽梵扩展自己并降临于世，通过一系列的化身让被系缚在物质世界重复生老病死的生物体更易接近他。阿笈摩文献[③]描述了这种“日益增长的可接近性”，以强调神像形体（*arcā-vigraha*）的重要性。梵文 *arcā-vigraha* 也称作 *arcāvatāra*，意思是可以用来崇拜的物化形象。就这一观点，室利毗湿奴派[④]学者室利尼瓦沙·查里作了恰到好处的解读：

可以用来崇拜的物化形象（*arcāvatāra*），构成神像崇拜的基础，被认为比神的其他化身（原文如此）[⑤]更值得关注。既然神只存在于超自然的领域，那么，其超验的形象就远远超出了人类可感知的范畴。神的维尤哈（*vyūha*）形象，即四位分身，或称四重扩展（即瓦苏戴瓦、桑卡尔珊、帕丢姆纳、阿尼茹达——译者注），对我们来说也是无法接近的。而维巴瓦（*vibhava*）形象是专为从

---

① 这是印度伟大的史诗《摩诃婆罗多》中描述的一件小事。“手持车轮的那一位”是指克里希纳。在库茹柴陀战场上，他以打破自己不参战的诺言为代价，展现了对其虔爱者的偏爱。

② 《薄伽梵往世书》第 1 篇第 3 章第 36~38 诗节。

③ 五夜派文献是阿笈摩中的一部分，无论是湿婆派还是毗湿奴派传统，都视其为与神像崇拜联系紧密的一套文献。毗湿奴派阿笈摩通常指的是五夜派阿笈摩。

④ 室利毗湿奴派：毗湿奴派的又一传系。据说自室利，或称拉克希米传递下来，罗摩奴阇是这一传承中主要的创始导师。

⑤ “化身（Incarnation）”是印度和西方学者翻译 *avatāra* 经常使用的一个术语。虽然约翰·卡曼充分意识到了二者之间的差异，但还是不时使用“化身（Incarnation）”这个术语指代 *avatāras*，这多少有些用词不当。关于这两个词的比较，参见卡曼《威严与柔和》第 10 章各处，包括该书第 196 页脚注 9，卡曼就其他学者著作中有关这一论题的研究成果作了综述。

> 事特定职责或逍遥时光而显现在尘世的形象，示现于遥远的过去。我们现在直接崇拜那些形象也是不现实的。居于我们内心，以最高我或称超灵的形式临在的神，尽管近在咫尺，但同样无法直接崇拜，因为物质的感觉器官察觉不到他。如此一来，临在于神像形体中的神，便恒常成为我们更易接近的崇拜对象。[1]

查里继续解释，依据神像外观上的起源，毗湿奴派文献将其分为四类[2]：斯瓦央瓦亚克塔（*Svayamvyakta*），“自显的”，被认为是凭薄伽梵的直接意愿而示现；提婆或称戴瓦（*daiva*），“与一位天神（*deve*）或称高等人类有关的”，据说是应某位宇宙事务管理者[3]的请求而显现的；赛达（*saiddha*），“与一位希达（*siddha*，圣人）有关”，是应一位苦行者的请求而显现的，这位苦行者有着高度专注的决心和强烈的愿望；还有玛努莎（*mānuṣa*），“与人类有关的”，是指依照圣典的具体说明和程序，使用八种物质材料中的一种[4]制作成型后被视为神圣对象来供奉。或许我们会反驳说，不管怎样，上面谈到的这些形象至少在某种意义上来说，都是由木头、金属或石头制成的，因此显然是易腐坏的。既然所有这些材料就其实质而言都是“物质的”，那么，由此而制成的神像当然也难免同等的“物质性”——粗糙、不洁和低等。此外，拥有特定外形的神像也暗示了不完美的人类形体。显然，他们丝毫没有展现“至高原人”（*puruṣottama*）的特点。然而，对外士那瓦来说，所有这些表面上的“不合格”，都被忠诚的虔爱者所认可

---

① 室利尼瓦沙 · S. M. 查里：《外士那瓦宗：哲学、神学与宗教秩序》，德里：莫逊拉尔 · 班那西达斯出版公司，1994 年，第 224 页。亦参见卡曼《威严与柔和》，第 195~196 页。

② 查里：《外士那瓦宗：哲学、神学与宗教秩序》，第 225 页。

③ “宇宙事务管理者”，是指为数众多的天神，诸如因陀罗、昌陀罗、阿耆尼和婆楼那，根据吠陀文献和宇宙古史的记载，强有力的个体生物因其杰出的虔诚表现，而被暂时授予这些职位。

④ 据《薄伽梵往世书》第 11 篇第 27 章第 12 诗节记载：“主的神像形体据说以石头、木头、金属、泥土、颜料、沙子、心意或宝石八种形式显现。”之前还有三个诗节说明了其他象征性的对象也可以成为薄伽梵的代表：“二次出生的人应该诚心诚意地崇拜我——他值得崇拜的主，以爱心向我的神像形体或我显现在地上、火中、阳光里、水中或崇拜者心中的形体供奉合适的用品。”

的一项基本资格，即“易于接近”所抵消。

约翰·卡曼引用一段追随罗摩奴阇的评论家的话，来阐明神的“至高无上性”与“可接近性”相辅相成的原理：

> 如果你跟一个跛足者说“请骑上大象”，那么他怎样才能骑到象背上呢？同样道理，对于一个身处不完美世界的微不足道的灵魂来说，他如何才能接近万有之主呢？解决之道当然在于“象”那一方，要是能请它迁就一下，弯下膝盖，这样跛足者就能爬到象背上。神也是一样，他放低自己，如此，在这个不完美世界中的灵魂就能够崇拜他了。①

罗摩奴阇认为②，作为化身，形体美是神的一个特质，既展示其威严壮丽，又展示其可接近性。③正如我们将要看到的那样，高迪亚－外士那瓦神学体系强调，这种品质构成了确认克里希纳为所有化身源头（*avatārin*）以及“最高神我”（*puruṣottama*）本人的一个基础。

第四节　克里希纳：最有吸引力的主

高迪亚－外士那瓦评论家广泛援引《薄伽梵往世书》来证实克里希纳的地位，认为他是“神本人”（*svayam bhagavān*），所有化身的源头。④他们所关心的是要向世人阐明，虽然克里希纳表面上以毗湿奴的一个化身显

---

① 瓦达库·提茹维达·皮莱：《部分》1. 3 前言。卡曼在《威严与柔和》第 93 页引用。

② 见罗摩奴阇《薄伽梵歌》评注的前言部分，卡曼在《威严与柔和》第 91 页引用。

③ 卡曼在其著作《威严与柔和》第 91 页列举了威严壮丽的至高者所具有的六项特性：知识、无尽的力量、最高统治权、永恒不变、创造能力以及辉煌灿烂。类似地，罗摩奴阇也用六项特性总结“可接近性”，即满怀怜悯、和蔼地屈尊、慈母般的爱、慷慨大度、关怀生物福祉、温情脉脉。显然，“形体美”可算作第七项特性。

④ 吉瓦·哥斯瓦米认为，这部典籍开头部分有一首重要诗节：“上面提到的所有化身，要么是至尊主的完整扩展，要么是完整扩展的部分，但其中的圣主克里希纳是第一位人格首神。每当无神论者制造混乱时，至尊主的这些化身就降临不同的星球，保护有神论者。”见《薄伽梵往世书》第 1 篇第 3 章《克里希纳是所有化身的源头》诗节 28。

现，然而事实上，正是他不仅成为毗湿奴的源头，而且也是五夜派经典中作为至高者被崇拜的薄伽梵的威严形象“那罗衍那”之源。毗湿奴女神派信徒与高迪亚－外士那瓦推崇的经典不同，这是二者之间的显著区别。前者奉《毗湿奴往世书》为尊，而后者追随柴坦尼亚，更加看重《薄伽梵往世书》，而非其他经典。但对高迪亚－外士那瓦而言，这并不是一个被简化到单纯区分经典权威性的问题。确切地说，他们将“威严”（*aiśvarya*）与“甜美”（*mādhurya*）视为截然对立的两极。我们可能会注意到，后者，即“甜美”，与罗摩奴阇表述的、后为卡曼所继承的“可亲近性”观点之间有着一定的亲缘关系，同时也存在显著的差异。

然而，“威严”被看作薄伽梵外围的或附属的品质（*tatastha-lakṣaṇa*），“甜美”则被称为他内在固有的品质（*svarūpa-lakṣaṇa*）。[①]不管这种论点或许表面上看来有多么藐视理性（亦即否定“威严”为神的一项主要特征），高迪亚－外士那瓦学者还是想要不仅就神的本质，而且就个我灵魂的本质作出声明。个我灵魂无疑是神永恒的从属部分，有着服务神的倾向。这一服务的倾向，以及由此而来的亲密地接近神的能力，并不是由神的这类“威严”品质所提供的，而是由神的审美特征——他的美丽和甜美所给予的。对于高迪亚－外士那瓦学者而言，克里希纳就是那位展示这些特征的至高存在。印度学者 O. B. L. 卡普尔，同时也是位实修的外士那瓦，他在某种程度上表达了这种信念：

> （克里希纳）不是像商羯罗和罗摩奴阇所认为的那样，是毗湿奴的化身，相反，他是毗湿奴和所有其他神明的本源。历史上的克里希纳乃是永恒的克里希纳降临人间，在他之中体现了至高的权力、无上的爱，还有无与伦比的妙乐。他既有具体的形象，同时又不断扩展自身。就其本质来说，他无限大，故能遍布整个宇宙。但其无限性却始终围绕着一个具体实在的形象而展开。他之存在本身乃有机统一体，一切尽在其中。尽管他的形象具体而实在，然而并不会因此限制或约束其自由，因为他调整其存在频度，使妙音散

① 卡普尔：《室利·柴坦尼亚的哲学和宗教：哈瑞－克里希纳运动的哲学背景》，第123页。

播各处，弥漫于浩瀚无垠的宇宙万有之中。他将无量无边的灵性与调制强度相结合；将动作之敏捷，与透彻的和谐还有温文尔雅的举止态度相结合；将永恒的平静、完美的沉着，与永远自我揭示的动力以及自我实现的创造性活动相结合。他的笛子唤醒我们的生命，让我们的内在调换到这样一种频率——我们对于爱、知识与和平的渴求，在完整统一的融合当中全部得到饱足。他为我们提供自由、弹性、和谐，以及导向最富裕、最完满的神圣精神生活所需要的一切。[①]

与他的“甜美”（*mādhurya*）一道，克里希纳的“具体实在性”也是高迪亚－外士那瓦宗关注的核心内容。[②]据史料记载[③]，克里希纳曾居住在温达文，也就是布阿佳（Vraja）那块方圆约 168 平方英里的土地上，包括位于今德里与阿格拉之间的马图拉城（Mathurā）。在这片神圣的土地上，有数百处经特别确认的地点，克里希纳从童年起，直到 11 岁，曾与他的同伴们一起在这些地方从事他的娱乐活动（*līlā*）。对于虔爱者而言，这片土地有着实实在在的、可触摸的具体特征。无论是在当时，还是现在，布阿佳的石头、树木和乳牛见证了克里希纳的“出席”。而成千上万安设在庙堂、神殿以及宗教社区的克里希纳“具体实在”的神像，每日里接受着当地居民和朝圣者的虔诚奉爱。

以上，我以关系范畴的角度，对化身理论作了简要而宽泛的概述。这一理论表明，对高迪亚－外士那瓦而言神像作为崇拜对象的意义所在，以及克里希纳作为最可亲近的至尊神的意义所在。接下来要考虑的是第二个

① 卡普尔：《室利·柴坦尼亚的哲学和宗教：哈瑞－克里希纳运动的哲学背景》，第 107 页。

② 伐罗婆阿阇梨耶的追随者们“普施提－摩尔伽”，还有尼跋迦的追随者“鲁陀罗传系”，或许亦持此说。

③ “据史料记载”，或许不适于西方学者，而对于毗湿奴派定是适用的。假如史料证实在某个历史时刻有可能发生了某些重大灵性事件，而对于受束缚的洞察力来说，这些史事可能是湮没不显的。有关这一论题，当代毗湿奴派有恰到好处的讨论。参见萨达普塔·达斯《理性的神话：一个理性的人会接受〈宇宙古史〉的故事为史实吗？》，1993 年在芝加哥世界宗教大会上的讲稿，《回归首神》1994 年 1/2 期合刊本。

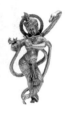

范畴：“程序”（*abhidheya*），即巴克提——奉爱服务。藉此臻达“目标”（*prayojana*）——对神纯粹的热爱。正是通过巴克提，神像崇拜的实践才得到滋养和维系。

第二章
作为途径和目标的巴克提

纯粹奉爱服务的表现是：一旦听到居于每一生命体心中的至尊人格首神超然的名字和品质，立即受到吸引。正如恒河水自然流向海洋，这般奉爱妙乐，不受任何物质境况干扰，径直流向至尊主。

——《薄伽梵往世书》3. 29. 11-12[①]

第一节　巴克提的定义

一、否定式定义：巴克提不是什么

基于对《薄伽梵往世书》的透彻理解，高迪亚 – 外士那瓦学者一向关注的是，将巴克提与他们认为[②]有别于巴克提的所有实践，特别是业报活动（*karma*）、知识思辨（*jñāna*）和瑜伽（*yoga*）区分开来。当然，这并不意

① 此处作者在其英文原著中给出了原梵文诗文，详见本书英文相关部分（译者注）。

② 正如小沃尔特 · G. 内维尔在另一有关早期毗湿奴派学者耶牟那阿阇梨耶的语境中所指出的，我们所关注的某些作者不认为自己往自己借鉴的出处里增添了什么。我在正文中说“他们认为”，是顺应当代强调个人独创性的先入为主的一种说法，如内维尔所指出的。其实，在六哥斯瓦心目中，他们的任务只是“恢复与清晰再现（他们的）源头的原意，以便提供给和（他们）同时代的人”。沃尔特 · G. 内维尔：《耶牟那论吠檀多与五夜派：整合古典与现代》，蒙大拿，米苏拉：学者出版社，1977 年，第 58 页。

味着完全摒弃后三者，而是要强调巴克提乃积极主动、完整统一的原则，由此臻达完美。①这里所说的业报活动（*karma*）指的是期待获得物质回报而进行的种种努力，不管这回报是马上就能到手的，还是经典上承诺在未来某一时点兑现的，诸如下一世吉祥的出生和物质收益等。而知识思辨（*jñāna*）跟出于一种从物质身体的存在状况中解脱的愿望，而渴求获得真知或灵性知识的抱负有关。其完美境界在于领悟到无有差别、“不具人格特征”的绝对真理。②这里所说的瑜伽，指的是阿斯汤嘎瑜伽练习——传统的八部瑜伽旨在领悟最高我，但从巴克提视角来看，这是受到批评的，因为想获得神秘力量的企图会导致自我膨胀，而这往往会使练习者无法专注于“领悟最高我”的目标。

对于后三种瑜伽练习——业报活动（业瑜伽——译者注）、知识思辨（智瑜伽——译者注）和阿斯汤嘎瑜伽，吠陀文献中不乏赞美之辞，高迪亚－外士那瓦流派并不完全持轻视态度，但也谨慎对待。在他们看来，此三者皆属“其他欲望”之列，而非真正有价值的、服务薄伽梵的灵性愿望。其结果只会让物质存在持续下去。服务薄伽梵的愿望，用巴克提来表示。③唯有巴克提才能引导人领悟绝对者的薄伽梵特征，尽管在巴克提灵性修习的初级阶段，其他三种瑜伽均可能起到辅助作用。④

高迪亚－外士那瓦对巴克提概念的强调，是将其置于多少有些游离于传统社会结构，即社会四阶层与人生四阶段制度（*varṇāśrama*，瓦尔那阿刷玛。晚近以“种姓”制度渐为西方人所知）的位置上。然而这一制度关注的是物质躯体方面的需要，故而主要满足上述三种较低层面的追求。但克里希纳－巴克提超越这一社会制度，从而实现四个职业阶层与四个生命阶段的真正目的。吉瓦·哥斯瓦米在其著作《论巴克提》一书中引用了《薄伽梵往世书》的观点：

---

① 卡普尔:《室利·柴坦尼亚的哲学和宗教：哈瑞－克里希纳运动的哲学背景》，第182页。

② 卡普尔:《室利·柴坦尼亚的哲学和宗教：哈瑞－克里希纳运动的哲学背景》，第177页。

③ 为了有利于克里希纳而行事，被称为巴克提。

④ 卡普尔:《室利·柴坦尼亚的哲学和宗教：哈瑞－克里希纳运动的哲学背景》，第180页。

因此结论是，通过履行按社会阶层和人生阶段制度规定给自己的职责，所能成就的最高完美境界，就是取悦人格首神。①

接着他作了详尽阐述：

在所有灵性路径中，纯粹的奉爱服务（殊达－巴克提）绝对是最佳的。因此，这个诗节说，奉爱服务优于按社会四阶层和人生四阶段制度从事的活动。接下来他（苏塔·哥斯瓦米）描述巴克提的本质。因为巴克提出于天性，所以是自发而充满喜悦的。同时，巴克提不含任何动机，换言之，除了“服务”本身之外，不寻求任何结果；而且它是不受干扰、永不间断的。也就是说，除了奉爱服务外，只要提及任何事物，那么或者快乐缺席，或者痛苦缺席，只有奉爱服务超越苦乐二元性。由此，它不被任何事物所中止，永远是绵密无漏的。当巴克提展示出“为主所吸引”的特征时，那么，以聆听有关主的事迹等为表现形式的奉爱实践，即萨达纳－巴克提，便开始了。②

与某些巴克提运动（比如卡比尔的）③不同，柴坦尼亚与六哥斯瓦米对既定的社会分层体系并非采取弃而不用的态度，而是将其置于达成更高目标，即克里希纳－巴克提的从属地位上。既然外显可见的巴克提灵性实践与庙宇神像崇拜有着明显的关系，那么，这种对待社会四阶层和人生四阶段制度（*varṇāśrama*）的态度就变得重要起来。据专门探讨毗湿奴派神学理论与实践仪轨的五夜派经典记载，哥斯瓦米们肯定，巴克提适用于每一个人，而不论其出身阶层，因为每个人都能够变得有资格接受启迪，从事这些实践，

① 参见《薄伽梵往世书》第 1 篇第 2 章第 13 诗节，《论巴克提》第 3 章第 3 诗节引用。

② 拙译著：《论巴克提》第 3 章第 3 节。

③ 拉宾德拉·库马尔·悉檀多萨斯垂：《穿越时代的外士那瓦宗》，德里：曼施罗摩·玛诺哈拉出版社，1985 年，第 168~171 页。

而实践便构成了对巴克提的耕耘——特别是吟诵曼陀罗，即神秘的真言[1]，以及崇拜神圣形象（*mūrtis*）。在普通社会交往层面，保留了等级差别，但同时在更高的巴克提层面，则又超越它。[2]

巴克提也不同于另一类人生追求——世俗的宗教信仰（*dharma*）、追求财富（*artha*）、满足感官欲望（*kāma*）以及解脱（*mokṣa*）。以上四种追求在社会四阶层和人生四阶段社会结构中得以促成。然而，印度几乎所有正式的宗教传统都将“解脱”视为人类的终极目标（包括大部分毗湿奴派体系，他们也强调巴克提是解脱的唯一途径）。但对高迪亚－外士那瓦来说，巴克提本身即是目标，因而自然涵盖了上文四个从属的目标，尤其是解脱。人类所有普通的目标与“殊达－巴克提”（*śuddha-bhakti*）——纯粹的奉爱相比，其重要性显得微不足道。

二、肯定式定义：巴克提是什么

如果巴克提被认为与人类大多数普通目标截然不同，那么其积极目标何在？或者说，如果它涵盖所有其他成就在内，那么其具体特征又是什么？高迪亚－外士那瓦认为，巴克提特指对克里希纳或他众多形象之一的虔信与奉爱，其宗旨只有一个：取悦克里希纳。[3]吉瓦·哥斯瓦米引用《薄伽梵往世书》第7篇第14章诗节34作为论据，证实这种看法的第一方面：

> 大地之王啊！学识渊博、经验丰富的学者们断定，必须为之献

---

① 曼陀罗：字面意思是思想的工具，神圣的诗节或言语，称呼某位个别神像的神圣方法。莫尼尔·威廉姆斯爵士主编：《新版梵英辞典》，牛津大学克拉伦敦出版社，1960年。

② 这在巴克提维诺德·塔库尔的译作《室利·柴坦尼亚八训规甘露》中也有论及。凯达尔纳特·达塔·巴克提维诺德译：《室利·柴坦尼亚八训规甘露》，马德拉斯：室利·高迪亚修院，1983年，第98~99页。

③ 请注意克里希纳·沙尔玛的论点，他认为目前（至少到1987年），学界对巴克提的界定不知不觉地采用了高迪亚－外士那瓦描述的巴克提概念。然而一段时间以来，关于这一点，或许有些属实，我认为，当今谨慎的学者会描述出一个更为微妙细腻的画面。参见克里希纳·沙尔玛：《巴克提和巴克提运动：一个新的视角》，德里：曼施拉玛·玛诺哈拉出版社，1987年。此论点文中多次出现，尤其是附录Ⅱ，第255~279页。

上一切的最佳人选，就是那位至尊人格首神克里希纳。[①]宇宙之内动与不动的一切都息止于他，万事万物都自他而来。[②]

既然神是“宇宙之内动与不动的一切之栖息所，万物自他而来”，那么，他就可被比作树之根。为了让整棵树长得枝繁叶茂，应该把水浇到树根处，保证根部有充分的营养。而服务神就相当于往树根处浇水。此外，服务神还可被比作进食而获取营养，由此确保身体新陈代谢系统将能量分配给全身的每个器官。“巴克提”这个词来自梵文动词词根“*bhaj*”，意即“分发”或“分享”[③]，常被简单地译为“虔爱”（虔信、信爱、奉爱）。高迪亚－外士那瓦强调其积极活跃的品质是对至高无上者恒常的服务实践。正如一缕阳光总是与太阳密不可分，既然个我的本质特征是服务，那么，服务和奉献的对象自然便是薄伽梵。

取悦薄伽梵，乃巴克提的宗旨。在茹帕·哥斯瓦米[④]（1488—156?）给出的巴克提高级阶段的定义中也有类似表述。他认为，巴克提高级阶段（*uttama-bhakti*）的宗旨是：让薄伽梵满意。在这一阶段，虔爱者为克里希纳做重复不断的、具有献身精神的顺意服务（*ānukūlyena kṛṣṇānuśīlana*）。所谓顺意服务，指的是顺从克里希纳的意愿。巴克提的这种本质特征是薄伽

---

① 参见格拉汉姆·M. 施维克《普遍的和机密的神之爱》，《毗湿奴派研究期刊》第6卷第2期，1998年春，第106页。该文对帕布帕德使用“至尊人格首神”这一表述方式翻译梵文词“薄伽梵”有精彩的解读。该梵文诗节使用“诃利”这一名字来称呼薄伽梵。

② 引自《论巴克提》第286章第44诗节。

③ 关于动词词根 *bhaj*，莫尼尔·威廉姆斯解释如下：“分开、散布、拨给或分给、同享、给予、赠予、装备、供应……［从这一语境中，提炼出巴克提（*bhakt*）的‘信爱’内涵：］服务、荣耀、敬畏、爱、崇拜。”在这一语境中，他将巴克提界定为：“依恋、奉献、对……喜爱、献身于……信任、效忠、崇拜、虔敬、信心、爱或奉献［连同‘工作’（*karman*）及‘灵性知识’（*jñāna*）一起，作为拯救的宗教原则或途径］。”

④ 六哥斯瓦米之一，茹帕在其著作《奉爱甘露之洋》一书中，将这一定义作为巴克提高级阶段的本质特征。

梵内在本质能量[1]（*svarūpa-śakti*）的功能。

同时，从天性上来看，巴克提也作为一种潜在的休眠状态存在于个我（正如第一章提到的，个我是中间能量的产物）之中，而个我受薄伽梵外在能量的影响和支配。换言之，由于生命体与薄伽梵有着永恒的关系，故对其怀有出于天性的自发奉爱。[2]但由于受到外在能量的吸引，而习惯于自私自利的追求，这种奉爱多少被屏蔽了。人如何打破习惯，唤醒奉爱，最终是一个恩典（*kṛpā*，*prasāda*，*vadānyatā*，*anugraha*）[3]的问题。这恩典通过一种或多种途径从薄伽梵那里获得，而这一切都是基于个我与薄伽梵之间本体论关系之上的。

16 世纪两位主要的柴坦尼亚传记作者之一的克里希纳达斯·卡维罗阇的著作被所有高迪亚－外士那瓦视为典范。他主张，巴克提的目标，即对神纯粹的爱，永恒存在于众生心中，有待于用恰当的方法唤醒：

> 对克里希纳纯粹的爱永恒存在于生物心中，并不需要从其他源头处获得。当心灵被聆听和吟诵净化之后，生物自然醒来。（《柴坦尼亚生平甘露》中篇第 22 章第 107 诗节）

“聆听”和“念诵”是两种练习（*sādhana*，萨达纳），帮助实践者唤醒潜在的克里希纳－普瑞玛（*Krishna-prema*），即对克里希纳不掺杂质的纯粹虔爱。《薄伽梵往世书》呈现了九种有助于达到巴克提完美境界的实践

---

① 桑玖克塔·古普塔将五夜派关于“薄伽梵能量”的一般概念解释为六种荣耀的总和：“神的这六种属性（原文如此），合起来构成他的能量（*śakti*），可译为他的能力、力量以及合而为一的潜在可能性……能量（*śakti*）是神的本质属性，是他的人格性或‘自性’（*ahaṁtā*）。”桑玖克塔·古普塔：《五夜派对曼陀罗的态度》，收录于哈维·P. 阿尔帕编辑的《曼陀罗》，纽约，奥尔巴尼：纽约州立大学出版社，1989 年，第 225 页。关于 *svarūpa-śakti*（神的内在能量），马宗达在《柴坦尼亚的生平与教导》一书中有详尽阐述。参见第 287~290 页。

② 巴克提维诺德译：《室利·柴坦尼亚八训规甘露》，第 170 页。

③ *kṛpā*，字面意思是“怜悯、亲切、同情”；*prasāda*，字面意思是“仁慈、好意、体贴的行为举止、恩惠、援助、调解”；*vadānyatā*，字面意思是“仁爱好施、心胸宽阔、慷慨大方”；*anugraha*，字面意思是“恩惠、好意、给予福利援助”（莫尼尔·威廉姆斯爵士：《新版梵英辞典》）。

方法。其中包括：从有资格的讲授者那里聆听有关神的话题（*śravaṇam*）；以谈论和唱诵的方式荣耀神（*kīrtanam*，克尔坦）。对神的正式崇拜（*arcanam*），尤其是通过服务神圣形象（*mūrti-sevā*）的程序，也包含在上述相互关联、彼此涵摄的九种实践当中。[①]而神像崇拜实践，是本书探讨的核心论题。因此，我们的下一个主题便是实践中的巴克提，梵文称之为萨达纳－巴克提（*sādhana-bhakti*）。

第二节　规范练习阶段的奉爱服务——作为途径的巴克提

一、控制感官

关于萨达纳（*sādhana*）这个术语，当代高迪亚－外士那瓦学者约瑟夫·T. 奥康奈尔给出了简要解释：

> 萨达纳（*sādhana*）主要是指宗教实践中的模式或程序。梵文字根 *sadh*，意思是"达成"或"获得"某事物。*sādhana* 是一种方法或程序，人藉此臻达其所向往的境界，达到一种完美或实现一个目标。在此情形下，目标本身又是一个更为完美的巴克提（对主的奉爱）的经验。而萨达卡（*sādhaka*）指的是一个正在努力达到这种完美的人。
>
> 萨达纳是一种程序……在这种程序中，外士那瓦不仅运用他/她的心意，也运用其物质感官——眼、耳、发音器官——将潜在的奉爱能力发展到更为完美的顶点。[②]

---

① 其他六项是：忆念神的名字、形象、品质和娱乐活动（*smaraṇam*）；*pāda-sevaṇam*，字面意思是"服务双足"，即为神和他的虔爱者作谦卑的服务；向神供奉祷文（*vandanam*）；"侍奉"，即参与神的使命（*dāsyam*）；培养和神之间的亲密关系（*sākhyam*）；完全向神臣服皈依（*ātma-nivedanam*）。

② 约瑟夫·奥康奈尔：《规范练习阶段的奉爱服务》，收录于史蒂文·罗森编辑的《外士那瓦宗：当代学者论高迪亚传统》，纽约：民间书籍出版社，1992 年，第 229~230 页。

茹帕·哥斯瓦米所著《奉爱甘露之洋》是高迪亚－外士那瓦社团中最重要的神学著作之一。书中将巴克提分为三类，其中萨达纳－巴克提（*sādhana-bhakti*），即练习阶段的奉爱服务，属于第一类巴克提。[①]而这又可细分为遵守规范和自发奉爱两个阶段。对于大多数实践者而言，遵守规范这条路径已经是既定规程，因为我们不难发现，从事世俗活动的习惯本身构成一种束缚，[②]使得一个人或多或少不能够在自发奉献的层面上，至少以一种持久不变的方式行事。巴克提实践者遵循古鲁（*guru*，上师），还有经典（*śāstra*）的指导，学习将自己所有的躯体和心智活动用于服务神。克里希纳达斯·卡维罗阇在引用茹帕·哥斯瓦米关于“高级奉爱”的定义（参见前文）后，详尽阐释了以所有的感官（由此可见，在印度哲学传统中，心意被视为内在的物质感官）练习做“顺意”服务的内涵。接下来他进一步引用茹帕的观点，而茹帕又为解读五夜派经典提供了参考：

> 巴克提意味着用自己的感官服务至尊主的感官。这种服务使人从所有短暂的物质名相中摆脱出来，并使其感官得到净化。[③]

克里希纳还有一个称呼叫“瑞希凯施”，即“感官之主”。迷幻性的物质能量摩耶（*māyā*）的作用，就是通过促成与感官对象相关的感官活动产生令人愉快的结果，来为受束缚的生物拥有“自我支配权”这一错觉提供支撑。在按规范守则做服务的实践（外迪－萨达纳，*vaidhi-sādhana*）中，实践者认识到薄伽梵在本质上是有知觉的，从而学习将所有感官活动献给“感官之主”克里希纳。因此，举例来说，人的视力被认为是神无限视觉能力的一个极微小的表现形式；同样，所有其他感官的功能都被看作是神有着无限感官能力的证据所在，而神恰恰希望生物以巴克提为标志，奉献其感官活动

---

① 另外两个阶段是巴瓦－巴克提（*bhāva-bhakti*），即超越规范练习的自发奉爱，以及普瑞玛－巴克提（*bhāva-bhakti*），即狂喜的纯粹奉爱。后文会有探讨。

② 有人可能同样会提到习惯于从事世俗活动所导致的“致盲效应”。由于习惯性地专注于世俗事务，一个人便无法洞察其与神的关系中自我的灵性身份，而最终结果就是被绑缚在物质存在（*saṁsāra*）中。

③ 《柴坦尼亚生平甘露》中篇第 19 章第 170 诗节，引用了《奉爱甘露之洋》第 1 篇第 1 章第 12 诗节。

作为对他的服务。而将感官活动献给神所得到的回报，恰恰构成了自我真正的感官满足。

《薄伽梵歌》受到大多数印度人，尤其是外士那瓦（毗湿奴派）所有传系的推崇，[①]被公认为一部强调巴克提重要性的典籍。高迪亚－外士那瓦将其奉为基本指南。《薄伽梵歌》是由克里希纳直接讲给他的朋友阿周那（Arjuna）的，其中第九章特别论及巴克提，在接近尾声的第 27 诗节中，表达了将一己之活动奉献给神的基本理念：

> 无论你做什么，吃什么；无论你供奉什么，施舍什么；无论你做什么苦行。琨缇之子啊！你都应该当作对我的奉献去履行。[②]

这节诗概括了前一诗节的内容：

> 以爱和奉献之心，无论向我供奉一片叶、一朵花、一个水果，还是一杯水，我都接受。[③]

这些简短的声明指出一个关键性的神学理念，那就是感官从事的活动可以作为奉爱服务直接献给神。就这一原理，《薄伽梵歌》以及《薄伽梵往世书》等经典都对其作了广泛而详尽的阐释，而五夜派文献是从更为专业性的角度，特别是作为正式的仪轨来探讨的。

对为数众多的有关巴克提规范练习的训喻进行归纳整理，使之系统化，是六哥斯瓦米承担的课题之一。茹帕·哥斯瓦米列出了 64 项对于规范练习阶段的奉爱服务极为重要的条款，所有这些都直接或间接地与神像崇拜有关。这些训喻所涉及的范围从基本原则，诸如“从一位有着恰当资格的古鲁那里接受弟子身份”，到更为具体的训示；诸如“要跟在便携式庆典神像被抬着走的游行队伍之后”。在这 64 项条款当中，可以发现关于每日神像崇

---

① 并不是说以《薄伽梵歌》独尊，这一点应该是显而易见的，因为我们频繁提及其他文献典籍。

② 《薄伽梵歌》第 9 章第 27 诗节。

③ 《薄伽梵歌》第 9 章第 26 诗节。

拜程序的训喻。而在另一部文献，哥帕拉·巴塔·哥斯瓦米所著的《哈瑞奉爱之美》中，根据崇拜程序又将供奉物品细分为 64 种。[1]

二、旨在奉爱的仪礼服务

对高迪亚－外士那瓦传统中神像崇拜实践的某些内容进行简要讨论也许是有裨益的。应该注意的是，这一传统在神像崇拜实践的基本框架和大体内容方面，均与外士那瓦的其他传承类似。学者们早就注意到了这一点，印度各传统当中的仪式程序有相当的一致性。所以，比方说，南印度的湿婆圣典派（湿婆悉檀多派）[2]，甚至是所谓“异教”传统，特别是耆那教和佛教[3]，在为各自崇拜的对象供奉物品时，顺序几乎是一样的。[4]

既然对于高迪亚－外士那瓦而言，《薄伽梵往世书》拥有核心经典的权威性地位，既然其中对于神像崇拜程序的具体描述简明扼要，相对来说不很繁杂，那么，我们可利用这部文献来了解崇拜的基本要素。

该书第 11 篇第 27 章引用了克里希纳亲自给他的亲密朋友乌达瓦（**Uddhava**）概括的程序：

---

① 萨纳坦·哥斯瓦米似乎在某种程度上参与了该文献的编辑工作。参见苏希尔·库玛尔·德《孟加拉高迪亚－外士那瓦早期信仰和运动史》，加尔各答：佛玛 **KLM** 出版社，1986 年，第 125~145 页。

② 戴维斯：《振荡宇宙内的仪式：中世纪印度的湿婆崇拜》，全书各处。

③ 探究耆那教崇拜及其与佛教、湿婆派、毗湿奴派崇拜的比较，请参见劳伦斯·巴布《缺席的主：耆那教仪式文化中的苦行者与国王》，伯克利：加利福尼亚大学出版社，1996 年。

④ 这也许表明，印度各传统当中，其宗教体系除了他们所宣称的差异性之外，在更深层面上是存在相似之处的。这又是另一篇论文的主题了！保罗·图米（第 5~8 页）指出了关于食物供奉与接受（大多数印度崇拜的一个重要方面）的一个有益的理论上的差异。然而一些人类学家根据“崇拜者与神像之间的关系等级进行交流”，来解释食物供奉与接受仪式。而其他人类学家（包括图米在内）似乎更加肯定巴克提的内在动因，对“菩莎达（*prasad*，供奉过的食物）是一种独特的文化理念”这一论点给予支持。接着图米对菩莎达与基督教的圣餐加以比较。保罗·**M.** 图米：《来自克里希纳口中的食物：北印度朝圣中心的盛宴与节日》，德里：印度斯坦出版社，1994 年，第 5~8 页。

关于这个议题，还有一种普遍存在的观点，就是将崇拜视为慷慨供养，这是许多亚洲崇拜形式的共同主题。

> 现在我要原原本本地讲解，一位通过相关吠陀原则获得再生[①]资格的人，当如何以虔爱之心崇拜临在神像形体中的我？请忠实聆听。[②]

《哈瑞奉爱之美》详细阐述了人要获得“二次出生”[③]身份必备的资格。人必须从一位有资格的上师那里得到恰当的启迪，并接受训练，举止态度恰当得体，拥有外士那瓦风范，这样，才可直接崇拜神像（*arcā-mūrti*）。[④]然后，这样一位“再生者”要严格遵守与服务神有关的日常行为规范。而代表神的，可能是一个被安置自己家中的小神像，也可能是庙宇中或大或小的神像。每一天的服务始于太阳升起前的一个半小时（*brahma-muhūrta*），这时人就立即起床，从身、心两方面做好准备以接近神。

> 崇拜者应首先清洁牙齿、沐浴、净化自己的身体。接着，他应一边吟诵吠陀祷文和坦特罗（密教——译者注）真言，一边用圣泥

---

① “再生（二次出生，twice-born）”这种表述方式是梵文词汇 *dvija* 标准的字面直译，指的是三个上等阶层成员，接受启迪（*upanayanam*）进入吠陀典籍的学习，这被视为由吠陀“母亲”而来的又一次出生。不应将其与西方基督教福音派相关表述方式混为一谈。

② 《薄伽梵往世书》第 11 篇第 27 章第 8 诗节，该文献第 11 篇所有诗节由 H. D. 哥斯瓦米译成英文。

③ 五夜派的体系为所有阶层成员通过培养恰当行为使自己具备资格崇拜神像，提供了可能性。

④ 克里希纳・柴陀・达斯编辑：《五夜派的启示》，收录于管理委员会－神像崇拜组：《日常服务》第一卷增刊。印度玛雅普尔：国际克里希纳意识协会管理委员会出版社，1995 年，第 11 页。“举止态度恰当得体，拥有外士那瓦风范”，特指以下四方面：（节制）饮食（素食），（规范）性行为（只允许以生育后代为目的的婚姻内的同居），完全避免麻醉品和赌博。

在身上涂抹标记，做第二次净化。①

上述及其他相关活动构成 *abhigamana*，也就是为接近神、崇拜神而做的准备活动。这些崇拜神的准备活动是用物品来举行崇拜仪式的普佳（*pūjā*）五步曲之一，见载于五夜派文献，此文献中有日常神像崇拜程序的相关论述。②普佳五步曲之二是收集崇拜用品，包括收集可用来供奉的鲜花、食物和其他物品，运用净化程序做好准备，以做供奉之用。至于食物，则需恰当的烹调。

人应该用品质上乘的用具崇拜我的各种神像形体等等（*pratimādiṣu*）。③但一位完全免于物质欲望的虔爱者，可以用他能够得来的任何物品崇拜我，甚至可以在内心通过想象，做成各种用品，崇拜他心中的我。④

普佳五步曲之三是瑜伽（*yoga*），意为“连接”，尤指从内在与自我相

---

① 《薄伽梵往世书》第 11 篇第 27 章第 10 诗节。

对婆罗门关注“纯洁”这一点，尽管从理论上有详细阐述（主要是西方），但这一传统内部相关的解释颇为简单明了，用我们西方一句箴言概括就是：“洁净接近于虔诚。”为了接近至纯至粹的神，需要洁净的品质，但是洁净（尤其是内心或知觉）终极而言是由神赠予的。然而人可以实践由神直接或间接规定的有助于洁净的活动，从其中最简单的沐浴开始。关于这一点可能会有争议。或许除了印度婆罗门典籍之外，在世界任何其他宗教传统当中，都不会找到有关斋戒沐浴方面周密而翔实的规定，故其重要性是显而易见的。可能毗湿奴派会强调说，其重要性不能被简化为仅仅关注与其他社会群体保持界限的问题。然而恰恰相反，受束缚的灵魂对洁净并无兴趣，尤其是内在的洁净——这使其永不能与神直接交往。

② 查里：《外士那瓦宗：哲学、神学与宗教秩序》，第 311~316 页。

③ *pratimā*，字面意思是，“一个形象、样子、符号、照片、雕像、外形、影像”；*ādi*，字面意思是“作为起始”，意即“等等”。如前所述（参见第 18 页脚注④），这里表明，神也可以各种具有象征意义的物质或元素受到崇拜。

④ 见《薄伽梵往世书》第 11 篇第 27 章第 15 诗节。

我们可能注意到，被公认的较低和较高崇拜资格之间的差别，在此被一带而过了。内在资格越高，对其高品质供奉的外在禁制约束就越少。《哈瑞奉爱之美》一书对哪些物品适合供奉，哪些不适合，有广泛而详尽的阐述。就可供奉和不可供奉的鲜花这一点，给出的细节可能最多，该书第 20 章用整整一章的篇幅来专门讨论这个问题。

连，将自己看成是神的一位仆人。从仪式上来说，会有一个“身体诸元素的净化”程序，[①]梵文称之为 *bhūta-śuddhi*；接下来是崇拜者按照经典描述，对其即将崇拜的神的某个特定形象作简短[②]冥想（*dhyāna*）；并在内心对崇拜程序进行演练（*mānasa-pūjā*）。[③]对于克里希纳形象的冥想，克里希纳本人在《薄伽梵往世书》中描述如下：

> 崇拜者当冥思我的精妙形象——这形象乃众生之源，现在居于崇拜者那经空气与火净化的躯体中。觉悟了自我的圣哲们，在神圣音节“唵”音振之末，体验到主的这一形象。

接下来的步骤是“呼唤神降临”，恰当的崇拜可以开始了：

> 最高我的临在充盈虔爱者的身体，虔爱者想着以跟他的证悟相应的形象显现的最高我。如此，虔爱者倾注全力崇拜主，全然凝注于他。虔爱者一边吟诵恰当的曼陀罗，一边触碰神像的各部位，以邀请最高我进入神像的形体。接下来，虔爱者当崇拜（住在那神像中的）我。[④]

普佳（*pūjā*）五步曲之四，是以特定的顺序提供服务并供奉几样物品，

---

① 阿笈摩文本描述了在心理层面“解构”其物质身体，然后再以净化了的物质要素将其“重构”的复杂程序。高迪亚－外士那瓦将其简化为一个要点，即只是简单冥想自己乃神的永恒仆人，摆脱所有社会阶层（*varṇa*）和生命阶段（*āśrama*）的名号。

② 在“依据规范进行崇拜”的语境下，冥想通常是简短的。更高级的实践者可能按照他 / 她认为合适的方式，相应延长冥想时间。这同样适用于 *mānasa-pūjā*，这是瑜伽（*yoga*）的下一个步骤。“*yoga*”这一术语通常与钵颠阇利古典瑜伽体系联系在一起。然而，根据语境不同，其含义也颇为广泛。

③ *manasa-pūjā* 涉及将每一样物品在内心里进行供奉，就像一个人在结束 *Manasa-pūjā* 后，会运用身体四肢实际地供奉它们一样。然而，在心意中，有可能对其程序进行修饰润色，尤其是想象出远远超过实际崇拜中会有的豪华程度。

④ 摘自《薄伽梵往世书》第 11 篇第 27 章第 23~24 诗节。其中，诗节 24 建议崇拜暂时的神像，而不是直接崇拜神永恒的灵性形体。尽管《薄伽梵往世书》的这个诗节似乎给出了也可崇拜暂时神像这一选择，但其实毗湿奴派真正崇拜的是神永恒的灵性形体。

同时吟唱恰当的曼陀罗，即神圣之真言。[①] 如前所述，《哈瑞奉爱之美》一书中描述了其中 64 种物品和服务（*upacāras*），所有这些合起来构成从清晨到夜晚一整天的崇拜程序，包括唤醒、沐浴、更衣、装扮、供奉食物、娱乐，以及服侍神休息。在提供一系列服务的过程中，神要么被看成是家中尊贵的客人，要么是在他自己宫中的气派十足的帝王。不管哪种情况，规范练习（*vaidhi-sādhana*）阶段强调的是小心翼翼地遵守规章守则。不过，个人在家崇拜神像不太可能每天履行这样复杂的程序；所有这 64 项（或更多）[②] 服务会在比较大的庙宇中提供，更加关注准时正点。而且这一切并非一人独立完成，而是有好几位仪式普佳瑞（*pūjārīs*，专家），轮流在一天中的不同时段作出恰当的服务。这种庙宇尼提亚 – 塞瓦（*nitya-sevā*），即每日服务程序，一年到头每周七天，每天都举行；而在家崇拜神像一周内大部分时间可以做得很简单，每周或每两周可以做一次更加精心细致的服务。

上面所说的第四步，以特定的顺序供奉物品，同时吟唱曼陀罗，这项服务在喜庆气氛中结束：

> 虔爱者应该跟其他人一道大声唱诵，载歌载舞，表演我超然的逍遥时光，聆听、讲述关于我的故事，以此，当有一段时间沉浸在这般喜庆气氛中。[③]

这段文字摘自《薄伽梵往世书》第 11 篇第 27 章。这一章的主题是神像崇拜，而且对神像的正式崇拜是九种巴克提实践之一，但是，歌唱、吟诵以及聆听有关神的话题这一训喻，不仅是神像崇拜的一个方面，也是九种实践中前两种最重要的奉爱服务——聆听和唱诵（*śravaṇam* and *kīrtanam*）的实质内容，我们曾在第二章第一节第二部分探讨过这一主题。这也与普佳五步曲最后一项 *svādhyāya* 有关，梵文 *svādhyāya* 字面意思是“自学”，指独自

---

① 本书第二章第三节第二部分，我会在神像崇拜（*arcanam*）语境下讨论曼陀罗吟诵。

② 有学者告诉我，《哈瑞奉爱之美》一书的评述者指出，虽然特别规定的条款列有 64 项，但神像崇拜服务具有潜在的无限可能性。因此，在遵守规范的前提下，崇拜领域内也存在自由发挥的空间。

③ 《薄伽梵往世书》第 11 篇第 27 章第 44 节诗。

一人而不是和别人一起，阅读、吟诵以及学习神圣典籍。自修乃神像崇拜实践中的一个反思环节，藉此涵养灵性，帮助实践者免于例行公事或过分专注于规范细节，而忽视了规范背后的本质目的，即通过服务的态度培养对神的自然奉爱。既然所研习的文本（对高迪亚－外士那瓦来说主要是《薄伽梵往世书》和《柴坦尼亚生平甘露》）强调与神像崇拜相关的其他类型的服务，那么，研习及吟诵经典的活动作为神像崇拜的一个步骤，表明了参与崇拜神像之外的其他服务项目同样是非常必要的。上述这些活动围绕以下内容展开：服务毗湿奴的虔爱者（*vaiṣṇava-sevā*）；服务神的圣名（*nāma-sevā*，而且是通过吟诵和歌唱的方式）；接待和服务来宾（*ātīthi-sevā*）；分发和进食圣化的食物（*prasāda-sevā*）；服务与神有关的圣地（*dhāma-sevā*）。通过认真练习上述服务（*sevās*），实践者有望从一个知觉不太成熟的阶段（这一阶段的特点是，以专注于神像为借口而忽视其他生命体）发展到意识、态度及行为举止比较成熟的阶段。神像崇拜的这一反思环节是非常重要的，因此需关注经典中的告诫，薄伽梵的一个化身卡皮拉（Kapila）在《薄伽梵往世书》中教导如下：

> 谁向我致敬，却嫉妒其他生物的躯体，谁就是分离主义者。由于他满怀敌意对待其他生命体，他心中永远无法获得平静。无罪的人啊！即使以恰当的仪式和物品崇拜我，却对众生心怀不敬，没有意识到我临在他们心中，这样的人永远不会通过崇拜我在庙宇中的神像而取悦我。[①]

第三节　作为目标的巴克提

一、引向神圣游戏：回应

以上对规范练习阶段的奉爱服务（*vaidhi-sādhana*）作了概述，现在我

① 《薄伽梵往世书》第 3 篇第 29 章第 23~24 诗节。

们可以回顾一下，高迪亚－外士那瓦神学体系所构想的奉爱（巴克提）实践的完整次第，尤其是茹帕·哥斯瓦米在《奉爱甘露之洋》一书中所阐明的。[①]他确认可从八个次第来实践巴克提。由于具备初步的信心，使人与其他实践者交往，一起从事规范练习，以此为开端。然后，在中止不良行为的阶段，人可体验到实质性的进展。在这一阶段，对巴克提实践的有效性产生坚定的信心，由此在修习当中变得稳定。

在下一阶段，开始体验到茹祺（*ruci*），即一种对巴克提真正的“品味”或爱好，特别是喜爱虔敬地聆听有关神的话题。由“品味（*ruci*）”发展出一种强烈的、不可动摇的对神之依恋（*āsakti*）。由此境界，超然的情感巴瓦（*bhāva*）便产生了。当这种巴瓦的情感体验强烈而深沉，普瑞玛（*prema*）便浮现于心中，这是对神最高的爱。正如我们前面提到的，这种对神最高的爱，被认为以休眠状态潜伏于一切众生的内心。

早于茹帕·哥斯瓦米 500 年左右的室利毗湿奴派学者罗摩奴阇在其著作《吠陀旨要》一书中阐释了类似的修习次第。在描述巴克提展开次第的结语中，他强调，经验神的恩典与经验巴克提本身，即是目标：

> 至高无上的人，充满怜悯，为这样的爱所取悦，将他的恩典播撒到这位有志者身上，摧毁其内在的所有黑暗。对至尊人的巴克提在这样一位虔爱者内心发育。巴克提本身就是无价之宝。发自内在的虔爱源源流淌，不会中断。这份虔爱本身就是绝对的妙喜，这份虔爱本身就是冥思，呈现最为生动鲜活的品质，即刻在内心屏幕上投放视频美景。通过这般虔爱——巴克提，人便臻达至尊。[②]

由此可见，巴克提被构想为既是方法，又是目标。它是臻达至尊人的途径和手段。不过目标达成后，仍不会放弃巴克提，因为正是它构成薄伽梵与吉瓦（*jīva*，个我）间互动关系的交流原则。从这个视角来看，巴克提被

---

① 《奉爱甘露之洋》第 1 篇第 4 章第 15~16 诗节。

② 参见克劳斯·K. 科罗斯特梅尔《印度有神论传统中的神话与拯救哲学》，加拿大宗教研究社编辑，安大略省滑铁卢：威尔弗雷德－劳里埃大学出版社，1984 年，第 105 页。《吠陀旨要》由 S. S. 拉伽瓦查尔译。

认为是超然生活的基本方式。唯此超然生活之方式，可确保直接经验神之临在。《拿拉达虔信经》语言风格简约凝练，是梵语文学诗歌体裁中典型的代表作。其中陈述道："当人在巴克提中臻达这种爱，那时，他目之所见唯有神，耳之所闻唯有神，心之所知唯有神。"[①] 正是在这一阶段，神的"可接近性"被完全经验到。如此，他庄严宏大的品质渐行渐远，变得不再重要，取而代之的是一种亲密感。关于这一主题，后面的章节会有更详细的阐述。目前我们只需注意到，毗湿奴派声明，当巴克提完全绽放之时，其本身可被看作结局或目标。在这一境界中，达成一种资格，藉此资格可以恰当领悟和全然经验到神的临在，不管神是为了发挥某一特定作用而以化身（*avatāra*）示现，还是以居住在心中的形象（*antaryāmin*），或是作为神像形体（*arcāvatāra*）显现。

二、交流的媒介：声与形

梵文 *śuddha-bhakti*（殊达－巴克提）是指纯粹奉爱。据说在这一阶段，一个人能领会"非物质的"[②] 声音与形象。传统的吠檀多不二一元论（*advaita-vedānta*）将一切声音和形象视为摩耶（*māyā*）和现象世界（*saṁsāra*）的展示，需要借助于称为 *upāsanās* 的各种技巧来冥想，以最终超越声音和形象。梵文 *upāsanās* 的意思是"用以接近的方法"。既然声音和形象都是感官的对象，那么感官活动（*karma*）必须停止，这时才能获得真知（*jñāna*）。一个有志于追求真知的人必须从感官活动上撤回其注意力。而由于中止诸如此类的感官活动极为困难，所以给出了各种"用以接近实相

---

① 见《拿拉达虔信经》第 55 节诗，*tat prāpya tad-evāvalokayati tad-eva śṛṇoti tad-eva cintayati*. 格拉汉姆·施维克译：《拿拉达虔信经：拿拉达关于奉爱本性及体验的简要教导》，载《毗湿奴派研究期刊》1998 年冬第 6 卷第 1 期，第 148 页。

② 威廉·H. 戴德惠勒：《虔爱者与神像：活在人格的神学中》，收录于乔安妮·蓬佐·瓦格恩、诺曼·卡特勒合编：《血肉之神，石制之神：印度神性的体现》，纽约：哥伦比亚大学出版社，1996 年，第 79 页。戴德惠勒批评不二一元论（*advaita*）哲学所认定的方程式"形象 = 物质"，并指出"无有形象"必然也是一种物质的观念，与"有形有相"的观念相互依存。"灵性形象"或"非物质形象"对虔爱者（*bhakta*）而言不是自我矛盾的措辞，对于拥有多种品质的绝对者来说，并非如不二一元论教义所说的，在任何方面都低于梵（*brahman*）——被构想成不具品质的绝对者（毗湿奴派将其解释为"没有物质的品质"）。

的方法和技巧”（*upāsanās*），作为通往完美之路上过渡阶段的修习。

与吠檀多不二一元论形成对照的是，毗湿奴派与印度其他有神论哲学流派一样，将神圣的声音与形象视为直接来自神的启示，并赋予其本体论意义上的核心地位。也许就这一点而言，高迪亚－外士那瓦较其他毗湿奴派传系走得更远，他们强调启示的纳玛（*nāma*，圣名）乃一种类型之“化身”的观念。藉由这一化身，神让自己变得最易接近，尤其在当今这个年代。[1]对此，克里希纳达斯·卡维罗阇引用室利·柴坦尼亚的话作为论据：

> 在这个喀历年代，由主的圣名“哈瑞－克里希纳”构成的这首伟大的曼陀罗，是主克里希纳的化身。仅仅通过吟诵这圣名，人便直接与主沟通往来。任何如是做的人一定获得拯救。[2]

继而，他将神圣的名字、形象、品格与普通的名字、形象、品格加以对比：

> 主的圣名、形象和品格都是同一的。在他们之间没有差别（*bheda nāhi*，不异）（非不一）。既然他们都是绝对的，[3]就都是超然妙乐的。在克里希纳的身体与他本人或者他的名字与他本人之间没有差别（区分，区分的基础）。但是，就受制约的灵魂（吉瓦）而言，这些（绝对）是各不相同的。一个人的名字有别于他的身体，有别于他的原本面貌，等等。[4]

---

① 古史文献将宇宙时间划分为四个年代（*yugas*）的循环周期，据此可知，我们现在正处于喀历年代（包括未来的 42 万 8 千年在内）。这是一个退化和堕落的年代，我们大多数人有很少的或根本没有耕耘灵性的倾向和能力。对于高迪亚－外士那瓦而言，吟诵哈瑞克里希纳摩诃曼陀罗（*harināma-kīrtana*）是巴克提修习的核心，尤其是以齐诵形式（*harināma-saṁkīrtana*）。贝克：《声音的神学》，收录于《外士那瓦宗》，第 275 页。

② 摘自《柴坦尼亚生平甘露》初篇第 17 章第 22 诗节。

③ 严格说来，“既然他们都是绝对的”不是韵文，却是对 *bheda nāhi*（无有差别）的解释。帕布帕德经常用“absolute（绝对的）”一词作为梵文 *advaya*（不二）的英文对应词，或许也可被理解为“不可约的、不可简化的”。

④ 摘自《柴坦尼亚生平甘露》中篇第 17 章第 131~132 诗节。我在括号内加上文字，我想，这有助于对这部分译文的理解。

接着他引用茹帕·哥斯瓦米所著《奉爱甘露之洋》一书来阐明，如何将此差异性运用于以有限的物质感官接近无限至尊人的问题：

因此，物质感官无法领会克里希纳的圣名、形象、品质和娱乐活动。然而，人只要热切渴望用自己的舌头（吟诵主的圣名并品尝主的祭馀）和其他感官（因为感官已被净化）作出服务，克里希纳本人便在世间显现。[①]

由上文可知，要领悟克里希纳作为化身（*avatāra*）降临现象世界，需要个体生物（*jīva*）激活感觉器官，从而对此作出回应。一元论者会争辩说，这意味着承担业报（*karma*），个体生物会由此更深地纠缠于虚幻存在中。对此，外士那瓦的回答是，这种感官活动即使看似业报活动，实际上是对神的奉爱服务（*bhakti*，巴克提），带来的效果是使人从物质束缚中脱身。《薄伽梵歌》第 9 章第 28 诗节紧跟着我前面引述的诗节（参见本章第二节第一部分），讲了这个问题：

如此（通过把活动奉献给我，你的主人），你便能摆脱工作的捆绑，免于吉祥或不祥结果的束缚。以这样弃绝的原则将心意凝注于我，你必会得到解脱，而臻达我。

正如我们前面已讨论过的，在奉爱服务中，人的感官被用来服务“神的感官”，而这成为与神交往互动的基础。藉由神的恩典，特别是通过神圣声音作为媒介，并不纯净的个体生物（*jīva*）在某种意义上回归其纯净的地位，而在纯净状态中与神交流是可能的。在这回归本性的过程中，舌头是所有被用到的感觉器官中最为重要的，因为它具有发音和品尝食物的双重功能。

五夜派文献详细阐述了神圣语言的复杂神学体系，认为这种神圣语言与

---

① 摘自《柴坦尼亚生平甘露》中篇第 17 章第 136 诗节。

天体演化过程及神的救世活动相互联系。[①]这涉及声音与形象之间的关系，与早期文献所表述的结论大体相同。对此，桑玖克塔·古普塔解释如下：

> 早期诸《奥义书》已经谈到，世界据说是由名字（*nāma*）和形象（*rūpa*）构成的。在系统哲学中，二者之间的关系成了言语及其所指对象之间的关系。如同所有坦特罗（密教——译者注）体系一样，在五夜派神学体系中，这种关系被应用于曼陀罗及其所指的神像：一个曼陀罗代表一尊神像。[②]

曼陀罗，即“有力的真言”和它所代表的神性之间的关系，要是以五夜派后期文献中出现的“巴克提”术语及奉爱实践的角度来看，便会得到愈发深刻的理解。在那种语境下，曼陀罗是神之恩惠的一种展示。早期五夜派文本指出，真心实意、准确无误地念诵从自己的古鲁那里得来的曼陀罗，被更多理解为是一种获得力量以及与曼陀罗所指称的神像相认同的方法。重点是在遵循瑜伽传统前提下的个人努力和冥思。五夜派后期文本将曼陀罗表述为“神之眷顾”的具体体现。念诵曼陀罗，凭借神之恩典，臻达与神交融之境。这是一种情感经历，而不再是简单的冥思体验。可见，五夜派早期与后期文本对于曼陀罗概念的解读迥然不同，而在该派的“皈依”修持法（*upāsanā*），即“结合崇拜的冥想法”中，存在二者的调和。“结合崇拜的冥想法”将曼陀罗的应用和物质形象的崇拜看作是同等重要的。[③]

高迪亚－外士那瓦强调曼陀罗吟诵的核心重要性，通过吟诵曼陀罗，舌头的发音吐字能力被用来从事对神的服务。虽然吠陀经和五夜派文献中有数个曼陀罗用于日常神像崇拜，但高迪亚－外士那瓦传系追随柴坦尼亚的教导以及他所树立的典范，最看重被称为“摩诃曼陀罗”（*mahā-mantra*）的首要真言。这首曼陀罗使用“哈瑞（*hare*）”“克里希纳”（*Krishna*）和“罗

---

① 古普塔：《五夜派对曼陀罗的态度》，第 225 页。关于这一问题，在五夜派之前和与之同时代其他学派的典籍中，已有大量语言学方面的思考，尤其是弥曼萨卡斯和语法学家们。但在《梨俱吠陀》赞美诗中早已有过关于神圣语言的讨论。

② 古普塔：《五夜派对曼陀罗的态度》，第 230 页。

③ 古普塔：《五夜派对曼陀罗的态度》，第 231 页。

摩”（*rāma*）三个神圣名字，以不同的组合重复这些名字，在语法上都属于呼格（而不像大多数曼陀罗适用于以与格崇拜的神）。① 在高迪亚 – 外士那瓦中产生了大量著作，包括克里希纳达斯·卡维罗阁所撰写的柴坦尼亚传记《柴坦尼亚生平甘露》（*Caitanya-caritāmṛta*），对怀着爱心虔诚唱诵摩诃 – 曼陀罗的重要性、练习方法、练习中需避免的障碍及其转化人心的功效等，都逐一进行了讨论。克里希纳达斯·卡维罗阁在其著作中记载，柴坦尼亚作为一名托钵僧（*sannyāsī*，桑尼亚西）居住在印度东海岸中部的佳甘纳特 – 普瑞（Jagannātha Pūrī），在那里度过他的后半生（直到 1533 年）。当时他亲身示范了如何将崇拜神像与吟诵哈瑞克里希纳摩诃 – 曼陀罗有机地结合起来，使之融为一体。柴坦尼亚的追随者们每天都在“宇宙之主”佳甘纳特宏大的庙宇中举行庆典活动，他们由柴坦尼亚带领大声唱诵摩诃 – 曼陀罗，在喜笑颜开的佳甘纳特及其同伴的神像面前热情洋溢地舞蹈。

这座古老的庙宇② 供奉的是统称为佳甘纳特的四个木制大神像，分别为佳甘纳特（Jagannātha）、苏芭朵（Subhadrā）、巴拉提婆（Baladeva）和苏达尔珊纳（Sudārśaṇa）。高迪亚 – 外士那瓦尊奉这些特别的形象分别为克里希纳、克里希纳的妹妹、克里希纳的哥哥巴拉提婆或巴拉罗摩，以及克里希纳炽热的神碟武器。在佳甘纳特神庙，柴坦尼亚（Caitanya）亲身示范哈瑞纳玛 – 桑克尔坦（*harināma-saṁkīrtana*），即通过齐颂神的圣名荣耀神，以此表明这是最简易、最有效的接近神、取悦神的方法。对于柴坦尼亚的追随者们来说，很显然，规制神的崇拜仪式的所有规范原则，都要从属于

---

① 这是有名的“哈瑞，克里希纳；哈瑞，克里希纳；克里希纳，克里希纳；哈瑞，哈瑞。哈瑞，罗摩；哈瑞，罗摩；罗摩，罗摩，哈瑞，哈瑞”。“哈瑞（*hare*）”既是对“诃利（*harī*）”，又是对“诃拉”（*harā*）的呼唤，前者是薄伽梵的一个名字，后者则是薄伽梵阴性能量的一个名字。

② 现今的庙宇可能建于公元 12 世纪。然而，关于庙宇起源及佳甘纳特的起源和祭仪的意义，众说纷纭。宇宙古史和其他文献中，存在着大量有关神像和庙宇的传奇故事。这些神像颇能打动人，因为他们不同寻常，在外貌上看只是一半形象。对此的解释是，由于虔诚的国王迫不及待地想看到神像雕刻工作的进展情况，所以违背了他不去打扰雕刻师的诺言。神于是传达了自己的意思：这个“未完工”的形象实际上是完整的，他一直渴望以这个特别的形象接受崇拜。参见哥琵纳特·莫哈帕特拉《奥里萨历史与宗教传统中的佳甘纳特》，奥里萨第 13 号研究项目，加尔各答：庞提 – 普斯塔克，1982 年，第 45 页，第 380~382 页。

一个首要原则，其包括两方面内容，即“时刻铭记主，片刻不忘记他”。[1]柴坦尼亚的极乐（esctatic）[2]表现也使他们确信，庙宇神像要被当作神的直接展示来崇拜。《柴坦尼亚生平甘露》记载了虔爱者们所经历的与神像之间互动交流的事件，向他们证实了神临在于这些形象中的事实。

在佳甘纳特－普瑞，柴坦尼亚的追随者们经验神之临在的一个重要途径是品尝菩莎达（*prasāda*），即按照仪式程序供奉过神像的祭馀。这座不寻常的庙宇颇具特色，其中一个特色就是，时至今日其仍保留了沿袭数世纪之久的一个传统，由婆罗门严格依据规范，遵循据说是自建庙以来就一直未变的食谱，准备和烹调大量食物来供奉神像。荟萃各种供奉过的食物的公共大餐，总是将柴坦尼亚每日里齐颂圣名的欢庆气氛推向高潮。用餐过程中，柴坦尼亚会鼓励他的追随者们要吃“到嗓子眼儿”。[3]由此看来，在高迪亚－外士那瓦传统中，舌头的第二个功能——品尝，被认为是必不可少的真正的愉悦，这是通过以食物为载体进行交流来实践巴克提的方法。如先前提到

---

① 语出《莲花往世书》,《柴坦尼亚生平甘露》中篇第 22 章第 113 诗节引用。

② 关于“极乐/狂喜（ecstasy）”一词，我已经在别处提过。为厘清奉爱的极乐（devotional ecstasy，ecstasy 指一种强烈的情感，经由身体上的表现展露于外）和瑜伽的极乐（yogic ‘enstasy’，此处，enstasy 亦指强烈的情感，却不流露于外）二者间关系，我们还应考虑前者与萨满教的极乐（shamanic ecstasy）之间的关系。米尔恰·伊利亚德在探讨萨满教与瑜伽的关系时，将萨满巫师的狂喜跟瑜伽行者的狂喜加以比较。他认为前者的特征是“极力致达某种精神状态以成就极乐之旅”，而后者以“完美的自主”，即“收摄入于内在解脱之境”为特征，梵文称之为 *jivan-mukta*，意为“在这一生中灵魂已获得解脱和自由”。参见米尔恰·伊利亚德《瑜伽：不朽和自由》，新泽西，普林斯顿：普林斯顿大学出版社，1969 年，第 339~340 页。由此不难理解，萨满教的极乐与奉爱的极乐也存在极大反差。朱恩·麦克丹尼尔在她的著作《圣人的痴狂：孟加拉极乐的宗教》一书中指出了这一点（芝加哥：芝加哥大学出版社，1997 年）。她在书中参考了米尔恰·伊利亚德提出的 ecstasy（狂喜、极乐）的词源学意义，即“站在外面”或“置身圈外”，进而强调奉爱的极乐是“知觉、情感或个性上根本性的转变，这将人带到距离其所认同的神圣对象更近的地方……”极乐中的心醉神迷之人通常经过一个分裂蜕变阶段，但最终体验到一种整合，将自我的各个层面融合在一起，或者说，在此境界当中，体验到自我与神圣者之间有了一种更加亲密的关系或结合为一体。然而，萨满教的极乐“展示的是灵魂与躯体的分离”，因而“提前体验了死亡经历”。而巴克塔（*bhakta*，虔受者/奉献者）的极乐涉及超意识，在超意识境界中，所有感官充满了对崇拜对象——神的知觉，或者说每一感官因盛满神知觉而处于“满溢”状态。肯尼斯·R. 华培:《神像崇拜：高迪亚－外士那瓦的瑜伽》，载德文期刊《明辨真理》，1996 年 10 月第 5 期，第 8~9 页。

③ 《柴坦尼亚生平甘露》中篇第 14 章第 23~46 诗节。

的，神在《薄伽梵歌》中允诺，他会接受怀着虔诚爱心献给他的食物。虔爱者们肯定，尽管被神像接受的供品也许并未发生物质上的转化，但是显然已经被神品味过了，留在供盘上的食物已经被注入他神圣的瞥视，使人的进食活动成了转化心灵、获得解脱的经历。对此，《薄伽梵歌》第 3 章第 13 诗节也有论及：

> 主的虔爱者免于一切罪恶，因为他们只吃事先供奉给主的食物；其他人烹制的食物只是为了个人的感官享受，实际上，吃下去的只是罪恶。①

修习者与其他同道之间互赠食物的同时，也使他与神之间的交流更加圆满。茹帕·哥斯瓦米在其著作《教诲的甘露》一书中，将赠与和接受食物列入神的虔爱者之间彼此交流爱心的六种方式之一。②

柴坦尼亚所亲身示范的，和“宇宙之主”佳甘纳特之间情感交流的高潮，在一年一度的檀车节（*Rathayātrā*）上被经验到。檀车节期间，四尊神像被安放在三辆巨型木质檀车上，沿城市主要街道巡游。③时至今日，这个节日庆典依然吸引了三十到五十万朝圣者。对柴坦尼亚及其追随者而言，檀车节有着隐秘的意义。解释这一点，须回到我们先前提到的布阿佳（Vraja）。那片土地被确认为是克里希纳童年的居所，是他与家人和朋友度过亲密时光的地方。正如《薄伽梵往世书》中所描述的那样，柴坦尼亚在极乐中，将自己认同为克里希纳的爱侣茹阿达（Rādhā），而在情感上与之产生共鸣。他用力拉动佳甘纳特檀车的情景，成为茹阿达在克里希纳离开她去了马图拉多年以后，尝试将克里希纳带回布阿佳一幕的再现。

《柴坦尼亚生平甘露》对此事有更为细节性的描述，有时虔爱者无法使

① 《薄伽梵歌》第 3 章第 13 诗节。

② 参见《教诲的甘露》诗节 4。其他四种交流爱心的方式是互相赠送与接受礼物、亲密地交谈与询问。

③ 根据“檀车节”这一事件，造出一个英文词“*juggernaut*”。《韦伯斯特词典》将其界定为：“（1）任何巨大的、压倒一切的、具有毁灭力的物体；（2）任何要求盲目奉献和无情牺牲的事物；（3）在印度奥里萨邦普瑞地区的克里希纳神像，每年被虔爱者载于大车上拉着巡游，据说有人曾不惜投身轮下，被碾压而过。”

佳甘纳特檀车继续前进，这被看作是由于佳甘纳特拒绝移动的结果。经柴坦尼亚好言相劝后，巨大的檀车竟在他一人之力下神奇地[1]运转起来。对于高迪亚－外士那瓦而言，这一事件展示了茹阿萨（*rasa*），即唯美的情感回应模式之卓越性。茹阿萨是支撑和维系神与他的虔爱者之间关系的实质。与上述隐秘的内在经验相反，神像崇拜作为巴克提实践，主要受外在行为规范的制约。而这种外在行为所指向的目标（*prayojana*），才是我们理解高迪亚－外士那瓦传统中神像崇拜理论的一个关键组成部分。这是第三章要探讨的主题。在第三章，高迪亚传统中有关神像崇拜更为具体的方面将被阐述得愈发清晰。

---

① 理查·戴维斯在其论文集《亚洲宗教传统中的神像、神迹与权威》（科罗拉多州博尔德：西景出版社，1998 年）里探讨了与神像有关的“神迹”这一概念。罗伯特·布郎的一篇文章中也讨论了“被期盼的神迹”，对理解檀车节那天也许发生在柴坦尼亚身上的事件富有启发意义。本书姑且接受《牛津足本大辞典》中“神迹”的定义：“在人类经历中所发生的不可思议的事件，以人类之力或任何自然力量的运作都不可能促成这一结果，因此应当归因于神或某一超自然体的特别介入。”

第三章
巴克提－茹阿萨：奉爱美学

当你日间离家去森林，片刻于我们犹如千年，因为看不到你。即便在我们热切地凝视你那被一头卷发衬托得如此可爱的美丽脸庞时，我们的快乐也被愚蠢的造物主所制造的眼皮妨碍了。

——《薄伽梵往世书》10. 31. 15[①]

第一节　再论克里希纳的能量

我们一直在讨论称为*arcanam*（神像崇拜）的奉爱服务模式，梵文*arcanam*指的是虔爱者（*bhakta*）向至尊人（*bhagavān*）献上正式的崇拜。然而，在高迪亚－外士那瓦传统中，克里希纳不是被单独崇拜的，而是和茹阿达（Rādhā）一起接受崇拜。茹阿达被称为*pūrṇa-śakti*，是克里希纳“能量”的具体体现和完满化身；而克里希纳被称为*pūrṇa-śaktimān*，是无限神圣能量（*pūrṇa-śakti*）的完全拥有者。关于茹阿达，卡普尔解释如下：

> 室利·克里希纳是神圣人格无限（在数量上）的局部展示的终极始源，而茹阿达是室利·克里希纳无尽神圣能量的终极源头。克里希纳与茹阿达之间的关系是不可思议的既同一又有差异的关系。本质上，他们作为同一实体而存在，为了享受神圣游戏而呈现两个

① 此处作者在其英文原著中给出了原梵文诗文，详见本书英文相关部分（译者注）。

> 不同形象。茹阿达与克里希纳是一体的，因为她与克里希纳喜乐能量展开的巅峰完全一致。但她又不同于克里希纳，因为她是被主宰的一半，而室利·克里希纳作为绝对者，是完全拥有主宰权的一半。基于这差异，室利·克里希纳以其内在固有的个性呈现一男性形象，而茹阿达则呈现一女性形象。然而，不可将他们之间的关系比作世俗男女的躯体关系。茹阿达的身体，与克里希纳身体一样，是由妙乐和知觉构成的，他们两人之间的爱属于灵性层面。①

正如克里希纳把自己扩展成各种不同的化身（通常是“男性”），茹阿达亦将自己扩展为无数的女性助手，作为牧牛姑娘（*gopīs*），协助茹阿达在布阿佳参与克里希纳恋爱的逍遥时光（*līlā*），以此取悦克里希纳。但在布阿佳，克里希纳也有其他类型的助手，尽管不被看作是茹阿达本人的扩展，不过仍然是克里希纳喜乐能量的展示，因为他们本着协助他娱乐时光这个唯一宗旨，而永恒地与他交往。这些虔爱者可能是克里希纳的朋友和亲戚，不过也可能作为动物（尤其是乳牛、猴子、孔雀和鹦鹉），甚至是不动的植物和树木——实际上他（它）们中的每一位都为神不断增加的快乐尽了一份力量。

克里希纳的每一位同伴，通过各自从事的奉爱服务，以及他（她）特定的茹阿萨——与克里希纳处于某种情感关系中所品尝到的种种滋味，而与他在一种独享的专有关系中相处。《薄伽梵往世书》中有一段著名诗节阐释了克里希纳是如何被视为各种关系之宝库的。下面这段话描述的事件，发生在

---

① 卡普尔:《室利·柴坦尼亚的哲学和宗教：哈瑞－克里希纳运动的哲学背景》，第98页。**A. K.** 马宗达对茹阿达身份问题所给出的又一种解释或许有助于我们理解这一点：“茹阿达是克里希纳的喜乐能量，但她既不是这能量的一部分，甚至也不是这能量的代表，她就是以最极致的满幅状态呈现的能量本身。”茹阿达是 *pūrṇa-śaktī*……茹阿达实现了最重要的情感，是最理想的喜乐能量的具体化形象。茹阿达事实上是喜乐能量的根基，在她那里，可认知的特性，或品质，或属性，或偶然事件，皆被认为是孕育或影响了玛杜尔－茹阿萨（*mādhurya-rasa*，情侣之爱）现象背后的最本质特征。在跳茹阿萨舞的现场……二元性的舞蹈以终极的结合为结束……终极的茹阿萨，从茹阿达－克里希纳的这一结合中浮现出来，露出真相。“事实上，他即是茹阿萨”（摘自《鹧鸪氏奥义书》)。克里希纳自己是“非二元灵知的真相”，和茹阿达一起的他是“非二元品味或情感的真相”。

克里希纳离开温达文前往玛图拉，面对恶魔国王康萨的挑战，并最终除掉他之后：

> 当克里希纳和他哥哥一起步入竞技场时，不同的人群以各不相同的方式看待他。摔跤手们看克里希纳恰似雷霆闪电；玛图拉的男人视他为最杰出的男性；女人们将他看作是丘比特本人；牧牛郎把他当作自己的亲人；没有虔敬之心的统治者认为他是惩罚者；在他的父母眼里他是孩子；博佳的君王视他为死亡；无知的愚者认为他是至尊主的宇宙身相；瑜伽行者视他为绝对真理；而维施尼（克里希纳的族人）把他看作值得他们崇拜的至尊神。①

《薄伽梵往世书》的早期注释者之一，室利陀罗·斯瓦米（公元14~15世纪）认为这段文本呈现了十种类型的茹阿萨（*rasa*），即关系。在他之后，茹帕·哥斯瓦米在其著作《奉爱甘露之洋》及《闪耀的蓝宝石》中，列出了12种关系，其中五种主要关系，七种次要关系。②茹阿萨学说的核心在于克里希纳是一切茹阿萨（关系）之甘露的具体体现和化身。一个人可能会在所有神明或半神人③当中作出选择和评价，但在启发茹阿萨情感方面，无论是就广度、深度，还是就庄严崇高的气质而言，没有任何一位非凡人

---

① 此处作者在其英文原著中给出了原梵文诗文，详见本书英文相关部分（译者注）。

② 七种次要的茹阿萨是：愤怒、惊异、幽默、骑士精神 、怜悯或仁慈、恐惧、恐怖或可怕。五种主要的茹阿萨是：平和的中性关系、主仆关系、朋友关系、父母与孩子的关系、情侣间的相互爱慕与吸引关系。茹帕以系统地将传统印度美学与神学相结合而著称，尽管在他和柴坦尼亚之前已经有某些思想和著述在朝这方向迈进。克劳斯·科罗斯特梅尔这样写道：关于美学的本体论，文学中不乏存在于终极实在的情感根基，由此形成了茹阿萨理论。柴坦尼亚的情感宗教便是如此，在当代文化中有着强壮的根系。同样，对两性爱情的礼赞，乃基于躯体层面的相互吸引，实际上，亦是基于灵魂层面的合而为一，在茹阿达和克里希纳这对神圣爱侣身上可以见到这一爱的投影，所有这一切在柴坦尼亚出场之前便已存在。克劳斯·K. 科罗斯特梅尔：《一个情感的宇宙》，收录于《室利·克里希纳·柴坦尼亚与巴克提宗教》，艾德蒙·韦伯、提拉克·拉杰·乔普拉编辑：《灵修研究》1988年第33期，法兰克福：彼得朗出版社，第115页。

③ 半神人（或天神），据吠陀经/古史文献记载，共有三千三百万。高迪亚－外士那瓦理论将其划归个我灵魂范畴，就其本体论地位而言，与人类、动物和植物相同。凭其虔诚行为，他们获得明显高于人类的“神授”资格和地位。然而，这一地位是短暂的，像任何个我生命体一样，这些天神也会死亡。

物可与克里希纳相提并论。更重要的是，除了克里希纳，没人能在任何方面，可以展示与之相媲美的玛杜雅－茹阿萨（*mādhurya-rasa*，两性间的爱慕），因为他所示现的是最原始、最基础的阿迪茹阿萨（*ādi-rasa*）——其他茹阿萨都与之有亲缘关系，并从中派生出各自的意义和功能。① 另一方面，克里希纳的卓越超群如其所是。这让人回想起，克里希纳不仅仅是众多化身（*avatāras*）之一，而且是所有化身的源头和宝库，梵文称之为 *avatārin*。就连克里希纳作为被造宇宙之始源这一事实，在他作为“情感之宇宙”的源头这一事实面前，都退居次位了。② 正如克劳斯·科罗斯特梅尔所表述的，③ 宇宙以永葆茹阿萨（*rasa*，关系）的和声为宗旨，每一生命体都在其中永恒地分享、品味着与至尊人的关系和情感。正是茹阿萨使克里希纳有别于甚至高于毗湿奴：

> 即使在幸运女神（Śrī）之主毗湿奴与克里希纳二者的真实本性之间无有差别（根据既定义理），通过茹阿萨（*rasa*），也使得克里希纳的真实本性愈加卓越。这便是茹阿萨的地位。④

因为茹阿萨（*rasa*）必然涉及关系，于是克里希纳的虔爱者在崇拜他的时候，就不把他当作“非二元灵知的真理”（*advaya-jñāna-tattva*），而是作为“非二元情感的真理”（*advaya-rasa-tattva*）。尤其对高迪亚－外士那瓦而言，这意味着把茹阿达与克里希纳合起来一道崇拜。

将男性神明与他们的女性伴侣或配偶合起来崇拜，在印度有着悠久的

---

① 印度的美学家历来都在争辩平和或怜悯哪个是核心情感。高迪亚－外士那瓦关注玛杜雅－茹阿萨（*mādhurya-rasa*，两性间的爱慕），认为它是和以下学说相伴产生的——它与克里希纳有关，是爱的最完美的表达。相反，世俗两性间爱的吸引以色欲为特征。

② 通过将克里希纳的身份确认为是外在世界创造者毗湿奴各种形象（*puruṣa-avatāras*）的源头，而进一步强调了物质创造的次要和从属地位。

③ 科罗斯特梅尔：《一个情感的宇宙》，第 113 页。

④ 尼尔·德尔莫尼科：《茹阿达：牧牛姑娘中的佼佼者》，载《毗湿奴派研究期刊》1997 年秋第 5 卷第 4 期，第 117 页。

历史。[1] 南印度的毗湿奴女神派传系遵循五夜派经典，主要崇拜以毗湿奴（Viṣṇu）或那罗衍那（Nārāyaṇa）的身份显现的克里希纳，将毗湿奴与他的配偶拉克希米（Lakṣmī），或者将那罗衍那与他的配偶幸运女神（Śrī，室利）合起来崇拜。拉克希米与毗湿奴之间的关系被看作是已婚夫妇关系，梵文称之为 *svakīya-rasa*。这与茹阿达和克里希纳之间的关系形成对照，茹阿达和克里希纳二人的关系更像是一种情侣关系，梵文称之为 *parakīya-rasa*。在 18 世纪神像崇拜领域，这一度成为高迪亚 – 外士那瓦的一个棘手的问题，因为他们对茹阿达 – 克里希纳的崇拜，受到另一个被称为罗摩南迪的外士那瓦团体的严厉批评。[2] 高迪亚 – 外士那瓦学者巴拉提婆 · 维迪亚布善和罗摩南迪数位学者，在拉贾斯坦邦加尔塔地区举办的一场辩论会，将这个问题推到了顶点。后者并不反对单独崇拜克里希纳，但他们坚持认为，把茹阿达也加进来和克里希纳在一起接受崇拜，是在纵容非宗教行为。高迪亚 – 外士那瓦传统告诉我们，后来巴拉提婆引用他本人对《梵经》的评注据理力争，挫败了罗摩南迪学者们所持的观点。[3] 巴拉提婆当时辩论道，茹阿达和克里希纳两人的关系合情合理、中规中矩，这不成问题。因为以本体论角度来看，他们二人永恒地联系在一起，一个是沙克提（*śakti*，能量），而另一个是沙克提曼（*śaktimān*，能量的拥有者和来源）。如果有谁获准和克里希纳来往，那么这个人必定是茹阿达，因为她是神圣戏剧的神圣女主角、

---

① 要了解与印度教的诸男神有关的诸女神的研究综述，请参见大卫 · R. 金斯利《印度教诸女神：对印度宗教传统中神圣女性的认识》，伯克利：加利福尼亚大学出版社，1998 年。

② 罗摩南迪是南印度室利毗湿奴女神派在北印度的一个分支，传承于 14 世纪宗教改革家罗摩南达。参见达亚南达 · 达斯《巴拉提婆 · 维迪亚布善：高迪亚 – 吠檀多学者》，载《回归首神》，1991 年 1~2 月合刊本，第 32 页。

③ 达亚南达 · 达斯：《巴拉提婆 · 维迪亚布善：高迪亚 – 吠檀多学者》，第 32 页（第二部分）。这一传统的原始资料是孟加拉文著作。室利 · 哈瑞达斯 · 达斯：《室利 – 室利 – 高迪亚 – 外士那瓦百科全书》，纳瓦兑帕圣地，哈瑞布 – 库提尔出版社，1955 年。当然，了解罗摩南迪传统对这一事件的说法也会很有趣。实际上，关于在高迪亚 – 外士那瓦（或在其他传系中，尤其是尼跋迦的追随者）庙宇中，茹阿达出现在克里希纳身旁一同接受崇拜的历史经过，并未见载于史料。S. K. 德指出，在哥帕拉 · 巴塔 · 哥斯瓦米所著的《哈瑞奉爱之美》一书中并未提及茹阿达。由此看来，茹阿达和克里希纳一同崇拜的仪式，显然是 16 世纪后形成的（苏希尔 · 库玛尔 · 德：《高迪亚–外士那瓦早期信仰和运动史》，第 508 页）。

对神之奉爱的最高典范，故而是完美贞洁的具体体现和化身。茹阿达和克里希纳表面上看似非法的关系，则给这幕戏剧平添了几分浪漫色彩，吸引崇拜者放下尘世的干扰因素，而进入那丰富多姿、动人心弦的超然茹阿萨的超验领域。[①]

第二节 布阿佳：甜美之地

在第一章第四节中，我曾简要提及克里希纳度过他童年和青少年时光的布阿佳（**Vraja**）。克里希纳在那里展示了他的具体实在性，还有他甜蜜而美妙的本质特征。甜美性与实在性在布阿佳完美地结合在一起，使得克里希纳，或更准确地说，是茹阿达－克里希纳这对神圣爱侣成为不拘小节的奉爱服务的接受者，让人更易接近。这就与为宇宙之主毗湿奴或那罗衍那（及其女性伴侣拉克希米或幸运女神）所做的更为正式的崇拜，形成鲜明对比。如果说克里希纳是茹阿萨（*rasa*）的具体体现和化身，那么他也应该是丽拉（*līlā*，神圣游戏）的具体体现和化身，可以说，克里希纳在布阿佳最充分地展示其逍遥时光的全部意义。对此，大卫·金斯利评论道：

> 在温达文（布阿佳），克里希纳远离尘世，没有必要出于实用性的考虑去做事。他用不着扮演某个角色，而只是自由洒脱地在一举一动中展露他的本性。在牧牛人的村庄，克里希纳远离他作为化身的使命世界，没有什么自由活动的禁区。温达文是一个游乐园，一个神奇的地方。在那里，克里希纳，那个爱玩耍的顽皮孩童，可

---

① 有学者提出，克里希纳和牧牛姑娘们“婚外的情侣之爱”这一学说直到六哥斯瓦米之后的一段时期才盛行起来。此前，六哥斯瓦米中的吉瓦·哥斯瓦米基于经典和美学标准文本《茹阿萨论》（*rasa-śāstra*）的推断，运用一个案例已经说明他们之间的关系属“婚内的夫妻之爱”，他说，他认为“婚姻内的风流韵事并无什么不当之处”（苏希尔·库玛尔·德：《高迪亚–外士那瓦早期信仰和运动史》，第 348~349 页）。又见简·布热津斯基：《克里希纳最终究竟有没有娶这些牧牛姑娘？》，载《毗湿奴派研究期刊》1997 年秋第 5 卷第 4 期。

以自由自在，不停地嬉戏作乐。[①]

当然，克里希纳在布阿佳的娱乐时光中也有漫无目的的成分，就这个意义而言，它不具有世俗的必要性，也不出于实用主义目的。[②]但在高迪亚－外士那瓦神学体系中，所有这些表面上看似缺乏目的性的游戏背后，却有着一个更为深刻的用意——就是要吸引受束缚的个我灵魂，使之从以谋求世俗成就为典型特征的昏睡状态中脱离出来。根据《薄伽梵往世书》所说，日益醉心于世俗名利之人，主要是渴求财富、学识、美丽的躯体以及下一世高贵的出身等。为了移除这些物质性的短暂追求，克里希纳通过他自己的超然魅力来吸引这些人。在布阿佳，他展现了他美丽迷人的形体和相貌（*mādhurya-rūpa*）。而正因为克里希纳在那里展现其美丽和魅力，布阿佳才变得如此令人着迷。就这一点，茹帕·哥斯文瓦米以诙谐的口吻警告他的读者：

> 我亲爱的朋友，要是你真的依恋世间的友情，那么，当主哥文达（克里希纳）伫立在凯西伽塔（位于温达文的一处特别的沐浴点）的雅沐纳（河）岸边时，最好别去看他的笑脸。他将他的笛子含在唇边，娇嫩的双唇美如枝头新芽。他微微偏头侧目瞥视着你，超然的身体弯成三度曲线，在月夜里熠熠生辉。[③]

由此可见，克里希纳在布阿佳所展示的美，对一个人全神贯注于俗世事务的现状构成威胁，因为后者并不能与克里希纳－巴克提－茹阿萨（Krishna-*bhakti-rasa*）交融在一起。如果一个人想要永处于俗务为先的状

---

① 大卫·R. 金斯利：《剑与笛：印度神话中的黑面形象——恐怖的卡利和美妙的克里希纳》，伯克利：加利福尼亚大学出版社，1975年，第76页。

② 克利福德·霍斯皮特尔在其所著《早期外士那瓦思想中的神圣娱乐》一文中，对*līlā*（神圣娱乐）及与之相关的梵文术语*krīḍā*在外士那瓦宗的各种不同意义作出有益探讨。见威廉·S. 萨克斯编：《游戏中的神：在南亚的娱乐时光》，纽约：牛津大学出版社，1995年。

③ 《奉爱甘露之洋》第1篇第2章第239诗节。《柴坦尼亚生平甘露》初篇，第5章第224诗节引用。

态中（并因而遭受反反复复的生、老、病、死之物质痛苦），那么，最好离布阿佳远一点。布阿佳是一个上演精彩戏剧的舞台，一个人进到里面，就如同被带到永恒的灵性国度，其内在会为不可预知的爱所转化。布阿佳的这种特质在约翰·斯特拉顿·霍利的论述中得到进一步凸显。在下段引文中，他将布阿佳与印度其他以“时空交叉之地‘提尔塔’”著称的圣地作了比较：

> 正如茹阿萨－丽拉（*rāsa līlā*，布阿佳各地上演的民间戏剧）中有首歌经常唱道的那样，温达文的街道上到处回旋着爱的洪流：那里是无章无序的。而一旦哪位粗心旅客一不留神被卷入这爱的潮水，那就没希望再逃脱了。指望在温达文找到一处安全通道，几乎是不可能的事。人来到温达文，不是为了（像在提尔塔那样）穿越时空，而是为了“被淹没”，淹没在未知的爱的神秘海域，于此“淹没”中，体悟到一种在陆地上从未经验过的静谧平和。[①]

克里希纳的虔爱者（*bhaktas*）渴望至少在布阿佳住上一段时间，以“淹没在未知的爱之海洋”。茹帕·哥斯瓦米将“居住在布阿佳”列为规范修习（*vaidhi-sādhana-bhakti*）阶段64项实践中的五项主要原则之一。居住在布阿佳，会使遵守诸多规范原则所获得的利益成倍增长。不单安放在庙宇里的神像，更有无数个与克里希纳娱乐活动有关的地点，都让人感受到他本人亲临的吸引力。同样地，甚至更重要的是，一个人会得到以温达文内湿瓦瑞（Vṛndāvaneśvarī，温达文首席女神）著称的茹阿达的祝福，以参与到神圣游戏中，为有着全然吸引力的克里希纳作服务。

不过，大多数人都没机会居住在布阿佳，对他们来说，去布阿佳及其周边地区朝圣是进入这超然地域的途径，这样至少可以有一段时间成为克里希纳娱乐活动的参与者。自16世纪以来，布阿佳一直是朝圣中心，时至今日，其每年接待的游客数目还是多于泰姬陵的。[②]有人独自前来，有的和家人一

---

① 约翰·斯特拉顿·霍利：《与克里希纳一起游戏：来自布瑞德万的朝圣戏剧》，新泽西，普林斯顿：普林斯顿大学出版社，1981年，第51页。

② 大卫·L. 哈伯曼：《解脱之途：自发练习阶段的奉爱之研究》，纽约：牛津大学出版社，1988年，第193页，第55页脚注。

起前来，有的则数百人甚至成千上万人组团而来。人们在温达文镇（需步行四英里）巡行，或绕拜哥瓦尔丹山[①]（需步行14英里），或是游览整个布阿佳（步行约200英里，需中途露营）。无论选哪一条旅游路线，沿途都会遇到克里希纳庙宇，每一处庙宇都坐落在与克里希纳某一特定丽拉（*līlā*，娱乐活动）有关联的特定地点，而这些特定丽拉都有权威经典的依据，或来自当地的古老传统。这样行进的时候（如果举止"恰当"，那么就会出于对圣地的尊敬而赤足），会一个接一个地达善（*darśana*，有幸觐见）克里希纳的神像。当人这样得见克里希纳之时，会被专心聆听他的娱乐活动所滋养，那些使人疏远神的世俗自我概念[②]（不如说是"错误的想法"）被无形中清除。感觉器官变得"克里希纳化"了，目之所视、耳之所闻、鼻之所嗅……所有感官对象都与克里希纳有关，沉浸于克里希纳亲临的经验当中。这时，便有可能领悟克里希纳的名字、形象、品质、娱乐、住所的超然本质。在这一知觉层面上，时空的局限性为超然情感的狂喜之洋（*bhāva*，巴瓦）所替代。

---

① 哥瓦尔丹山是布阿佳地区的一座神山，据说曾被克里希纳像擎一把伞那样，举了七天七夜，以保护温达文居民免受因陀罗的狂怒及其暴雨的伤害。

② 正如史蒂文·吉尔伯格所指出的，人类学家维克多·特纳呼吁我们从社会边缘性、阈限性及社群后续经历等方面，关注朝圣体验中的共同主题。吉尔伯格强调："去温达文朝圣（居住在那里，更是如此）如果没有一个根本上的阈限体验，就没有意义。"去温达文朝圣不只是一次远离社会的度假，而是远离尘世的度假。史蒂文·J. 吉尔伯格：《温达文：神秘经历的所在地》，载《毗湿奴派研究期刊》1992年秋第1卷第1期，第23页。大卫·哈伯曼在其著作《穿越12座森林之旅：同克里希纳不期而遇》（纽约：牛津大学出版社，1994年，第69~71页）一书中，对特纳关于朝圣，尤其是去布阿佳朝圣的论点作出评论。又，A. W. 恩特威斯尔所著的《布阿佳：克里希纳朝圣中心》（格罗宁根：爱格伯特 – 弗斯腾出版社，1987年，第105~107页），探讨了布阿佳朝圣的特别之处，同时反对人类学的泛化推理。E. 瓦伦丁·丹尼尔所著《流动的符号：做一位泰米尔式的人》（伯克利：加利福尼亚大学出版社，1984年，第7章），是又一部印度语境下很有趣的著作，不过是从"一元论"角度探究朝圣主题。丹尼尔在亲身经历一次朝圣之旅后，依据查尔斯·S. 皮尔士所提出的现象范畴为"第一性"，经验范畴为第二性和第三性的理论，对朝圣现象作出分析。

第三节　通往完美的互补路径：薄伽梵道与五夜道

高迪亚－外士那瓦崇拜茹阿达－克里希纳神像，不过他们这样做的时候，是把自己看成室利·柴坦尼亚的仆人，在他们心目中，室利·柴坦尼亚正是茹阿达和克里希纳“合而为一的形象”。克里希纳尽可能使自己容易让人接近，但在这个灵性退化的宇宙周期喀历（Kali）年代里，大多数受束缚的个我灵魂（*jīvas*）未能意识到他，未能将自己内心的忠诚和热爱直接倾注于他身上。为此，正如克里希纳达斯·卡维罗阇告诉我们的，克里希纳示现了一次特别的降临，以向个我灵魂提供一个更容易接近他的途径。这一次，他作为室利·克里希纳·柴坦尼亚·摩诃帕布（Śrī Krishna Caitanya Mahāprabhu）化身前来，扮演一位他自己的虔爱者（*bhakta*），以便亲身示范一位克里希纳的虔爱者在情感、态度以及行为举止等方面的所有细节。

> 室利·茹阿达和克里希纳之间的爱情是主的内在喜乐－给予能量的超然展示。尽管茹阿达与克里希纳从其身份上来说是一体的，可他们还是永恒地分为两个个体。现在这两个超然的本体再次以柴坦尼亚的形象结合为一。我向他顶礼，他就是克里希纳本人，却以室利妈媞·茹阿达茹阿妮（Śrīmatī Rādhārāṇi）的情感和肤色展现自己。[1]

由此可知，在高迪亚－外士那瓦神像崇拜实践中，至少从过去的两个世纪或更长时间起，[2]就已经通常把柴坦尼亚的神像与茹阿达－克里希纳神像一道崇拜。不过很多时候，人们看见柴坦尼亚的神像会和他最亲密的同伴室利·尼提阿南达帕布的神像在一起。尼提阿南达帕布被确认为克里希纳在

---

① 《柴坦尼亚生平甘露》初篇第 1 章第 5 节诗。

② 正如追溯茹阿达神像崇拜的历史一样，要对柴坦尼亚神像崇拜的历史追根溯源也是困难的事。苏希尔·库玛尔·德在其著作《高迪亚－外士那瓦早期信仰和运动史》（第 227~230 页）中认为，将柴坦尼亚认同为茹阿达－克里希纳合而为一的形体，是在六哥斯瓦米著作出现之后发展起来的理论。然而，这可能会是在克里希纳达斯·卡维罗阇于其著作《柴坦尼亚生平甘露》中颇为全面而清晰地阐述这一学说之后不久才发生的事，显然克里希纳达斯·卡维罗阇与六哥斯瓦米有过交往。

温达文娱乐时光中的哥哥巴拉罗摩。[①]从外观来看，两人通常双臂高举，呈起舞姿势。他们同时以传道说法的精神而受到后世的纪念。按《薄伽梵往世书》记载，他们四处旅行，有力地教导克里希纳 – 巴克提（Krishna-*bhakti*，对克里希纳的虔爱），强调“齐颂克里希纳名字”（*harināma-saṁkīrtana*，哈瑞纳玛 – 桑克尔坦）的重要性。此外，在如何服务克里希纳的虔爱者方面，他们亦为后世树立了完美的典范。

在高迪亚 – 外士那瓦神学体系中，柴坦尼亚和尼提阿南达现身说法，展现了克里希纳 – 巴克提的神圣精神生活，强调以下三种实践活动：其一，学习和教授《薄伽梵往世书》及相关经典；其二，齐颂克里希纳的名字；其三，为外士那瓦（Vaiṣṇavas，克里希纳的虔爱者）服务。以上三项实践构成了梵文所称的巴嘎瓦塔 – 摩尔伽（*bhāgavata-mārga*），字面意思是“薄伽梵的仆人之路”[②]（简称“薄伽梵道”——译者注）。与这条“路径”联系在一起的还有对巴克提实践的强调，这一点受到克里希纳亲密同伴的启发和激励，并以其为楷模，练习自然而发地从事奉爱服务（*rāgānugā-bhakti-sādhana*）。这里所强调的是自发的奉爱服务，与遵守经典规范阶段所做的奉爱服务（*vaidhi-bhakti-sādhana*）颇为不同，不过，仍然属于练习（*sādhana*）阶段的奉爱服务。由此可知，自发的奉爱服务（*rāgānugā-bhakti-sādhana*）在超越规范化练习阶段（*vaidhi-bhakti-sādhana*）的同时，仍会存在某些规范的因素。

---

① 本观点在《柴坦尼亚生平甘露》初篇第 5 章各处均有提及。

② 史学家们追溯到早在公元几世纪或更久远的年代，就存在两个多少有些区别的外士那瓦宗，一个称为薄伽梵派（*Bhāgavatas*，巴嘎瓦塔），而另一个称为五夜派（*Pāñcaratras*）。有学者指出：“二者主要区别似乎在于，尽管那罗衍那的虔爱者巴嘎瓦塔已接受了婆罗门的社会阶层，而五夜派对此却漠不关心，甚或持反对态度。”参见苏维拉·贾斯瓦尔：《外士那瓦宗的起源与发展：公元前 200 年至公元 500 年的外士那瓦宗》，德里：穆恩施罗摩 – 玛诺哈拉出版社，1981 年，第 46 页。然而，在商羯罗所作的《梵经》注释中，也将五夜派文献的追随者们称为巴嘎瓦塔。参见斯瓦米·甘比拉南达译：《室利·商羯罗阿阇梨耶的梵经注》，加尔各答：阿兑塔修院，1965 年，经文 Ⅱ. ii. 42，第 440 页。总之，此处所使用的两个术语 *bhāgavata-mārga*（薄伽梵道）和 *pañcarātra-mārga*（五夜道），着重点各不相同。至于我个人的研究，我通过电子邮件询问数位巴克提 – 瑜伽哲学的学者，得出以下结论：本书中对 *bhāgavata-mārga*（薄伽梵道）这一术语的使用方式，是 20 世纪初期印度毗湿奴派学者巴克提希丹塔·萨拉斯瓦提所特别强调的。

与薄伽梵道相辅相成的是五夜派之道（*pañcarātrika-mārga*，简称“五夜道”——译者注），后者以规范化的练习（*vaidhi-bhakti-sādhana*），尤其是以规范化的神像崇拜实践为特征，这一点我曾在第二章中有所论及。《柴坦尼亚生平甘露》记载了历史上许多奉爱服务的事例，包括某些公认的在灵性层面地位崇高的灵魂与克里希纳神像之间的沟通，有助于更好地理解这两条“道路”是如何达成互补关系的。而且，对于那些阅读或聆听常含有某些“神迹”因素的文本的高迪亚－外士那瓦来说，这些“神迹”恰恰证实了认真实践巴克提的有效性，以及神临在于被崇拜的神像中所给予的回应。

其中有一个故事足以说明这两条“道路”是可以做到相辅相成的。这个故事是以玛达文陀·普瑞（约 1420—1490）为中心展开的。他是一位深得高迪亚－外士那瓦（Gauḍīya-Vaiṣṇavas）尊崇的苦行者，是柴坦尼亚的古鲁的古鲁。他在布阿佳崇拜称为哥帕拉的克里希纳神像。一次梦中，他得到他神像的命令，要他去佳甘纳特－普瑞弄些檀香木①。于是，玛达文陀·普瑞便独自踏上漫长的旅程。他在接近目的地的途中，顺便拜访坐落在瑞沐那（Remuṇā）的哥琵纳塔（Gopīnātha，克里希纳又一个名字）神庙。他想，为了给哥帕拉神像做更好的服务，可以在那里作番调研。

> 玛达文陀·普瑞心想：“我要向祭司打听一下给哥琵纳塔供奉什么食物，这样我们的厨房里也可以做同样的安排，为室利·哥帕拉神像献上类似食物。”当婆罗门祭司被问及这个问题时，他详细解释了给哥琵纳塔神像供奉什么样的食物。这位婆罗门祭司说道：
>
> “傍晚我们给神像供奉用 12 个陶罐盛放的甜奶饭。因为它的味道美如甘露，故得名阿密瑞塔－凯利。这甜奶饭以哥琵纳塔－祺罗②享誉全世界。在世界上任何其他地方都不供奉这种甜奶饭。”
>
> 就在玛达文陀·普瑞和婆罗门祭司谈话的时候，甜奶饭被作为

---

① 把檀香木研磨成浆，涂在身上，有清凉之效。它是印度供奉神像或献给尊贵之人的标准物品之一。

② 祺罗（*Kṣīra*）是一种牛奶或炼乳。“甜奶饭”是为人喜爱的甜品，把米放入煮浓的牛奶里，加糖慢慢小火熬熟。更准确的叫法应该是“*kṣīrānna*”（牛奶加谷物/米），不过，一般简称为祺罗（*Kṣīra*）。

一道供品摆在了神像面前。听了祭司一席话，玛达文陀·普瑞这样想到：

“如果不用我开口，就能给我一点甜奶饭的话，我就能品尝一下，然后给我的主哥帕拉制作同样的供品。”

玛达文陀·普瑞意识到自己内心产生了想要品尝甜奶饭的想法，感到无比羞愧。他立即转念，开始冥想主毗湿奴。就在他这样想着主毗湿奴之时，供奉完毕。阿尔提（*ārati*）仪式[①]开始了。仪式结束后，玛达文陀·普瑞顶拜神像，然后离开了神庙。他没有对任何人再说什么。

玛达文陀·普瑞不行乞。他完全无所依附，对物质事物不感兴趣。如果不用他乞讨，有人给了他些食物，他就吃；否则他就戒食。一位像玛达文陀·普瑞这样的帕罗摩汉姆萨（*paramahaṁsa*，至尊天鹅）[②]总是满足于对主的爱心服务。物质的饥渴不会妨碍他的活动。当他内心产生了想要品尝一点给神像供奉的甜奶饭这一念头时，他觉得自己作出了冒犯的行为，因为他竟想要吃正在给神像供奉的食物。玛达文陀·普瑞离开了神庙，坐在村里空荡荡的集市上。他坐在那里开始念诵圣名。与此同时，庙里的祭司服侍神像躺下安歇。[③]祭司完成他的日常职责后，就去休息。在睡梦中，他看到哥琵纳塔神像来跟他说话，主这样说道：

“祭司啊，请起床，打开庙门。我为那位托钵僧（玛达文陀·普瑞）留了一罐甜奶饭。这罐甜奶饭就在我的布帘后面。因为

---

① 阿尔提（*Ārati*），又称为 *ārātrika*，是一个向神像供奉各种物品的简短仪式。站在神像面前，一手摇铃，一手舞动着供品。供奉的主要物品有灯（点燃樟脑丸或浸泡在纯净黄油或油中的棉灯芯）、盛满水的海螺。大多数庙宇，这种仪式一天中会举行五到八次，在仪式之前要供奉食物。这是公共活动，观众可以借此机会静静观礼，同时献上祷文，或者吟唱适合特定神像的颂歌。欲了解从一个基督徒的有趣视角对这一仪式作出的考察，请参见普拉桑拿拜神父：《耶稣：仪式的化身——作为我们伟大阿尔提的圣祭礼》，载《维迪亚玖提神学反思期刊》1997 年第 60 期，第 192~199 页。

② 帕罗摩汉姆萨：天鹅般的崇高人物，对一位灵性造诣极高的苦行者的称谓。

③ 萨亚那 – 塞瓦（*Śayaṇa-sevā*）：安歇服务。傍晚时分，将神像放置在小床上。要是神像太大太重，在这种情况下，就用一个 *utsava-mūrti*，也就是更小一点儿的神像，通常是金属制成的，作为大神像的翻版，将其放在床上，代表大神像。

> 我耍了个小把戏，所以你没有看到它。一位叫玛达文陀·普瑞的托体僧正坐在空无一人的集市里。请从我后面把这罐甜奶饭取出来，交给他吧。”
>
> 祭司从梦中醒来，立即从床上起身，按照惯例，进入神像房前，他沐浴了一下。然后按照神像的指示，在布帘后找到了那罐甜奶饭。他把罐子取走，又把原来放罐子的地方擦干净。接着走出神庙，关上庙门，带着这罐甜奶饭来到村子里，在每一个货摊前大声喊着，寻找玛达文陀·普瑞。祭司托着那罐甜奶饭，呼喊道：
>
> “谁叫玛达文陀·普瑞？请来接受这罐子！哥琵纳特为你偷了这罐甜奶饭！请过来，取走这罐甜奶饭，无比幸福地享用祭馀吧！你是这三个世界中最幸运的人了！”[1]
>
> 玛达文陀·普瑞听到这一邀请，便走出来自报家门。祭司于是把那罐甜奶饭交给他，在他面前直挺挺地倒下，五体投地顶拜他。祭司详细讲述了甜奶饭的来历，玛达文陀·普瑞立即沉浸在对克里希纳的狂喜之爱中。[2]祭司一看到玛达文陀·普瑞展现出来的极乐之爱的征象，不由得大为惊叹。于是明白了为什么克里希纳对他（玛达文陀·普瑞）深怀感激，他看到，克里希纳的行为与玛达文陀·普瑞的奉爱境界是相称的。祭司向玛达文陀·普瑞顶拜后，返回神庙。与此同时，玛达文陀·普瑞在心醉神迷的喜乐中，享用了克里希纳留给他的甜奶饭。

故事结尾说，之后这位苦行者急忙上路，以免第二天清晨当地的虔诚居民成群结队来围观他。

这段记载中，一位专注于规范化庙宇神像崇拜的祭司，赢得了克里希纳的恩典，得以洞悉神与他灵性造诣高深的虔爱者之间的亲密往来。这位苦行者玛达文陀，有着崇高的奉爱情感与敏锐的知觉，甚至为自己在神像正接受供奉的食物时产生了品尝的想法而深感羞愧，尽管他这么想实际上没有什么不当之处（因为他的想法是等供奉结束后再品尝）。平时，克里希纳看似以

---

① “三个世界”：印度普遍的宇宙观，指地球、天堂及其中间的宇宙地带。

② “沉浸于狂喜之爱中”，梵文称作 *prema-āviṣṭa*，字面意思是“充满爱”。

他的神像形体（*arcā-mūrti*），在被动地接受着崇拜和供品。而这次，他突然间变成一位积极主动的施事者，“玩了一个小把戏”，以此向他的虔爱者保证：这想法不算冒犯。那位知晓一切的神哥琵纳特（Gopīnātha，后来便以 Kṣīra-cora-Gopīnātha——“偷甜奶饭的主”而闻名），察觉到玛达文陀想要品尝甜奶饭，动机只有一个，那就是，提升对“以哥帕拉形体显现的他自己（克里希纳）”的服务质量。在这种情况下，他抓住时机，充当了一次他虔爱者的仆人，满足了他虔爱者心中的愿望。他打破常规，可以这么说，他成了“甜奶饭的偷盗者”，以其行为证明，他的虔爱者非但没有违反任何规范原则，相反，想品尝甜奶饭的心态本身，最好地诠释了整个规范原则背后的真正目的，即一个人不该想着享受任何东西，除非为了神的享乐，已经将其供奉给神了。与此同时，克里希纳也充当了他的祭司仆人的古鲁，向他透露了玛达文陀的崇高灵性地位。[①]最后一个要点，从这段引文，我们也理解到，那位祭司未能领会透露给他的一切意味着什么；倒是他忠诚恭顺地[②]履行职责（包括细节之处，例如，即使在不同寻常的情况下，接近神像前也要沐浴），使之有资格获得这一祝福。

上述引文，除了呈现“奉爱之路”和“规范之路”如何在神像崇拜的语境下互为补充外，同时，又是众多例证中一个典型范例，以向虔爱者证实——神“活跃地临在于”其神像形体中。正如该故事所描述的一样，经典中也有其他类似的记载，神有时会“打破自然律法的常规”。他这样做，与其说是为了展露他的能力和力量，不如说恰恰相反——是为了向人展示他的“易接近性”——他随时准备成为他仆人的仆人，从而打破了他永远是主人的“常规”。

---

① 这个特别故事的后文，也是意味深长的。玛达文陀只是继续他的使命，去为他的神像哥帕拉找檀香木。尽管很显然，他已达到灵性完美境界（他被称为“至尊天鹅桑尼亚西”），而且那种完美已通过“哥琵纳特事件”得到进一步确认，但他没有因此而退隐无为，远离尘世。相反，不二一元论学派传统托钵僧的追随者们一般来说会放弃一切努力，试图终止业力作用。而毗湿奴派托钵僧一直保持积极活跃，把解脱当作是“永恒服务于神的起点”。即使在解脱状态中，一位外士那瓦仍会遵守神像崇拜的规范原则，以身作则教导那些正在成长中的后来者。

② 祭司的恭顺之处，文中已有暗示。尽管他于梦中接收到来自神的特别策划，也未表现出丝毫骄傲。

第四节 故事中微妙的临在

根据高迪亚－外士那瓦理论，正如神以其神像形体出席，而让自己变得可亲可近一样，茹阿萨（*rasa*）以其反面——“神的缺席”营造一种微妙的临在感。自玛达文陀·普瑞时代起，[①]高迪亚－外士那瓦就把“情侣之爱”的心绪（*mādhurya-rasa*）从前述五种主要的茹阿萨中单列出来，作为对神“顶级之爱”的范式。“情侣之爱”中还有一个独特的方面，就是“与所爱之人的分离感”（*vipralambha* 或 *viraha*）[②]，或称“心上人缺席的感觉”，这是高迪亚－外士那瓦诗人和神学家一直关注的主题。玛达文陀·普瑞因为以这种心境向克里希纳供奉了一段简短而又富有创意的祷文，而再次得到高迪亚－外士那瓦的颂扬。他因此被誉为“神爱的播种者”，以最崇高的情感播撒克里希纳－普瑞玛（Krishna-*prema*，对神纯粹的热爱）的种子。后来，这神爱的种子，到柴坦尼亚·摩诃帕布（Caitanya Mahāprabhu）时代，以他本人为标志，已长成一棵参天大树。

> 啊！我的主！最仁慈的主人啊！玛图拉之主啊！我何时再与你相见？因为见不到你，我一颗焦灼的心躁动不安。我最钟爱的人啊！现在我该如何是好？[③]

玛达文陀·普瑞为他的哥帕拉神像服务，他感觉到克里希纳就在他的神像中。他的感受如此强烈，所以把一个梦境的内容看作是直接来自克里希纳本人的讯息——吩咐他为了神而踏上一段充满艰难险阻的旅程。在最后一段祷文中，他表达了与神的分离之情。神临在每一个当下，但从某种意义上来

---

① 弗莱德海姆·哈迪认为将玛达文陀·普瑞的生卒年份定在 1420 至 1490 年之间似乎是可信的。参见弗莱德海姆·哈迪：《玛达文陀·普瑞：孟加拉－外士那瓦与南印度巴克提之间的纽带》，载《英国皇家亚洲协会期刊》1974 年，第 23~41 页。该文对下面所引诗节作了细致的分析。

② *vipralambha* 字面意思是“欺骗，失望，情侣的分离，分开，分裂”；*viraha* 字面意思是“抛弃，遗弃，分手，分离（尤指恋人之间），离开，缺少，缺乏”。莫尼尔·威廉姆斯爵士：《新版梵英辞典》，牛津大学克拉伦敦出版社，1960 年。

③ 《柴坦尼亚生平甘露》末篇第 8 章第 35 诗节。

说，他又不是“充分地亲临”。

与此类似，一位汇编了毗湿奴派仪轨《哈瑞奉爱之美》的南印度婆罗门哥帕拉·巴塔·哥斯瓦米，极其渴望直接见到克里希纳，就像克里希纳以“圣石”（*Śālagrāma-śīlas*，被视为那罗衍那或毗湿奴直接展示的神圣小石头）形象展现在他面前一样。在这一事例中，神后来以“自显的”神像形体“茹阿达罗曼”（Rādhāramaṇa，给予茹阿达快乐的人），满足了他的愿望。①

关于神临在神像形体这一点，还有一精妙之处在于凸显柴坦尼亚作为克里希纳本人的身份，此类故事所呈现的基本主题是，克里希纳的神像形体无疑直接就是神本人，不过，从某种意义上来说，柴坦尼亚·摩诃帕布“更是如此”，或者说，“这一点尤为重要”。我们正在探讨的是巴克提的目标以及基于这一目标而从事的神像崇拜理论，在结束这部分内容之前，我想简要叙述两个故事。

第一个故事同样涉及食物供奉，含有恶作剧的成分，却呈现不同的一面。发生的时间是在柴坦尼亚还是孩童的时候（当时叫“尼迈”），地点是在纳瓦兑帕（今西孟加拉境内）他父母家中。一位行乞化缘的婆罗门客人受到尼迈父母的殷勤款待，结果他们精心准备的食物却被这位淘气的孩童在同

---

① 这一故事以柴坦尼亚在南印度旅行期间遇到年轻的哥帕拉·巴塔为开端。哥帕拉·巴塔成为柴坦尼亚的追随者，切实履行导师对他的指示，经过艰苦的长途跋涉，来到位于今尼泊尔和西藏边界，喜马拉雅山中的卡利－甘达基河的发源地。他要从那里带回几块圣石（śālagrāma stones）——黑色的小圆石，被外士那瓦奉为毗湿奴的神像形体，然后去温达文加入到其他哥斯瓦米们的行列，每天从事专门适用于此类神圣象征物的崇拜仪式。哥帕拉·巴塔就这样数年如一日地崇拜圣石，等待有一天柴坦尼亚能够兑现对他的承诺——他最终会得到他（柴坦尼亚）的接见（*darśana*）。直到 1542 年春天的一个清晨。头一天晚上，据说哥帕拉·巴塔因为自己尽管做了种种努力，怀着奉献精神做了种种恰当的仪式，还是不配直接见到克里希纳，而悲伤得失去知觉。第二天早晨，他醒来时，注意到安放圣石的篮子盖一夜之间歪斜到一边，心想一定是有蛇钻进篮子里了。他轻轻推动扣着的盖子，没能打开，就用了根棍子撬开，结果发现，一尊美丽的十一又八分之一英寸高的克里希纳神像取代了那些圣石，他的身体呈著名的三度曲线站立，吹奏着笛子，带有一处独特的标志——肩上嵌入一块圣石——表明这是一尊“自显的”（*svayam-vyakta*）神像。这是六哥斯瓦米留在温达文的唯一一尊克里希纳神像，由于害怕穆斯林的攻击，没有从温达文被转移到布阿佳境外的其他城镇（其他绝大部分神像最终安顿于拉贾斯坦邦的斋浦尔）。对茹阿达罗曼（Rādhāramaṇa）的崇拜一直沿袭至今（在 1826 年建造的庙宇中），很大程度上还是沿用由哥帕拉·巴塔确立的同一个崇拜标准。恩特威斯尔：《布阿佳：克里希纳朝圣中心》，第 79、185~186、413 页。

一个晚上“捣毁”了两次。每一次，当这位婆罗门就要给他的克里希纳神像（圣石）供奉完米饭的时候，尼迈都会闯进房来，抓起米饭就往嘴里塞，以此为乐。尼迈父母一再道歉，因为害怕婆罗门有力的诅咒，便向他保证会准备好第三次供品。当婆罗门第三次供奉时，全家人都进入了梦乡——当然除了尼迈，他又一次重演了他的恶作剧。克里希纳达斯告诉我们，这一次，尼迈在这位虔诚的婆罗门面前展现了他作为克里希纳的真实身份，以此让他明白了，他面前的这个人恰是以圣石形象接受爱心供奉的神本人。①

第二个故事讲的是柴坦尼亚第一次拜访佳甘纳特神庙的经历。他年轻时，就进入了弃绝阶层（*sannyāsa*），成为一名托钵僧。在寡母的要求下，他同意将总部设在佳甘纳特－普瑞镇上，这样，他母亲就能得到有关他的讯息。他比朋友们先到了普瑞。一到那儿，他立即去庙里觐见佳甘纳特。

通常一位来庙宇参观的普通访客，会在礼拜之后②起身，双手合十地站在神像面前，献上祷文，或者只是聚精会神地注视神像，留意当天神像身着的衣裳和饰物比平时有什么特别之处。有的虔爱者会在顶礼后走上前来，献上供品，诸如水果、鲜花、甜品等。祭司会在这些物品上洒水净化，再吟诵恰当的曼陀罗，献给佳甘纳特。然后，这位虔爱者会加入到其他人的行列，和他们一道歌唱赞美神的颂歌，或在庙堂静静坐上一阵，只是为了与他们的“主”在一起，感受他的临在。

但这一次与众不同，经典告诉我们，室利·柴坦尼亚一看见“他的主”便心醉神迷，失去知觉。在场所有祭司和其他人不知该如何是好。后来，最资深的皇家宫廷学者萨尔瓦包玛·巴塔查尔亚，意识到这不是一位普通的桑尼亚西（*sannyāsī*，托钵僧），于是将这位不知名的托钵僧带回自己家中。数小时过后，柴坦尼亚苏醒过来，恢复了知觉。又过段时间，他同意从萨尔瓦包玛那里，接受吠檀多哲学的教导。课程历时七天，这期间年轻的桑尼亚西一直沉默不语，直到萨尔瓦包玛主动问他学到了什么，柴坦尼亚才诚恳地直言相告：

---

① 这个故事见载于温达文达斯撰写的孟加拉文著作《柴坦尼亚－至尊人格首神》，上篇，第5章。

② 遵照经典训令，妇女顶拜时，应双膝跪倒，以头触地。

我能清楚地理解【《梵经》】中每一条格言的含义，但坦白地说，您的解释扰乱了我的心思。格言的含义本身明确地反映其主旨，可您呈现的有别于原意的主旨只不过如乌云般覆盖了经文本义。您没有解释《梵经》的直接意义。实际上，您所做的似乎是要掩盖他们的真实内涵。（《柴坦尼亚生平甘露》中篇，第 6 章第 130~132 诗节）

柴坦尼亚接下来就吠檀多哲学发表自己的见解，驳斥了他刚刚从老师那里听来的一元论观点。最后，他就《薄伽梵往世书》中一段著名的“阿特玛罗摩－诗节”给出精湛的分析，作为他发言的结论：

所有满足于灵性本我的人（*ātmārāmas*），尤其是那些稳定地走在觉悟自我路途上的人，尽管已摆脱各种物质束缚，还是渴望为至尊主献上纯粹的奉爱服务。这表明至尊主拥有超然品质，由此吸引每一个人，包括解脱的灵魂。①

萨尔瓦包玛变得谦卑恭顺，猜想他的学生不可能是别人，必是神本人，因为除他之外，无人能呈现如此渊博的学问和深刻的认知。萨尔瓦包玛拜倒在地，恳求原谅。柴坦尼亚向他示现了自己作为至高神的真实身份。首先展现了不可一世的毗湿奴形象，接着展示了克里希纳的形体，接受他供奉的祷文。

故事接近尾声的时候，又一次涉及“神与其虔爱者之间以食物为载体的交流”这一主题。第二天清晨，柴坦尼亚从佳甘纳特庙带回了祭馀。当时萨尔瓦包玛刚起床，还没来得及履行婆罗门初步净化仪式，就愉快地品尝起佳甘纳特的祭馀。他表现出对柴坦尼亚刚刚萌生的信心和自发的奉爱：

从那天起，萨尔瓦包玛·巴塔查尔亚除了柴坦尼亚·摩诃帕布的莲花足外，不知还有别的什么，而且从那天开始，他能够只按照

① 《薄伽梵往世书》第 1 篇第 7 章第 10 诗节；《柴坦尼亚生平甘露》中篇第 6 章第 186 诗节引用。

> 奉献服务的程序解释启示圣典。①

由此可见，这段文本再度涉及 *arcā-mūrti*（神像形体）这一术语，并且将佳甘纳特与《柴坦尼亚生平甘露》一书的男主角柴坦尼亚·摩诃帕布并列起来。我们可以说，唯有凭借神本人的仁慈，才能充分领悟佳甘纳特所昭示的神性。在此，神以两个形象出现，一是作为“主人”（*sevya*）的佳甘纳特；一是扮演“仆人”（*sevaka*）角色的柴坦尼亚·摩诃帕布。萨尔瓦包玛·巴塔查尔亚受到柴坦尼亚启发，能够体悟克里希纳作为“薄伽梵”的本体地位，这优于对绝对者的非人格概念“梵”的认知。那时，他便能明白柴坦尼亚恰是克里希纳本人。在那一认知阶段，他才有可能通过恰当进食以及对神像的菩莎达（*prasāda*，供奉过的食物）表示敬意，而彻底领悟佳甘纳特神像形体的身份和特性。神通过神像形体，让人可以接近他。不过，要臻达与神亲近的圆满境界，唯有通过他的纯粹虔爱者（*śuddha-bhakta*）这一渠道。

前三章中，我依据柴坦尼亚对吠陀文献主题的三分法，即关系（*sambandha*）、程序（*abhidheya*）和终极目标（*prayojana*），就高迪亚－外士那瓦神像崇拜理论，作了简要梳理。最后一章，将从西方的一个宗教传统，也就是犹太教传统的视角，审视这一神学体系，看一看高迪亚－外士那瓦传统中所敬奉的看似物质的形象，如何被认为是可以崇拜的？

---

① 《柴坦尼亚生平甘露》中篇第 6 章第 237 诗节。

第四章
神像崇拜与偶像崇拜

我亲爱的主，您不是一尊雕像；您就是南达王的儿子（克里希纳）。现在，为了那位年迈的婆罗门，您可以做您以前从未做过的事。

——《柴坦尼亚生平甘露》中篇第 5 章第 97 诗节[①]

中东主要的一神论宗教传统——犹太教、基督教和伊斯兰教，其不言而喻的显著特征之一，就是反对偶像崇拜[②]——不合礼仪地崇拜神或崇拜神以外的其他生命体。通过阐释“什么是偶像崇拜”以及“避免偶像崇拜的必要性”来实现对它的关注，成为上述宗教传统内“一神论”的概念构想中必不可少的要素：在神被恰当崇拜的地方，必然不存在偶像崇拜的空间；而一旦产生偶像崇拜，必然意味着未能名副其实地崇拜“唯一真神”。这种态度以 19 世纪基督教新教在印度的传教士为典型代表。他们构想的主要目标是将他们所认为的偶像崇拜从南亚次大陆上彻底清除。[③]对他们来说，似乎无处不在的庙宇神像崇拜，就是印度人所有错误宗教观的缩影，应该受到谴责，

① 此处作者在其英文原著中给出了原梵文诗文，详见本书英文相关部分（译者注）。

② 乔纳森 · Z. 史密斯的文章《宗教，诸宗教，宗教的》，对“宗教”一词的源流及其分类作了极好的概括，又追溯了“偶像崇拜”的范畴。收录于马克 · C. 泰勒编：《宗教研究的批评术语》，芝加哥：芝加哥大学出版社，1998 年。

③ 关于这一点，参见弗雷德里克 · 马格林《佳甘纳特 – 普瑞》，收录于史蒂文 · J. 罗森编：《外士那瓦宗：当代学者论高迪亚传统》，纽约：民间书籍出版社，1992 年，第 214~215 页。该文提及 19 世纪早期英国人和佳甘纳特神庙间的有趣博弈。

并尽一切办法予以根除。当然，他们更多是非难，而几乎没有或根本没有花精力去理解神像崇拜的实践或与此相关的神学反思。如果仅仅出于习惯上的迷信和敌视，何谈对种种实践进行“理解”？所以需要理性。

可以说，当人类进入公元后的第三个千年，宗教家以及宗教学者的态度发生了显著变化[1]（至少在某些领域内）。较之于 19 世纪在印度有可能发生的宗教对话，基于来自不同宗教传统的人士之间的相互尊重，实现对话的可能性大大增加。不管是作为新形势带来的结果，还是导致新形势产生的条件，[2]“偶像崇拜”这一术语都不大可能被应用于当代关于非西方宗教的讨论中。然而，这个术语没有销声匿迹，因为它在西方一神论宗教中的确有着深远的影响。因此，为了更好地理解神像崇拜实践，本着对话的精神，对“偶像崇拜”的概念进行探究，允许这一概念对本研究课题——高迪亚 - 外士那瓦传统中的神像崇拜实践提出质疑和挑战，是颇有价值的。[3]作为一种反思性实践，神学研究通常是一项定义边界活动，以回应反方观点的挑战。也许有人会问，如果高迪亚 - 外士那瓦宗的追随者被指控进行偶像崇拜，那么，他们将如何从神学角度回应这种挑战？

我认为，对这个问题简短的回答是，正如任何宗教实践一样，高迪亚 - 外士那瓦传统中的神像崇拜若不合规范，亦有退化的倾向，甚或变质而成某种类似于犹太 - 基督教所摒弃的“偶像崇拜”的事物。再一个简短的回答是，对或多或少不被近东宗教传统所赞同的诸多观念或实践来说，“偶像崇拜”是一个极为轻蔑的字眼。那么，以我们的研究课题，来抵御近东诸多宗

---

① 有关基督徒态度的转变，我猜测，近两个世纪以来的传教士著作或传教士书面培训资料，会有这方面的备案记录。通过查阅这些文件，可以看出“偶像崇拜”这一术语的使用频率。关于学术史与“偶像崇拜”的范畴，请参见第 67 页脚注②。

② 马克 · C. 泰勒在其著作《宗教学研究的批评术语》（芝加哥：芝加哥大学出版社，1998 年）一书的引言中，简要介绍了宗教的相互关联性及其现代性，这对学界颇有裨益。

③ 关于发生在不同宗教传统间的某种反思型对话模式，我的灵感主要来自于耶稣会的弗朗西斯 · X. 克卢尼，以及他的两本主要著作《吠檀多之后的神学》（奥尔巴尼：纽约州立大学出版社，1993 年）、《透视文本》（奥尔巴尼：纽约州立大学出版社，1996 年）。我不敢说自己的这个小课题在质量上接近于他所做的比较研究工作，也不敢声称是得其研究之精髓。不过，我力求效法其范式，从自己的传统出发，走出去面对其他传统，然后，再回过头来，以一种崭新的视角，对自己的原有传统进行反思。

教传统观念，便是不很现实的冒险做法，难以取得任何成效。相反，尝试在中东最古老的犹太教传统中，考察偶像崇拜的概念，如其所是地领会某些系统化的、分析性的文本中对这一概念的阐释，定位二者的交集以及不一致的领域，才是理解高迪亚－外士那瓦传统最富成效的做法。

通过分析犹太教传统中用以解释偶像崇拜概念的五种不同方式，正如在《圣经》文本中被表述的以及在拉比的著作——尤其是迈蒙尼德的著作中被详细阐释的，可以达到这一目的。背叛、象征物、神话、谬误、不当实践是构成偶像崇拜概念[①]的五个综合性因素。对此我将结合主题一一考察，出发点不是期待本书会成为比较神学领域的力作，而是呼吁学界对高迪亚－外士那瓦义理的特色给予关注。如果有学者想要了解围绕神像崇拜的概念结构，希望能起到投砾引珠的作用。

第一节　偶像崇拜与背叛

摩西·哈尔博塔与阿维赛·马格利特认为，将偶像崇拜视为背叛这一理念，尤其在《希伯来圣经》中有最为成熟的表述。在那种文本或祷文集中，偶像崇拜的观念主要基于对上帝与以色列人之间存在独特关系的理解之上。这种关系用人类家庭结构义务的语言来描述的话，就是一夫一妻制的单配婚姻。

> 这种一夫一妻制的范式体现在，上帝只与以色列人结婚，并且只把以色列人带出了埃及。由此，传记体的“罪”的概念也对那些不适用“罪”的人给予界定：它不适用于那些与制定专有义务者没有历史渊源的人。这条关于偶像崇拜的禁令并非通用和万能的，因

---

① 摩西·哈尔博塔与阿维赛·马格利特合著的《偶像崇拜》一书，对犹太教传统中的偶像崇拜概念作出分析研究。这里需要关注的五个主要范畴就是引自这部著作。其中每一范畴都有助于考察高迪亚－外士那瓦神像崇拜的理论体系。然而，鉴于犹太教所理解的偶像崇拜，其适用范围非常之广，因此对高迪亚－外士那瓦义理中哪怕是稍微涉及神像崇拜之处进行一定程度的考量，亦是颇有必要的。摩西·哈尔博塔、阿维赛·马格利特：《偶像崇拜》，马萨诸塞州，剑桥：哈佛大学出版社，1992 年。

为它成型于一种独有关系的暗喻。[①]

这种关系的排他性，通过阐明不履行它的后果而被放大。如果整个以色列民族[②]或个人敬拜“其他神明”，或与其他政治权力（通过订立条约等方式）“相勾结”，会被视为通奸。[③]在通奸之罪十恶不赦的社会环境中，甚至会被处以死刑。[④]崇拜其他神明，而对上帝不忠，就是在为自己招致上帝本人所施加的苦果。不管是已经遭受严厉的惩罚，或者至少被以惩罚相威胁，最终和解达成了，专一独有的关系被重新确立。[⑤]

背叛神的偶像崇拜，引起道德沦丧，从而使这一问题复杂化。《所罗门智训》第 14 章列举了各种邪恶的个人行为，最后得出结论：“崇拜邪恶的偶像是万恶之源，众恶之首。”（《所罗门智训》14：27）有评论家认为，《所

---

① 参见哈尔博塔、马格利特合著的《偶像崇拜》，第 22~23 页。不过，就像耶海兹克尔・考夫曼在其著作《以色列的宗教》一书中所指出的，虽然伊赛亚与其他先知一样，并不认为其他族群的偶像崇拜是罪恶，可实际上“他设想有那么一天，这些族群会放弃偶像崇拜，转而忠于以色列的神”。的确，考夫曼注意到，第二圣殿时期的态度与第一圣殿时期普遍流行的态度相比，完全是一个逆转。以色列从“外人眼中的未知领域”到成为一个使命的中心，担当着把偶像崇拜和异教信仰从世界上铲除的使命。耶海兹克尔・考夫曼著，摩西・格林博格译：《以色列的宗教：从开端到巴比伦的流亡》，芝加哥：芝加哥大学出版社，1996 年，第 449、450 页。

② 考夫曼论道：“虽然在人们当中发现犯有某些偶像崇拜的罪过，但整个民族从来不会背弃上帝。”尽管如此，所有人被认为要为少数人的罪过而负责。比如，拜金牛犊的罪过就被视为整个民族的罪过，虽然据说只是一小部分人为此而受到惩罚（出处同上，第 230 页）。西奈山之约的新颖之处在于，它是藉由一个人——先知摩西，传达给整个民族的。由此说来，“摩西律法的所有规章原则都是颁给整个民族的，而整个民族要为他们的背信弃义负责”（出处同上，第 234 页）。通奸这个比喻如此频繁地被用来描述偶像崇拜，这一视角本身使得上述情形格外耐人寻味。通奸涉及的是发生在两个个体之间背信弃义的行为，但关系到偶像崇拜的观念，则适用于一个人或一个民族。在这种情况下，整个民族被看作“一个人”（或许更进一步，“个体性”被重新界定为仅仅为了彰显“集体性”而存在的事物）。

③ 参见哈尔博塔、马格利特合著的《偶像崇拜》，第 16 页。引用《以西结书》16：15~26、28~34.

④ 出处同上，第 30 页。作者指出，只有在通奸被认为是相当严重的不道德行为时，《圣经》中将其与偶像崇拜相提并论才奏效。而在当代社会中，对于通奸的态度有所缓和，结果“弱化了这个比喻”。

⑤ 出处同上，第 18~20 页。正如作者所阐释的，神与以色列人之间的和解，涉及婚姻 – 通奸比喻的延展和嬗变。

罗门智训》中的这段话，表明了偶像崇拜最本质的邪恶特征，即对“小我”的关注，而“小我”因与神切断联系而变得毫无生气（新译本《圣经》第5卷）。为了重建与神的关系，那种既作为偶像崇拜的原因，又作为其结果的道德滑坡现象，一定要被彻底清除。

神及其虔爱者之间“排他性的独有关系”这一表述，也见载于毗湿奴派典籍。不过，通常是就个人而言的，而非一个群体或一个民族。同时一直在强调通过奉爱服务（*bhakti*，巴克提）与神建立密切关系的强烈感受。例如，在《薄伽梵往世书》第九篇，毗湿奴宣布：

> 纯粹的虔爱者一直在我内心深处；而我也一直在纯粹虔爱者的心中。我的虔爱者除我之外，不知任何其他事物；而我除他们外，也不知任何其他人。①

我们注意到，有趣的是，就在说这番话之前，毗湿奴将自己比作一位忠心耿耿的丈夫，听命于忠贞而贤淑的妻子。在此，转而将萨杜（*sādhu*），即虔爱者，比作一位贤妻。上段引文将虔爱者描述为是“除了神之外，不受任何人、事、物的吸引”，对于他们，神以自己全部的爱和情感相回报。由此可知，“排他性的专有权”这一术语，是依据不被打扰的人类关系来描述的，而非以背叛或通奸相威胁。即便存在以背叛相威胁的情况，那么，考虑到神作为无上独立的存在，免于一切义务的本体身份这一点，有权发出这种威胁的也只可能是神，而非虔爱者。室利·柴坦尼亚在其《八训规》中表达了他对神无条件的奉献精神，而神被描述为，虽处于情侣心态当中，却对他的情人不承担任何义务：

> 除了克里希纳，我不会将任何人接受为我的主。即使他拥抱我时，粗暴待我；抑或离开我时，教我心碎，他一直都是我的主。他完全自由，喜欢怎样便怎样，因为他永远是我毫无条件崇拜的主。

① 摘自《薄伽梵往世书》第9篇第4章第68诗节。

（《八训规》第 8 诗节）[①]

与追求今生或来世利益者（*karmin*，求福报者）、追求真知者（*jñānin*，知识思辨者），及追求完美的神秘主义者（*yogin*，瑜伽行者）形成鲜明对比，巴克塔（*bhakta*，虔爱者）对神没有任何要求。而尽管神没有什么义务可承担，却从来都不会忽略他的虔爱者。《摩诃婆罗多》记载了一个发生在库茹柴陀大战期间的著名事件。克里希纳的虔爱者认为这是一个有力证据，可以证明克里希纳并非反复无常，而总是恪守对其虔爱者的承诺。在克里希纳看来，与虔爱者之间的关系（这一事例中是朋友关系），比维护自己“信守承诺”的名声来得更为重要。[②]

克里希纳（或毗湿奴、那罗衍那）的忠实虔爱者，也许并不存在成为“潜在通奸者”的问题。不过，外士那瓦如何看待崇拜其他神明？对这一问题，《薄伽梵歌》提出了基本概念：虽然克里希纳从来不是“妒忌成性的神”，[③]但如果谁与他的意愿相违，他也的确表达了对此的不悦。这一点，《薄伽梵歌》特别用了两段文字来表述：其一是在第 11 章中，描述了神的显现（阿周那看到，一个可怕的宇宙巨人简直在吞噬着所有众生，除了忠诚的般度五兄弟外）；其二是克里希纳对恶魔品性的描述，他这样告诫道：

那些胸怀嫉妒、为害世界之徒，那些最下贱的人类渣滓，我把

---

① 《柴坦尼亚生平甘露》末篇第 20 章第 47 诗节。

② 克里希纳作出承诺，在库茹柴陀那场同室操戈的战斗中，他不会亲自拿起武器参战，毗湿摩（彼士玛）将这一点看成是他与阿周那作战的优势。当阿周那危在旦夕时，克里希纳不由得对毗湿摩采取激烈反攻（这样，毗湿摩想要看到他崇拜的主对他展现愤怒的愿望得到满足。《薄伽梵往世书》如是说）。这一事件促使 18 世纪高迪亚 – 外士那瓦著述家维施瓦纳特 · 查夸瓦尔提指出，在《薄伽梵歌》中，当克里希纳命令阿周那“大胆宣布：‘我的虔爱者永不毁灭’”时，他预见到了自己将失去“信守诺言”的美誉：要是克里希纳自己这样宣布，可能没人相信他，但想必同样的话出自阿周那之口会被当真。

③ 《柴坦尼亚生平甘露》中有一段关于柴坦尼亚与阿兑塔阿阇梨耶（Advaitācārya）关系的描述，暗示了就柴坦尼亚一方而言有些“吃醋”的心理：柴坦尼亚在年龄上较阿兑塔阿阇梨耶年轻得多，后者为了不让柴坦尼亚把自己尊为长者，于是表面上假意宣传一元论观点，有意激起柴坦尼亚的愤怒。根据克里希纳达斯 · 卡维罗阇的说法，阿兑塔阿阇梨耶视柴坦尼亚为至尊主，因此，他为受到柴坦尼亚的尊敬感到难堪。见《柴坦尼亚生平甘露》初篇第 17 章第 66~69 诗节。

他们无休止地投进物质存在的海洋，投入种种邪恶的生命种族中。这些人轮转于邪恶的生命种族，永远不能接近我，而且逐渐堕落到最令人厌恶的存在之中。①

《薄伽梵歌》第9章第23诗节提及其他神明的崇拜者。克里希纳明确指出，这种人实际上是在崇拜他，但所借助的方法错了。一般而言，这类崇拜的问题在于，使人永处于受捆绑的存在状态中。虽然有时也会体验到短暂的愉悦感，但最终仍导致不断重复的死死生生。同时《薄伽梵歌》也说，不管怎样，即使崇拜的方法错了，也会因其努力从事崇拜的活动而得到相应的回报。这些其他神明的崇拜者会"去到"（*yānti*）他们所崇拜的对象那里。

对神的错误形象的错误崇拜，会引发更多严重后果。《薄伽梵往世书》第5篇记载了一个有趣的故事，以此表明，如果企图把毗湿奴的虔爱者作为"活人祭"，供奉、讨好帕德拉－卡利女神的话，其后果会怎样：

安排崇拜卡利女神的所有恶棍和盗贼，都是心智低下、被激情和愚昧属性束缚的人。②他们都被发财的欲望所征服，竟敢胆大妄为地违背《吠陀经》的训喻，以致准备杀死出身于婆罗门之家、觉悟了自我的灵魂佳德·巴拉塔……无论如何都没理由将佳德·巴拉塔杀死，卡利女神不能容忍这一行为。她能立刻明白这些罪恶的歹徒就要杀害主的伟大虔爱者。于是神像突然间爆裂开来，卡利女神本人以闪烁着强烈耀眼光芒的身躯，从裂成碎片的神像中显现。③

在故事结尾处，局势得到扭转，帕德拉－卡利实施了非凡的正义之举，

① 据《薄伽梵歌》第16章诗节19~20可知，这类"定罪"可能持续相当长的时期，但绝不是永久不变的。最终所有众生都会获得至高福气，尤其是藉着神的虔爱者的仁慈。而且，就在受束缚的灵魂于生死圈中轮转之时，神作为"永远居于其内心的管理者、指挥者和调控者"，一直陪伴着他。

② 印度古典哲学数论体系按照三种形态，即 *sattva*（启明、善良）、*rajas*（激情）、*tamas*（黑暗、惰性、愚昧），来分析这个现象世界。可以知道，人根据其性情倾向，以这三种形态或精神状态，来定位自身所有活动及世界观。

③ 《薄伽梵往世书》第5篇第9章第17~18诗节。

杀死了想拿这位圣人作牺牲的邪恶之徒。由此可见，《薄伽梵往世书》这段文本与《圣经》中不赞成偶像崇拜的某些表述，大体上存在相似之处（如果说不反映在内容上，至少在语气上）。有一点除外，那就是在《圣经》作者看来，偶像崇拜非但反映出人自身的堕落，而且说明他不够聪明，因为那些偶像被认为完全是毫无生气、无能无力的。我将在本章第三、四节进一步探讨高迪亚传统中不恰当崇拜的问题。

第二节　偶像崇拜与象征物

我选择犹太教作为代表西方一神论对偶像崇拜的批判传统，一定程度上是一位非常有影响力的犹太思想家摩西·迈蒙尼德（1135—1204）的缘故。尽管他关于偶像崇拜之象征物的观点，并不一定来自圣经犹太教，却在形而上学中占有重要的一席之地。其著作《迷途指津》的问世推动了否定神学的发展。[①]迈蒙尼德阐述了激进的二元论观点，认为神与世界截然不同，任何有关神的绘画、图示甚或语文表征，都是错误和误导人的。这种观点与我们正在讨论的毗湿奴派传统大相径庭，因此值得特别关注。[②]如果我们以更宽泛的角度考量犹太教的话，会发现就神圣的象征物而言，它与印度的若干宗教传统之间存在一个共性元素，因为二者都认为神是可以借助某些恰当或不恰当的手段被描述和被表现的。但犹太教（伊斯兰教也如此，基督教诸传统很少见）对以形象化的方式表现神，一向持彻底否定的态度，认为仅凭相似

① 无论如何，这并不是说，他是“否定神学”理论的首创者。

② 从《圣经》文献的各种描述中可以看出，其中并未否定“神有形象”这一观念。不过，很显然，出于崇拜的目的而以图形、绘画等视觉形式代表神是被严格禁止的。可是，在迈蒙尼德看来，“神的任何象征形式都是违禁物，因为根据形而上学理论，神没有形象。所以，任何神的代表性形象，以及对这类代表性形象的任何崇拜行为，自然构成了对‘假神’的崇拜。这种做法无疑是有问题的，原因是任何基于相似性的代表性形象都是误导人的，凡是看到或崇拜这类代表性形象的人，会产生对神的错误观念”（哈尔博塔、马格利特合著的《偶像崇拜》，第45~46页）。哈尔伯特和玛格利特二人引用C. S. 皮尔士的观点，将“基于相似性的代表性形象”（以相似性为基础，用某物代表另一物）与“有着因果关系的代表性形象”（像“借代”修辞手法一样，涉及关系而非相似性）、“符合传统习俗的代表性形象”（由于约定俗成，用一事物表示另一事物，正如用“茶杯”这个词代表我们用来喝饮的器皿）加以辨析。

性而将神表现为物化形象的尝试是错误和不恰当的。[①]

梅纳赫姆·凯尔纳认为，迈蒙尼德主要依据两个标准界定宗教的原则，一是上帝的统一性，一是禁止偶像崇拜。[②]两个标准彼此涵摄。迈蒙尼德强调，上帝的统一性排除了其物质形体化的可能性。而如果对上帝的统一性不甚了解，那么，偶像崇拜便乘虚而入。之所以看起来经典中似乎暗示了上帝有物质形体，是由于对 *zelem*（形象）这一词汇的误解造成的。迈蒙尼德在《迷途指津》的一开篇，便就 *zelem* 一词的含义发表了自己的见解，认为它有别于希伯来语中的 *toar* 所表达的 form（形体）的普通含义。

> *toar* 这个词根本不适用于神。另一方面，*zelem* 一词象征某种特定形象，即构成一事物之本质的那种形象，该物藉此如其所是；一事物的真实性在于它是独特的存在。以人而论，“人体”是那个赋予人类洞察力的构成要素：基于这种理性的认知，*zelem* 一词被用于如下表述——“神以自己的形象（*zelem*）创造了他”。[③]

同样地，迈蒙尼德也就数个《圣经》术语的双关含义作了解释，这些词表面上是指身体特征，比方说，*panim*、*aḥor* 和 *leb*，分别指“脸庞”“后背”和“心”，实际上有着更为深刻的内涵。[④]就这样，迈蒙尼德将注意力转向上帝的统一性 / 无形无相，认为上帝独享专有权，即他只接受遵照他的命令所作的崇拜。虽然迈蒙尼德相信“偶像崇拜者”不会认为石头或金属形象本身就是世界的创造者，但他断言，这些人的问题在于，他们“只注重仪式，而未能理解其内涵，也未能理解被崇拜者的真实角色和品质”，于是他们“放弃上帝存在的信仰”。[⑤]

由此可见，迈蒙尼德认为，一个人对经典的肤浅（错误）理解，促使他

---

① 哈尔博塔、马格利特合著的《偶像崇拜》，第 45~46 页。

② 梅纳赫姆·凯尔纳：《迈蒙尼德论人类的完美》，乔治亚，亚特兰大：学者出版社，1990 年，第 23 页。

③ 摩西·迈蒙尼德著，M. 弗里德伦德尔译：《迷途指津》，纽约：乔治·劳特利奇父子出版社，1947 年，第 13 页。

④ 同上，第 52~54 页。

⑤ 同上，第 52 页。

制作神像，最初是想将其作为与神沟通的媒介。但因为全神贯注于此类形象的崇拜仪式，结果竟“以假乱真”。一张图片或一尊雕像，要是作为神的象征物被崇拜，也许很容易成为崇拜者唯一关注的中心，而非这形象所代表的那位“人物”本身。由于这个错误，一个由物质元素构成的有形象征物很可能变成偶像，“人们将其并不具备的力量归于他”。尤其是，由于上述错误导致这个象征物因而获得“对其崇拜者的控制力”。[①]一旦产生替代物，那么在崇拜者心目中，其形象便取代了本应受到崇拜的神的地位。由此，迈蒙尼德认为，在这种情况下，崇拜的真正对象便失去了所有的价值和重要性。在其编纂的《犹太法典》中，他以下列文字总结了偶像崇拜的渊源：

> 随着时间逐渐流逝，上帝那受到尊崇与荣耀的名字被人类遗忘，从他们的唇间和心田消失，不再为人所知。所有普通民众和妇女儿童，知道的仅仅是木像、石像，还有宏伟的圣殿。他们从童年起就被训练朝拜圣殿，匍匐拜倒在这些形象面前，做礼拜，并以其名义发誓。甚至他们中的智者，诸如牧师及地位与之相当者，除了星辰和苍穹之外，也想不出还有什么别的神明存在。由于这一缘故，便仿照这些形象，制作了崇拜的形象。然而，没人知晓宇宙的创造者，没人认可宇宙的创造者，除了寥寥几位独居的隐士之外……（《偶像崇拜法律及异教徒法令》1：2）[②]

如果说在《圣经》传统中，形象化的象征物是危险的，那么，或许有人说，在印度有神论传统中，尤其对外士那瓦宗而言，形象化的象征物几乎

① 哈尔博塔、马格利特合著的《偶像崇拜》，第 42 页。

② 伊萨多·特维尔斯基：《迈蒙尼德的一位读者》，收录于尼尔·科佐多伊编辑：《犹太教研究图书馆》，新泽西，西橘：贝尔曼出版社，1972 年，第 72~73 页。

是必需的。[①]正如前文曾探讨的化身理论，薄伽梵降临世间，所带来的形象化象征物就像语言象征物一样多，这或许一点都不令我们感到意外。[②]既然他以这个物质世界的参与者身份显现世间，既然他的一个特别目的是让受束缚的个我灵魂更易接近他，神就允许，甚或鼓励形象化的象征物作为其化身降临的自然结果，尤其对于灵性层面较高的灵魂来说，是可见或可想象的对象。

虽然薄伽梵作为化身（*aratāra*）降临世间，所有人都能够看见他，但只有在灵性方面称得上行家里手的圣人（*ṛṣi*）或纯粹虔爱者（*śuddha-bhakta*），才能获得那种视域，如其所是地达善（*darśaṇa*，见到）神的形

① 为什么在印度教，尤其是在虔爱传统中，不存在偶像崇拜的问题？彼得・班尼特在其论著中有充分而明确的阐释。然而，主体与客体、象征物与被象征本体之间的二元对立，在西方学术界崇拜话语中占主导地位（如，埃德蒙・利奇爵士、保罗・蒂利希、罗伊・艾伦、维克多・特纳以及其他学者提出的模式），这类对立“在印度很容易化解，根据灵魂（*jīva*）、神像（*mūrti*）与天神（*deva*）都是神性的具体方面这一原理。他们之间的差异性不会被简化为绝对的二元对立。更确切地说，在诸多虔爱传统中，差异性使觉悟了的灵魂，在得享一种与仁慈的人格神之间高度亲密和爱的关系之时，意识到体验神圣妙乐——阿南达（*ānanda*）的天赋能力。”他接下来指出西方的一个偏见，“神圣象征物这一观念的本质”，乃植根于“人－神、人间－天堂、世俗－神圣、具体－抽象”的二分法。这种象征物因而充当了“中介代理”的角色，“通过指向并因而参与到其所代表的实相当中”，拥有特别的身份和地位。班尼特引用 E. H. 冈布里奇的观点，后者认为，危险就是由此产生的：我们都“有这样一种倾向，随时可能复归到本原状态，体验图像及其模型，或者名字及其持有者之间的融合为一”。对此，班尼特反驳道，“但是，无疑在宇宙中，将两个世界分开的明显界线是不存在的（谁会说这样的宇宙是‘原初的’？）”或许反之亦然。只有当我们于潜在的统一性中，亲身体验“形象与原型、具体与抽象、人与神、象征物与被象征本体”之时，才有可能得到启迪而有所悟。在西方正统哲学传统中，神圣形象（*holy image*）是一种象征或符号，代表了一种更高的、不可捉摸的无形存在。然而，对于崇拜者而言，始终存在着一种倾向——把这形象看成有其自身的神圣美德。相反，在普施提－摩尔伽（瓦拉巴的毗湿奴派追随者，与高迪亚－外士那瓦颇为类似）当中，存在着一种观念，认为从根本上来说，物质形象与至高神之间无差别。新柏拉图主义或经验主义也认为，将某形象称为一种象征物，就是在贬抑其内在固有的神圣性。象征物是转喻说法，而非隐喻。从某种意义上来说，象征物即为其所代表的事物。在瓦拉巴的毗湿奴派追随者看来，神圣形象，毫不夸张地说，就是克里希纳本人的形体。彼得・班尼特：《克里希纳本人的形体：神像崇拜与瓦拉巴的毗湿奴派追随者》，载《毗湿奴派研究期刊》1993 年夏第 1 卷第 4 期，第 114~116 页。

② 从艺术史角度也可看出，文学上的化身象征物与图形化身象征物是并行发展的。参见 **T. S.** 麦克斯威尔《亚洲的神：形象、文本及其意义》，德里：牛津大学出版社，1997 年，第 10~11 页。

体，并能将其所见传达给他人，以便后者聆听、复述、冥思，并将那一形体雕刻出来。对雕刻好的形体，如果忠实于启示圣典（《阿笈摩论》，或称《工巧论》，被认为忠实记录了这些“异象见证者”的描述。其中，*śilpa-śāstra* 为《工巧论》，此译法出自中国社会科学院孙晶研究员——译者注）的规范说明，① 那么可按指定的程序进行崇拜。若做得恰当，实践者便能获得与“直接”见到神的圣人或虔爱者同等的视域。②

此外，对于神像形体的理解，涉及启示、语言象征物、形象化的象征物，以及在一位导师指导下对形象化象征物的规范崇拜。当人通过巴克提各个阶段循序渐进时（正如第二章第三节第一部分所概述的），随着心意和感官越来越多地从事对神的奉爱服务，看见神性超然形体的能力便得到充分开发。“见”的过程即为再认知的过程——从这个意义上讲，人在自己心中意识到至尊人的超然形象。在那一阶段，神像的价值并未减弱（而在某些严格的一元论传统中，神像完全是个工具）。更确切地说，因为巴克提本身即为目标，当人在神像中发现了真正的“代表”的存在，那么通过巴克提的力量，不断吸引神的注意力，这种感觉便愈发强烈。虔爱者（*bhakta*）会声

---

① 适用于造像师的指导方针主要涉及形体比例、标准特征和姿势（站姿、坐姿或卧姿）。参见吉腾德拉·纳特·巴内杰《印度造像的发展》，德里：曼施罗摩 – 玛诺哈拉，1974 年，特别是第三章“造像标准”。就造像标准来说，现今主要沿袭南印度造像作品的规格。若论高迪亚 – 外士那瓦的实践，至少现在，似乎于经典训令关注较少，也许更多依靠自己古鲁的指示。不管哪种情况，都需服从传统，正如海因里希 · 齐默所指出的：任何虔爱者都不准凭一己想法，随心所欲地自行塑造神的形象，因为只有神本人才能见证何为神性。神示现于哪个特别展示物中，是他自己的决定。甚至与他被感知和被表现的传统方式（这是神圣传统的核心）哪怕有一丝一毫的背离，显然都是荒谬的。就高迪亚 – 外士那瓦传统而言，正如其文本所证实的，完全是口述形式保存下来的神的自显故事。海因里希 · 齐默著，吉罗德 · 察伯尔和詹姆斯 · B. 罗森合译：《印度神像的艺术形式和瑜伽》，新泽西，普林斯顿：普林斯顿大学出版社，1990 年，第 50 页。有关依照“模型”雕刻神像，18 世纪孟加拉文著作《奉爱的宝珠》一书中，记载了与柴坦尼亚同时代的高瑞达斯 · 潘迪特的一个有趣实例：他恳请柴坦尼亚（和尼提阿南达）不要离开他在孟加拉的家去普瑞，二人满足了他的愿望，同意为他摆足够长时间的姿势，以便他能雕刻出据称是他们二人的第一对木质神像。他尽其余生保管并崇拜这对神像。他们是完全相同的形象。他的后人告诉我们，至今在纳瓦兑帕附近的同一个镇上，这对神像依然在受到崇拜。

② 参见齐默《印度神像的艺术形式和瑜伽》，第 53~64 页。书中探讨了“外在视域和内在视域”，认为印度造像有利于一种冥想式的观看，辅之以正确地专注于恰当曼陀罗的吟诵，自然而然地导向“内在视域”。

明，他/她并没有犯崇拜“替代物的错误”，而是以纯净的感官和心意，在洞察中不断修正——身处物质世界而感知不到神，这一缺憾和错误为巴克提程序所纠正，使人能够在见到神圣形体的视域中获得神的祝福。①

历史上的圣人和虔爱者直接认识到了克里希纳的形象，这是高迪亚－外士那瓦学说的核心。关于这一点，高迪亚－外士那瓦特别推崇被认为是这个宇宙始祖的造物主——梵天（Brahmā）在其著作《梵天本集》（*Brahmā-saṁhitā*）中用梵文诗节描述的神示异象。梵天在经历漫长的苦行（*tapas*）后，接受克里希纳对他的启蒙。由神的名字组成的一首神圣曼陀罗，将其引入有关超验存在的秘传知识体系中。他凭借恰当地聆听和重复这首曼陀罗，最终被授予神圣视域，得见哥文达（Govinda，克里希纳又一个名字）。接下来，梵天开始详细描述他所见到的哥文达，非但一一列出他的“身体”特征，而且强调他的形象不含任何尘世属性：

> 他总是吹着笛子，眼如盛开的莲花瓣，头上饰有孔雀羽毛，美丽的形体泛着云朵般的蓝。那绝无仅有的美轮美奂吸引了百万个丘比特——原始的主，哥文达，我崇拜您。
>
> 他的颈上围绕着森林鲜花串成的花环，飘来荡去。他佩戴着孔雀羽毛，手持饰有珠宝坠链的笛子。他永恒沉浸于爱的逍遥中。他那夏玛逊达尔的三度曲线形体，是他永恒的魅力——原始的主，哥文达，我崇拜您。
>
> 我崇拜原始的主哥文达，他的形体充盈妙乐、全知和真理，因而散发最为璀璨的光芒。那超然形体的每一部位都具有其他感官所有的功能。他永恒见证、维系和调控着无限的灵性和物质宇宙。②

上面三节诗中的前两节，形象生动、细致入微地描述了哥文达（Govinda）的身体特征，着重强调他的美——用以吸引其配偶们的魅力所

---

① 例如，《薄伽梵歌》第 11 章第 8 诗节描述了克里希纳将“神圣视力”赐予他忠诚的朋友阿周那，允许他看自己的宇宙身相。而且克里希纳还在《薄伽梵歌》第 9 章第 2 诗节中论及“通过直接感知而领会”。

② 萨格尔译：《梵天本集》第 5 章第 30~32 诗节，第 81~85 页。

在。而第三诗节给出了一个更为抽象的描述，提醒听者，虽然如前文所示，神的容貌特征实在而真切，但较之于普通人的身体特征，具有更高本性。他有一个“身体”，不过，他身体的每一“部位”都能行使与任何其他“部位”一样的功能。这后一节诗与其他吠陀文本的描述（所有吠陀文献都被视为天启圣典，即圣人或虔爱者的“幻觉异象”）[1]有异曲同工之妙，《白骡奥义书》描述如下：

> 他无有手足，行动起来却最为迅疾，万物皆在他掌控之中。他无有眼耳，却视听无碍。无人熟知他，可他通晓一切。他亦是知识的对象。圣者称他为至上，为原初的人格首神。[2]

上段引文中自相矛盾的语言，在“有形”与“无形”间制造了张力，[3]更偏重于神的王者气派和最高权威，而非高迪亚－外士那瓦传统中所偏好的易接近性和亲密关系。高迪亚－外士那瓦通过对“物质形体”与“灵性身相”作出区分，力求解决这一矛盾。前者以被束缚的个我灵魂所能理解的时空有限性为特征；而后者以分享神的本质属性“永恒－全知－妙乐的身相”（*sac-cid-ānanda-vigraha*）为特征。

对柴坦尼亚的追随者来说，梵天诗节的启发意义在于，《白骡奥义书》中所否认的不是像这样长着肢体器官的形象或身体。更确切地说，其否定的是，将神的形体看成与我们平常所经历的形体有着相同的有限性。这样，在

---

① 拉金德拉·P. 潘德亚在其所撰《吠陀先知的视域》一文中，就吠陀先知的视域这一主题有简明的论述。该文收入希瓦拉曼所编《印度的灵性》一书中，纽约：十字街出版社，1989 年。

② H. D. 哥斯瓦米译：《薄伽梵往世书》第 10 篇第 87 章第 28 诗节要旨。收入《巴克提韦丹塔全集》。

③ “有形－无形”间的张力与“有限－无限”间的二元对立，有些相似之处。罗伯特·卡明斯·内维尔所著《破碎的象征符号之真相》（奥尔巴尼：纽约州立大学出版社，1996 年）一书对此有过探讨。在就象征性符号的神学分析中，他认为，形象或符号可以看作有限与无限之间的边界限制或边界标记，在二者间发挥着调和作用（第 69 页）。当这些形象或符号未能精准地标示边界时，象征物就成了偶像崇拜的工具：“宗教象征物一旦为偶像崇拜所用就成了假的，也就是说，将某种有限的、非神圣的或世俗事物的涵义，加之于其所指代的对象，并且没有指明此类含义何以不足以诠释所指对象。”（第 20 页）

保留了神之无限性的同时，在其全能性方面也未做任何妥协。[①]对外士那瓦而言，神的全知全能，通过他授予纯粹虔爱者神圣视域以及将异象传达给他人的能力这一点，而得到进一步证明和展示。

毫无疑问，这种支持“灵性身相”的论点以及领会它的可能性，不会是迈蒙尼德所喜欢的，因为他坚持认为，凡用来描述神的语言一定要被理解为只是一种比喻性的说明罢了，因此语言使人联想起的人体特征或人类品质不应被看成是代表了神的。关于这一语言透明度的问题，《薄伽梵往世书》是以另一种不同的角度提出的：

> 室利·帕瑞克西特说道：“婆罗门啊，吠陀诸经怎么可能直接描述那难以言状的至高绝对真理？吠陀诸经仅限于探讨物质自然属性，而至尊之人没有这些属性，超然于所有物质展示及其成因。”[②]

实际上，在后来的讨论中，吠陀文本有这样的表述——将那些对神怀有抵触心理的、“像动物一样的”人捆绑起来。帕瑞克西特王问题的答案，其要旨在于，神完全有能力向他想要给予祝福的人展现自己，并且吠陀诸经本身有时也受到他的祝福以呈现他的娱乐时光（*līlā*）。《奥义书》再度强调，

① 这里可能会让我们想起迈蒙尼德的观点，即虽然“神充满智慧”一句在字面上没有什么认知意义，但出于施教目的这样说，也比说“神不具智慧”（认知上同样无意义的对立面）要好。第一种表述引发对神的尊敬心态，而第二种表述导致不敬心态（参见哈尔博塔、马格利特合著《偶像崇拜》，第153~154页）。有人也许会争论说，宣称物质形象是神的形象乃是对神的无礼。毗湿奴派的回答或许是，如果那形象仅仅是物质的，这种说法很可能成立。既然圣典中宣布它们是非物质的（至少不单纯是物质的），如《莲花往世书》有云：“一个认为毗湿奴那令人崇拜的形象只不过是石头的人，有着地狱般阴暗的心态。”那么，领悟了这句话的内涵，便去除了冒犯无礼的可能性。斯瓦米·帕布帕德也曾指出，克里希纳将世界的物质元素视为“与他隔离的本性”。尽管物质形体由神的外部能量构成，不过还是他的能量，他可以按自己的意志将其转为内在能量。以另一视角来看，涉及基督教观点，认为上帝作为化身乃是令其蒙羞之事，这一观点是由约翰·卡曼在其著作《威严与柔和：上帝概念反差与和谐之比较研究》（第195页）中提出的，“被奉为神圣的形象是神‘化身降临’的最终结果……降至甚至比神的人类崇拜者还要低的层面。神圣仁慈的‘真实临在’表现在神的恩典，他以柔弱的物质之躯，任凭那些人用手触碰他——甚或是不当对待他。”从这一视角来看，如果物质形体是对上帝尊严的极度轻视，那么他选择来接受这一形体，为的是祝福受束缚的灵魂。

② 《薄伽梵往世书》第10篇第87章第1诗节。

神拥有向他择定的那个人揭示自己的特权：

> 辩论、独自思考或研习诸经，皆不能臻达最高本我。相反，唯有最高我选择向谁施恩，那人才会达到最高我。对那人，最高我展示他自己真实的个人形象。[①]

20 世纪早期高迪亚－外士那瓦宗最主要的学者之一巴克提希丹塔·萨拉斯瓦提，在与美国学者阿尔伯特·E. 苏哲思教授的访谈中，反驳偶像崇拜的指控，为神像崇拜进行辩护，曾论及根据“纯粹灵魂”的接受能力，展现“神的真正形象”：

> 如果一个纯粹的生命体或无瑕的灵魂见到神的那个永恒形象，便会将其接纳在自己纯净的身心之中，然后再把这超自然的形象从他的内心放到尘世，以神内在固有的、原本真实的形象启迪世人。这决不应被冠以“偶像”之名。甚至就在神向下来到这个现象世界之时，他依然凭其难以了解的神秘力量，保持原样，未受摩耶之力的影响或触及。他的原本形象亦复如是。正如一度透露给他纯粹虔爱者的那个形象，即使被向下带到这个尘世，依然超越此现象世界……外士那瓦哲学中的“神圣的形象”，必然是神根本形象的直接化身。经由不完美的比较，它或许被说成是超越于物质视力感知范畴的神之根本形象的“代理”，就像在艺术与科学领域，用未经加工的天然“象征物”表示不可见的物质一样。[②]

---

① H. D. 哥斯瓦米译：《羯陀奥义书》第 2 篇第 2 章第 23 诗节和《秃顶奥义书》第 3 篇第 2 章第 3 诗节。

② 鲁跋·维拉斯·达斯：《毗湿奴之光：被赋予力量的化身室利·室利摩德·巴克提希丹塔·萨拉斯瓦提·哥斯瓦米·摩诃罗阇·帕布帕德传记》，密西西比，华盛顿：新斋普尔出版社，1988 年，第 93 页。巴克提希丹塔·萨拉斯瓦提，孟加拉本土人。说一口流利英语，也可以用英文流利写作。引文是长篇对话（始于 1929 年，地点是西孟加拉的克里希纳纳加尔）的一部分，后来由一位被认为具有听记能力的弟子记录下来。总之，这个记录得到讲话人的认可。

这里提出的“代理”概念也暗示了象征物，但其含义有别于“形象化的”或“语言上的”象征物。代理是指能够代表另一个人行使特定职能的人，基于所代表之人的授权，担任代理角色。既然外士那瓦宗强调神像崇拜是私人的交流，那么或许有人说，除非代表者与被代表者完全是同一关系，否则他们所崇拜的就是替代物。外士那瓦认为，这当然不会被看成是受缚吉瓦（*jīva*，个我灵魂）一方的过错，更确切地说，是全能的神为了受缚吉瓦的利益着想，所做的一种变通，以促成交流的实现。[①]

值得注意的是，在犹太教内部，与迈蒙尼德的激进二元论相制衡的，是中世纪的卡巴拉神秘传统。该传统设定了神性的两个层面，其一为不可知的无限，其二为启示的十项大能。约翰·卡曼指出，印度教发展了这些观念，并断言在神与哈西德派神秘主义者之间有一种亲密的个人关系。[②]

第三节　偶像崇拜与神话

根据耶海兹克尔·考夫曼的研究，犹太教偶像崇拜观念与异教观念密不可分。然而，他指出，《圣经》“并未就异教信仰的本质与内涵作出彻底诠释”。[③]相反，《圣经》只构想了“最低水平的”异教信仰，这反映在其针对偶像崇拜的论辩中——指责异教诸神不啻“人造工艺品”或“木头石块”（《申命记》4：28；28：36，64）。考夫曼认为，《圣经》并未就所谴责的诸神，给出任何有关神话学特征的知识。《圣经》中反对偶像崇拜的论辩，只是基于盲目崇拜的说法。其中没有一处经文，否认了正以某形象（images）

---

① 或许此处可与 9 世纪正统基督教传统中，和反对崇拜圣像者相对立的捍卫圣像崇拜者的态度作一比较研究。需要明确的是，“崇拜”（*worship*）”和“敬奉”（*veneration*）是有区别的，与印度虔爱传统相比，卫护圣像者心目中“象征物”的确切涵义和价值可能有所不同。在印度虔爱传统中，神像、神的名字、神的虔爱者同样值得崇拜，因为他们同样能够将神的“临在”传递给虔诚的灵魂。或许有人说，用来崇拜的神像（*arcā-vigraha*）作为象征物，并非罗伯特·内维尔所说的“已经破损的象征物”，而是“导致破碎的象征物”——换言之，这类神像足以摧毁使人持续物质捆缚状态的一系列外在名相。

② 卡曼：《威严与柔和》，第 256~258 页。

③ 考夫曼：《以色列的宗教：从开端到巴比伦的流亡》，第 7~20 页。

被崇拜的诸神的存在，也没有对其神话故事的真实性持有异议。“《圣经》文本当中，没有一处否认诸神的存在；《圣经》只是对他们不予理会。”考夫曼接着阐述：

> 《圣经》对异教信仰涵义的不了解成为最基本的问题，同时也成为理解《圣经》信仰最重要的线索。这凸显了《圣经》信仰与异教信仰之间的分歧。承认这种分歧对认识《圣经》信仰至关重要。这不仅构成《圣经》对异教信仰特有的歪曲，也构成以色列宗教史的基本事实。①

考夫曼的这一主张，如果说不能代表《圣经》宗教学者的典型观点，那么，或许就是犹太人典型的歉意表达，因为他们在犹太教一神论与假定的所有其他宗教“神话多神论”之间加以对比。看来外士那瓦宗可能不是世界上唯一不符合考夫曼所归纳的颇为广泛的异教信仰传统。不过，异教信仰可能是对高迪亚－外士那瓦传统中的神像崇拜持有异议（*pūrvapakṣa*）②的一个典型表述。鉴于此，我们会简要分析异教信仰的所谓特征，进而思考高迪亚－外士那瓦宗何以不具备这些典型特征。

此外，既然高迪亚－外士那瓦宗的神像崇拜涉及仪式活动，那么我们最好考察一下为哈尔博塔与马格利特两人所追随的学者考夫曼，在《圣经》式的敬拜神与异教崇拜的差异方面所呈现的主张。实际上，在他们看来，异教崇拜必然涉及神话，③这使偶像崇拜从单纯的拜物教扩展到完整的世界观。

---

① 考夫曼：《以色列的宗教：从开端到巴比伦的流亡》，第20页。

② *pūrvapakṣa*，字面意思是“最初的主张”，印度哲学辩证法中的通用术语，用来指“将受到驳斥”的观点。

③ 在此语境中，哈尔博塔与马格利特似乎将神话界定为“传统社会的集体科学”，社会藉此呈“闭合”之势，与允许不同理论对峙和争鸣的现代“开放”社会形成对比。“神话与现代理论的区别，并不在于神话明显失真而理论具有依据原则的正确性；甚至也不在于神话原始简单，而理论先进发达。二者间的差异是社会性的。神话服务于一个“闭合的”社会，而现代科学理论服务于一个开放的社会……从神话到理性的过渡，因而并不是在这样一种近似性的前提下，从一个显然失真到一个正确理论的转型。这是从一个闭合的社会到一个开放社会的转型。差异不在于理论讲了什么，而在于讲说的内容所处的社会背景。《偶像崇拜》第85~86页。

《圣经》式的敬拜神与异教崇拜之间的差别之一在于，异教诸神能力有限，而上帝拥有绝对意志。异教诸神受天命和自然所局限，而上帝“通过他的言语而非战争”[①]创造世界。考夫曼论道：

> 一神论的标志并非神作为创造者，永恒，慈祥，甚或全能的概念，这些观念在异教世界也随处可见。与此相反，神的概念应该是作为万物的源头，并不受制于宇宙秩序，也不是从某一预先存在的领域突然显现的……原始部落的最高神并未体现出这一观念。[②]

差别之二，根据这一观点，上帝的绝对神圣性决定了仪式的性质，与异教诸神崇拜仪式的性质截然不同。而后者以巫术为其仪式特征，借此获得控制神明的某些手段（这些神明受到原初本性的约束，通过仪式，人巧妙地操控这本性）。《圣经》仪式则在契约语境下发挥作用：“上帝同意应人的要求行事，是因为人遵行了上帝的旨意，而不是因为上帝迫于外在的巫术或仪式手段，才为了人的利益去行动。”考夫曼发现在异教信仰中存在“场域混淆”的问题，他认为诸神与世界皆从“同一子宫”显现，由此移除了“（诸神）与人类乃至其他生命体之间的固定界限”。[③]

差异三，人神之间中介渠道的类型不同：异教预言要求先知或祭司具备一定技能；相比之下，《圣经》预言是由上帝择定一位信使，以传达他的旨意。

差异四，异教道德植根于自然天性之中，与此形成对比的是，《圣经》

① 参见哈尔博塔、马格利特合著的《偶像崇拜》，第68~69页。

② 考夫曼：《以色列的宗教：从开端到巴比伦的流亡》，第29页。

③ 考夫曼：《以色列的宗教：从开端到巴比伦的流亡》，第35页。

道德则源于上帝的意志。[①]在哈尔博塔与马格利特看来，异教神话可进一步以大量的独立生物参与神圣故事为特征，这一点与一神论的故事有所不同。在一神论故事中，不存在大量“决意限制神圣意志”的生物。[②]

根据前文有关高迪亚－外士那瓦宗本体论学说的颇多论述，可以看出，上述异教神话故事的种种特征，并不完全适于描述毗湿奴派的薄伽梵概念以及包括创造宇宙在内的他的娱乐活动（*līlā*），亦不能描述直接针对他所做的那种崇拜——巴克提。关于神或薄伽梵的地位，我曾在第一章第二节第三部分引用《薄伽梵往世书》中蜘蛛和蛛网的例子，来类比神与他的创造。神具有独立性，《薄伽梵往世书》从开篇第一诗节起，便对这一主题作了充分而详尽的论述。全书的四个核心诗节出现在第二篇中，亦探讨了同一主题。其中第一核心诗节，克里希纳对梵天说道：

> 梵天啊，在创造之前，只有我——人格首神存在。除了我自己之外，什么都没有。既没有物质自然，也没有创造的原因。你现在看到的也是我——人格首神，毁灭之后剩下的还是我——人格首神。[③]

从神的独立性来看，克里希纳－巴克提与其他类型的崇拜方式形成对比。正如第四章第一节所提及的，克里希纳在《薄伽梵歌》中指出，对“其他诸神”的崇拜，其实是在崇拜他，可是由于缺乏真正的理解而导致实施的

---

① 参见哈尔博塔、马格利特合著的《偶像崇拜》，第 69 页。作者论及这些差异时，引用了耶海兹克尔·考夫曼的观点。同恩斯特·雷南和亨利·法兰克福一道，他认为神话传说乃“异教信仰独特的表现形式”。哈尔博塔和马格利特二人认为，不论这个评价是否公允，或者不论《圣经》本身是否为虚构神话，通常都会得出以下结论：不管考夫曼是否给出了神话的最佳定义，他“事实上已经明确指出两个世界间的本质差别。虽然它并不类似于神话学文献与非虚构文献之间的差异，但这种差异性还是存在的”（第 71 页）。二人接下来陈述自己观点，即《圣经》中的上帝更多以其人格性，而非绝对意志为特征，包括他在与世界的复杂关系中所表现出的“情感相互依附性”，因而使《圣经》故事呈现神话维度，即使根据考夫曼本人的说法，也是如此……我们这里所说的“依附性”，就如一个人依赖他所钟爱之人，或依赖之前一直承担的义务（第 73 页）。

② 参见哈尔博塔、马格利特合著的《偶像崇拜》，第 79 页。

③ 《薄伽梵往世书》第 2 篇第 9 章第 33 诗节。

“方式错了（*avidhi-pūrvakam*）”。[1]这种间接崇拜所获得的结果有限而短暂，崇拜者缺乏良好的判断力。[2]鉴于这类崇拜者追求的是负责宇宙事务的诸天神的恩惠，由此在某种意义上说，履行仪式的用意就成了通过巧妙的操控手段，使天神感到必须满足其愿望。而克里希纳对那些一心直接接近绝对之神的人表示宽容和仁慈，唯以“不含操控心态的”巴克提为途径，才能恰到好处地实现目标——臻达绝对的神克里希纳：

> 人唯有通过奉爱服务（*bhakti*），才能领悟我作为至尊人格首神的实相。如此虔诚奉献，全然体悟我，便能进入神的国度。[3]

《薄伽梵往世书》强调，对神的奉爱服务不应混同于买卖交易：

> 啊，我的主！啊，整个世界至高无上的导师！此外，您对您的虔爱者如此仁慈，您不会诱使他做任何无益于他的事。另一方面，人若希望以奉爱服务换得某些物质利益，那么他不可能成为您纯粹的虔爱者。实际上，他这样做，就成了用服务换取利润的商人。[4]

这种主张与迈尼蒙德关于阅读《摩西五经》的恰当心态的表述不谋而合：

> 谁要是为了求得回报或消灾避难之目的，从事《摩西五经》的学习，那么，就不是为了自己而学习。谁要是既非出于恐惧，亦不希冀报酬，而纯粹出于对普天下之主的爱，为了让他高兴而去专心研习《摩西五经》，才是为了自身利益而学习，因为他喜欢我们这

① 《薄伽梵歌》第 9 章第 23 诗节。

② 《薄伽梵歌》第 7 章第 23 诗节。

③ 《薄伽梵歌》第 18 章第 55 诗节。

④ 《薄伽梵往世书》第 7 篇第 10 章第 4 诗节。

么做。[1]

外士那瓦认为，通过向有资格的巴克塔（*bhaktas*，虔爱者）学习，真正意义上的巴克提便可成就。在《薄伽梵歌》中，将这样的巴克塔按字面意思称之为“明心见性者”或“见到真理者”，其灵性理解力已被神的恩典唤醒：

> 今天我（克里希纳）向你（阿周那）讲解这门古老的与至尊人关系的瑜伽科学，因为你既是我的朋友，又是我的虔爱者，故能领会这超然科学的奥妙。[2]

这些“见到真理的人”不一定与《圣经》所说的先知概念，即“为上帝所择定的信使”相符，同时他们既非巫师术士，亦非传达祈福者的欲求的熟练祭司。灵性导师的资格，受到广泛的关注，尤其是在注重神像崇拜仪轨方面的五夜派文献中。其中最基本的资格是，不专注于物质事务，完全摆脱其影响，而稳处于梵（*brahman*），即有关绝对者的知识中。就这一点，《薄伽梵往世书》论道：

> 因此，谁若诚心渴望真正的快乐，就该寻找一位真正的灵性古鲁（*guru*，导师），托庇于他，被他启迪。真正古鲁的资格是，他经过深思熟虑，体悟到经典的结论，并能使他人信服这些结论。如此伟大的人物，已托庇于至尊首神，抛开所有的物质事务。要知道，他们就是真正的灵性导师。[3]

---

① 特维尔斯基:《迈蒙尼德的一位读者》，第 86~87 页（《律法新诠》1，“忏悔”10. 5）。当代毗湿奴派学者可能会在这种表述中，辨识出巴克提的成分，他们认为这种理念或多或少地存在于全球宗教传统中。从犹太教的源头处收集这类表述，与毗湿奴派的巴克提表述两相对比，是比较神学研究的又一个潜在主题。显然，《雅歌》会是一个起点。

② 《薄伽梵歌》第 4 章第 3 诗节。

③ 《薄伽梵往世书》第 11 篇第 3 章第 21 诗节。

就薄伽梵与其他生命体交流互动的道德维度，我们在探讨神之“伴侣”的完美典范（*pūrṇa-śakti*）——茹阿达的身份时，简要论及过这一主题。道德秩序最初由吠陀文献确立，而毗湿奴派神学认为，吠陀文献起源于薄伽梵的“呼吸”。根据这一理论，神既是伦理道德秩序的创始者，同时亦是其维系者。特别是，作为居于个体生物心中的“超灵”（*paramātmā*，前文亦称为“最高我”——译者注），其从内在发挥着控制、管理等作用。不过，除此之外，他还通过各类化身，行使其伦理道德秩序创立者和撑持者的职能。当神的一位化身与魔性生物发生冲突时，他会与之“打斗”。但事实上，他从来不会受到恶魔们的真正威胁，因为后者在其真正身份上，只不过是他的仆人，接受特别委派，扮演“打斗玩伴”的角色，与他实际交锋，以此逗他开心。① 如此看来，在神的上述消遣活动中，并不存在“大量独立的生物”。对于神的意愿，他们不持对立或限制态度，而是参与实现神圣意志的过程，并增益其魅力与品味。

最后，作为神之独立性的一个必然结果，宇宙创造，即薄伽梵外部能量的表现形式，显然是从属于他的；神从不受制于原始的自然本性。相反，他以化身形式进入尘世，为的是扩展其丽拉（*līlā*，娱乐活动），并维系达摩（*dharma*，法，宗教原则）。至于神的物化形象——神像，一般认为，是由物质元素构成，易于腐坏；然而，正是因为这些元素隶属于薄伽梵，所以，据称他可以凭自己的意愿“进入”该形象，接受他虔爱者的崇拜，并与之互动交流。如此，神以神像形式，对崇拜他的人给予回应。②

将“异教信仰”视为“神话”的观点本身存在诸多问题，不过，对此的分析并非本书主旨。可以这样说，仅仅将神话定义为“想象”，并因而认定

---

① 有关神圣打斗娱乐理论，《薄伽梵往世书》中有详尽阐述，尤其是关于毗湿奴与两恶魔黑然亚克沙和黑然亚卡西普之间的冲突。这类“恶魔”实际上是毗湿奴的虔爱者，暂时遗忘其作为虔爱者的真实身份，以便推动打斗丽拉（*līlā*，神圣游戏）的进展。他们最终使神的意志得到彰显。不过，正如所有吉瓦（*jīvas*，个我灵魂）那样，他们亦持有微小独立性。他们根本不是尾随的影子，也不是反光或回声，亦非不具一己情感和愿望。

② 毗湿奴派和印度其他传统，通过修复或更换方式来解决神像的自然腐坏问题。通过一定仪轨程序，神受邀暂时驻留在一个容器内，直到修复完成或新的神像准备停当。以佳甘纳特（Jagannātha）木制神像为例，每 12~14 年，有一个周密复杂的“身体更新”程序，“木形的梵（*dharu-brahman*）”从旧神像被转移到新神像中。接下来，举行仪式，将旧的木制形象埋在庙宇庭院内。

它是“不真实的故事”（对“异教”的批评可能类似），这对于克里希纳-巴克提的实践者来说并不受用。他们不可能将经典中所提到的受人崇敬的神圣故事，看成是虚构的。这些经典的确包含寓言体故事，显然需要理解其背后的深刻寓意。但一般而言，不必担忧将历史考据学的批判性眼光强加于经典之上。[①]对经文的解读，历来被限制在上师传承世系（*guru-paramparā*）的经典诠释学母体之内。对于历代上师而言，经典的宗旨就是使人成就对神的纯粹奉爱，这一宗旨自始至终得到维护和贯彻。

第四节　偶像崇拜：谬误与不当实践

我在第四章第二节中论及，迈蒙尼德对肤浅地阅读经典，导致造像来崇拜这一结果，表示担忧。迈蒙尼德认为，这种不当行为源于不正确的信仰，本质上来说，是由构想上帝多样性和复杂性的哲学和概念上的谬误所致。很难指望迈蒙尼德这样一位激进的二元论者，会为“限定不二论者”（*viśiṣṭādvaita-vādin*）或“不可思议即一即异论者”（*acintya-bhedābheda-vādin*）提出的观点所打动，他们将世界多样性的存在或多或少与神的存在相认同。由于对迈蒙尼德而言，“尽善尽美”乃上帝的本质特征，故而他对形象化及语言表现形式的要求才极为严格，以保持上帝的“完美性”。[②]

毗湿奴派巴克提理论（及毗湿奴派的吠檀多哲学）也承认，有必要维护神的完美性，但并未受到不完美的语言或形象将有损于神在人心目中的完美性这种观念所困扰。相反，他们认为有必要在心目中同时保有两种观念——神既超越于世界，同时又参与其中。正如《薄伽梵歌》中克里希纳所言：

> 我以未展示的身相，遍透整个宇宙。众生皆在我中，我却不在他们中。然而，一切受造之物又不处于我之内。看啊，这就是我玄秘的富裕！虽然我是一切众生的维系者，虽然我无处不在，我却不

---

① 需要提到的是，有些西方学者从事对印度神像崇拜的研究，可能并未将西方视角不恰当地强加其上。参见班尼特著作，书中各处。

② 参见哈尔博塔、马格利特合著的《偶像崇拜》，第 111 页。

属于这宇宙展示的一部分，因为我自身便是创造之源。[①]

毗湿奴派巴克提传统通过包容现象世界表面的不完美，使神之完美性得到维护和彰显：如果说拥有身体和形象是不完美的，那么，克里希纳以其永恒－全知－妙乐（*sac-cid-ānanda*）的身相（*vigraha*）[②]挫败了这一观点。如果说尘世的活动表现出不完美性，那么，克里希纳以他的丽拉（*līlā*，娱乐活动）展现他作为完美的主人、朋友、儿子和爱人的角色，挫败了这一观点。如果说根据上述所有被视为启示的特征来描述神的尝试，被认为是谬误，那么，克里希纳的虔爱者会把那种“谬误”接受为是深刻洞见的核心——“情感宇宙”的真谛即是巴克提。[③]

哈尔博塔与马格利特两人特别提到，在迈蒙尼德那样的哲学家与12世纪犹太思想家兼诗人R. 犹大·哈列维（1075—1141）之间，存在研究视角上的反差。迈蒙尼德关注谬误，而哈列维关注不当崇拜。作为哲学家，前者注重通过哲学推理确定恰当的崇拜对象，因而，对恰当的崇拜方式关注较少。而哈列维正好相反，他认为，既然对于拉比犹太传统来说，崇拜对象视传统而定（依据哈拉哈律法），那么，主要的关注点应是建立恰当的崇拜模式，这“通常取决于崇拜者的意图、诚恳和认真的程度”。[④]且不论哈列维

① 《薄伽梵歌》第9章第4~5诗节。

② *vigraha*：动词词根 *kṛ*，意为“做，制造”。*vigraha-kṛ* 意为“分离，即个体形象或形体、外形、体型、身体”（莫尼尔·威廉姆斯：《新版梵英辞典》）。《梵天本集》中用 *sac-cid-ānanda-vigraha* 描述克里希纳的身体，意思是，“他永恒的形象，充满全知与妙乐”。

③ 丹尼尔·谢里顿在其关于《薄伽梵往世书》的评述中指出，从这部文献中可以看出“印度的特别智慧”，在于将深奥的智者话语、深沉强烈的情感共鸣与令人振奋的意象结合起来。“本书所唤醒的深沉情感，对于理解力是极为重要的。如果读书时有所领悟，却未激发强烈情感反应，则几乎不被视为真正的洞见。”丹尼尔·P. 谢里顿：《〈薄伽梵往世书〉的不二一神论》，德里：莫提拉·班那西达斯出版公司，1986年，第八章。关于“神圣的错误”，《薄伽梵往世书》频频强调克里希纳在温达文的伙伴——这些最崇高的灵魂的失误，以此凸显克里希纳的神性。并非因为这些人愚痴，而是因为他们在神的能量——瑜伽摩耶（*yogamāyā*）的影响下，扮演各自角色，发挥各自作用，以此使神的丽拉（*līlā*，神圣游戏）成为可能。瑜伽摩耶（*yogamāyā*）与摩诃摩耶（*mahāmāyā*）形成对比，后者亦为神的能量，其功能是使受束缚的灵魂遗忘自己与神的关系。

④ 参见哈尔博塔、马格利特合著的《偶像崇拜》，第189页。

这一观点本身是好是坏，但他得出的这一结论却是将犹太教与其他《圣经》一神论传统隔离开来，其他传统因偏离犹太教所传达的启示，均被视为偶像崇拜的宗教信仰。①

高迪亚－外士那瓦神像崇拜的经典和口述传统，对神像崇拜的正确实践方法和错误做法均有详细说明。②正如第二章第一节第二部分论及的，神像崇拜是《薄伽梵往世书》中所列九种互有交叉的奉爱实践中的一种。这九种奉爱实践，作为培育巴克提的过程，涉及以感官和心意从事目标明确的活动，旨在取悦神。神像崇拜是其中最为正式的奉爱实践，因此，茹帕·哥斯瓦米引用古史文献，列出崇拜中要避免的不下 64 项“冒犯”（*sevā-*

---

① 参见哈尔博塔、马格利特合著的《偶像崇拜》，第 190 页。

② 确定神像崇拜中何为正确、何为错误，可能涉及多种因素，这样一来，恰当运用规则就成了一门艺术。18 世纪高迪亚－外士那瓦最重要的诗人之一纳柔塔玛·达斯，提出一个由亲近经典（*śāstra*）、上师指导（*guru*）、与同修交往（*sadhu*）三要素组成的制衡体系。虔爱者要做的就是，运用其辨别力找出合适的方法，在前述三者的指导下进行修习，如此可避免茹帕·哥斯瓦米提到的过失——或者教条地拘泥于规则，或随心所欲忽略规则的失衡状态。毗湿奴派可能会赞同下面的观点，即这种失衡情形会导致不恰当地崇拜神，因而流于“崇拜偶像”。当失衡占了上风，崇拜动机便呈现多元化，而非单纯出于服务神的目的。一旦想要神成为自己的仆人，而不是让自己成为神称职的仆人，整个神像崇拜的宗旨便迷失了。因此，有关规范化练习阶段的奉爱服务（*vaidhi-bhakti-sādhana*）的原则方面，要不断努力找到一个恰当的平衡点，强调小心谨慎，尊敬的心态与假定的更为亲密的服务心态（朋友、父母及情侣心态）相比应置于第一位。因此举例来说，当崇拜茹阿达－克里希纳（Rādhā-Kṛṣṇa）神像时，建议修习者以崇拜拉克希米－那罗衍那（Lakṣmī-Nārāyaṇa）的心态去做。拉克希米－那罗衍那不是别人，正是茹阿达－克里希纳，但他们展现的是作为已婚夫妇的王者气派和华丽庄严，而非不为社会所认可的乡村纯朴爱情魅力。有人可能会问，那么为什么不直接崇拜拉克希米－那罗衍那的形象，而是以崇拜他们的心态崇拜茹阿达－克里希纳？高迪亚－外士那瓦可能会这样回答，因为他们追随的是柴坦尼亚·摩诃帕布，他特意降临世间，为的是教导世人将崇拜茹阿达－克里希纳作为人生最高目标。同时，柴坦尼亚也强调念诵神的名字，尤其是将念诵“哈瑞－克里希纳”摩诃曼陀罗，作为崇拜神像实践中最为重要的活动。他们通过遵循柴坦尼亚的教导，同样找到了平衡崇拜的基石。事实上，神像崇拜的所有程序与作为核心活动的哈瑞纳玛－桑克尔坦（*harināma-saṁkīrtana*，在神像面前集体唱诵神的名字）相比，被认为处于第二位，并对后者起支持作用。柴坦尼亚居住在佳甘纳特－普瑞期间，亲身示范了集体唱咏圣名这种崇拜方式，他的追随者继续遵行这一实践方式。

aparādha）。[①] 所有这些冒犯都与某类品质的缺失有关，诸如，不够纯洁、不够尊敬、不够努力、不够虔信等等。在高迪亚－外士那瓦传统中，这被解释为多少忽视了直接临在神像中的神。就像在人类社会中，在上级或长者面前，举止态度可能失礼一样，前文所列大部分冒犯与此类似，这样就容易理解了。例如，在不洁状况下，不可来到神像面前；不可在神像面前流露出傲慢态度；不可忽略向神像供奉新鲜应季水果；等等。当然，通过控制六种感官冲动——言语、心意、愤怒、舌头、肚腹和生殖器的冲动，这些冒犯多半可以避免。此类冒犯通常被看成是较严重的，但通过真诚从事经典规定的赎罪苦行，无疑会得到纠正。[②]

较上述更为严重的是“对圣名的冒犯”，梵文术语称之为 *nāma-aparādha*，即对神的神圣名字在信心、态度、言语或实践方面所做的冒犯。就其中的十项冒犯，《莲花往世书》中给出了详细阐述。既然神的名字与神本人是等同的，那么，忽视圣名的吟诵或在发音上粗心大意，则反映出一个人对待神的态度。十项冒犯中最严重的冒犯有三：其一，不尊敬神的虔爱者，特别是在言语方面。其二，不服从古鲁。只有在他的指导下，才能学习并实践巴克提。其三，沉溺于罪恶心态和行为，企图通过更多的冥思圣名抵消过失。可以预料，初习者会有冒犯圣名（*nāma-aparādhas*）的倾向，解决这个问题的关键在于，继续练习唱诵－冥想。同时，培养摆脱冒犯的真诚愿望。

最严重的冒犯是“对外士那瓦的冒犯”，即以自己的身体、言语或心意，得罪了一位在练习克里希纳－巴克提的同道。纠正这类冒犯的唯一途径是，恳请被冒犯者的宽恕。正如我们被警告的，即使神本人也不能抵消这类

---

① *aparādha*，字面意思是“冒犯、犯规、过错、错误”（莫尼尔·威廉姆斯：《新版梵英辞典》）。高迪亚－外士那瓦学者从词源学角度，指出其含义为“偏离崇拜”。参见巴克提·婆莫德·普瑞·哥斯瓦米《克里希纳的心：外士那瓦的冒犯与灵性的谨慎之途》，旧金山：曼荼罗传媒，1995 年，第 1 页。

② 拉比犹太教与毗湿奴派印度教实践者，都在规范原则体系下做事。不过，应当承认，由于二者起源于不同范畴的启示，故而在各自规范原则的性质上体现出差异性。《摩西五经》的律法，作为契约的实质内容，与我们在此讨论的由毗湿奴派印度教传统中所尊崇的往圣先贤的“记忆”所构成的规则，二者在特征方面存在差异。在某些情形下，针对某些对神像或涉及神像崇拜的冒犯后果，有颇为严厉的警告，尤其是针对偷窃珠宝等属于神像的物品这类冒犯行为。

冒犯。[①]

我们可能注意到，所冒犯的对象越是接近神性，或者说，越是“与神同一”，那么冒犯的结果也愈发严重。因而，虽然在神与神像之间存在着同一性的原则，可是，应当承认，在神与他的名字之间有着“更大的同一性”，而在神和他纯粹的虔爱者之间存在着“最大的同一性”。[②]我们可能还记得，毗湿奴在《薄伽梵往世书》中（9. 4. 68）宣布，他将虔爱者看作是他的心：“我的虔爱者除我之外，不知任何其他事物；而我除他们外，也不知任何其他人。”

以上论及的所有不同种类的冒犯，都与以某种形式表现出来的缺乏尊敬有关。而这些都被认为是源于要么对尊敬和崇拜的对象的本质全然无知，要么拒绝领会和赞美这种本质。《莲花往世书》对错误态度概述如下：

> 谁要是认为毗湿奴的神像是石头做的；谁要是认为灵性导师是位普通人；谁要是认为外士那瓦属于某一种姓或某一宗派信仰；抑或，谁认为沐浴毗湿奴神像或外士那瓦双足的水，或恒河水，都是寻常之水；谁认为毗湿奴的名字或他的曼陀罗，尽管能够摧毁喀历年代的罪恶影响，还是属于普通的词汇；谁认为毗湿奴并不高于，而等同于他所创造的世间万物，这样的人无疑是地狱里的居民（*nārakī*）。[③]

---

① 参见《薄伽梵往世书》第 9 篇第 4 章第 69~71 诗节。另见普瑞·哥斯瓦米·摩诃罗阇《克里希纳的心：外士那瓦的冒犯与灵性的谨慎之途》，第 13~18 页。

② 但此处“最大的同一性”，不应被曲解为本体论上的身份同一性，这完全有悖于毗湿奴派所公认的，吉瓦（*jīva*，个我灵魂）作为神之仆人的永恒身份。一个是神，一个是神之仆，是完全不同的两码事。

③ 另一个关于视神像仅仅为物质元素的严厉警告来自 14 世纪毗湿奴女神派传统中的两位圣者——皮莱·楼卡阿阇梨耶和玛纳瓦拉·玛穆尼卡。他们的警告是针对看重一位虔爱者出身或种姓的语境发出的。瓦苏达·那罗延在其论著中提到他们二人的警告：“强调一位虔爱者的种姓，就像对构成神像化身的成分进行质疑和分析一样，该受到谴责。这两种情形就像视自己生母的生殖器官（约尼）为普通性对象一样，是卑鄙和庸俗的。”瓦苏达·那罗延：《神像化身：在地如在天上》，收录于乔安妮·庞佐·瓦格纳、诺曼·卡特勒、瓦苏达·那罗延编辑：《肉身里的神，石头中的神：印度神的化身》，纽约：哥伦比亚大学出版社，1996 年，第 62 页。

引文中的“地狱居民”可作如下理解：尽管由于神的仁慈为其提供了诸多从事奉爱服务的机会，可总的来说，在培养对神的虔爱和奉献方面未有任何进展。正如前文在即将开始偶像崇拜的讨论时曾提及的，神对一再漠视他指导的人表示不悦。他的回应是，让这类不听话的生命体反复出生在恶魔物种，作为最严厉的处罚。但是高迪亚－外士那瓦历代宗师向我们保证，与惩罚相反，神更倾向于通过以身作则的合格导师（*ācāryas*）和天启圣典（*śāstra*）予以指导。对于外士那瓦而言，有规律地从恰当的来源处恭顺聆听启示的知识，是必不可少的实践，可避免偏离正道，而落入不当崇拜之列。

美国学者苏哲思教授在与巴克提希丹塔·萨拉斯瓦提的访谈中，一定被他坚定而自信地回应自己所持的外士那瓦崇拜偶像的观点所震惊。谈话过程中，萨拉斯瓦提主动出击，而非被动防御，谴责了几类西方和印度的宗教人士为“偶像崇拜者”，恰如其分地运用了这一《圣经》术语，给任何不从事巴克提实践的人定了名：

> 热爱神是灵魂的真正职责，是关于实相真正知识的科学，[①] 那些心中没有神爱的人怎能不把神像当偶像？外士那瓦哲学成熟审慎，完美无瑕。而那些没有神爱的宗教人士，经过真正的科学分析表明，在不同程度上都是偶像崇拜者，要么宣称自己拥护“神无形象”的说法，要么拥护“神有物质形象”的主张。正如那些将神性归属于物质并加以崇拜的人，比方说在未开化族群中有火的崇拜者；或者众多拜星者，像希腊人崇拜木星、土星等星体，都是肤浅幼稚的崇拜者。与此类似，另有一些人宣称超越于物质之外的一切皆无形无相，他们成为无二无别义理的倡导者，这些人同样是偶像崇拜者，甚至是“更大的”偶像崇拜者。单一主神的崇拜者，或只崇拜某位吠陀神明者，或五位神明的敬奉者（称为

① 萨拉斯瓦提使用“科学”一词很可能是用来呈现梵文词“*vijñāna*”，这一术语在梵文中有着与“知识、智慧、理解、识别、洞察”相关的多重含义。我认为他在此处所表达的意思类似于“被恰当运用的智慧”，这也相当于梵文词“*prajñā*”。之后的“真正的科学分析”一词，指的是“在被公认的圣典权威基础上，由被公认的神学家所作的分析”。

> *Panchopasakas*）崇拜想象出来的偶像，认为他们是神。根据其说法，神没有永恒－全知－妙乐的形体（*sat-cit-ānanda-vigraha*），正因为神不存在某种形象，所以不可能有用来冥想的主题。而为了便于冥想神，需构想出某个形体。他们都是偶像崇拜者。某些瑜伽行者和其他人的行为也被认为是盲目崇拜，为了净化心灵或提升心智功能，想象出一位神，并练习冥想他的某一虚构形象，等等。而那些将个我灵魂看作神的人，则是最亵渎神的偶像崇拜者，因为凡是将任何俗世事物或形象想象为神的，均属偶像崇拜。
>
> 为外士那瓦哲学所建构的神像崇拜理论，与其他思想家所持的神有形象或神无形象的学说，存在着天壤之别。摩诃帕布·室利·柴坦尼亚·提婆驳斥形形色色的偶像崇拜，教导世人服务于拥有神秘力量的、无限仁慈之神的神像化身。①

由此，可以说，心中拥有“神之爱”，是确定何为恰当崇拜，何为不当崇拜的首要条件。而“成熟审慎，完美无瑕”，这一标准使进一步对其甄别成为可能。当然，外士那瓦（Vaiṣṇavas）无意指责他人为“偶像崇拜者”，而是要对“无论谁崇拜哪个形象，必被谴责为偶像崇拜”这一思维模式提出质疑，同时表明，高迪亚－外士那瓦（Gauḍīya-Vaiṣṇavas）本身并不认同所有形式的物化形象崇拜。确切说来，在神像崇拜的各个神学体系之间，以不同方法进行崇拜时，会产生哪些不同程度的差异？其中，又有哪些不为高迪亚－外士那瓦所支持？这一主题本身，值得另撰一文，深入探讨。

① 鲁玻·维拉斯·达斯：《毗湿奴之光：被赋予力量的化身室利·室利摩德·巴克提希丹塔·萨拉斯瓦提·哥斯瓦米·摩诃罗阇·帕布帕德传记》，第94页。

结　语

我在序言部分提出本书核心议题——“根据高迪亚－外士那瓦神学理论，一个显然毫无生气的物质形体，在何种意义上，被视为神圣并因而受到尊崇？这种正式的神像崇拜实践，在哪些方面被认为是解决了接近至尊者或为至尊者所接近的问题？”这一问题暴露出对崇拜“有形物”的质疑，这种质疑在反对制作与崇拜任何种类的形象的《圣经》禁令中有充分表述。《圣经》禁令符合《圣经》一神论观念的本质：膜拜“独一的永恒上帝”意味着，首先，至少从反面的训令上讲，不得敬拜偶像，无论是唯一神的形象，还是“其他神”的形象。

与《圣经》传统形成鲜明对比的是，一般而言，外士那瓦宗尤其是高迪亚－外士那瓦宗，对崇拜神的圣像持热忱鼓励甚或指导训示的态度，以作为虔信之士的外在举止与内在精神生活不可或缺的一个组成部分。不仅如此，所有宗派的外士那瓦都认为自己也属一神论。不过，当然，他们的“一神论”观念与近东诸宗教的一神论观念存在着本质差别。或许有人会下断语说，用“偶像崇拜”一词来论外士那瓦传统，未免有失精准，因为它不能描述外士那瓦传统究竟是怎么一回事。本书尝试运用另一类阐述方法，允许这一传系的经典代表那些致力于这一实践的人说话。

正如犹太教是依据经典的宗教，高迪亚－外士那瓦宗亦以传统经典为取向。[①] 在前文的论述中，我尝试提请关注作为克里希纳崇拜经典依据的某些文本，以此表明，崇拜克里希纳并非一个欠考虑的粗浅实践，亦非无经验的

---

① 不应忽视的是，两种传统在经典形成方式上有着天壤之别。其中第一点是，犹太人强调书面文本，而印度人注重声音即吟诵文本。参见芭芭拉·A.、霍尔德里奇《吠陀经与摩西五经：超越经典之文本性》，奥尔巴尼：纽约州立大学出版社，1996年。两种传统之间有一个重要的共同点，那就是，他们都在很大程度上以各自圣典为依据，可以说，圣典在犹太教与外士那瓦传统中皆占据着某种绝对权威的地位。

混淆范畴的案例。相反，支撑它的是一套系统的神学理论，解决了神的至高无上以及由此产生的表面上难以接近的问题；一方面考虑到以物质形式呈现的“存在”之本质，另一方面，也顾及神无所不能的基本特征。

正如神像崇拜并非出于草率肤浅、幼稚无知的想法，在实践上它也不是反复无常、违背道德的行为。与此相反，崇拜克里希纳的仪礼程序受到经典训令、古鲁指导以及传统惯例的严格约束，旨在始终保持纯粹与礼仪，以此作为必要的前提条件，从而使真正的奉爱互动能够在崇拜者与神像之间发生。①

我们也可看到，高迪亚－外士那瓦神像崇拜在实践方面，为人类的不完美提供了解决之道，对人类在奉爱的完美层面上行事并体悟的潜在可能性予以肯定，使人能够超越肉身存在所施加的局限性。巴克提（*Bhakti*，奉爱服务）是交流的中间媒介，通过这一渠道，巴克塔（*bhakta*，虔爱者）被允许进入“情感的世界”，在那里，克里希纳作为灵性情感茹阿萨（*rasa*）的源头，统御着那片领域。在高迪亚－外士那瓦传统中，当奉爱服务达到被称为“巴瓦”（*bhāva*）的巴克提较高阶段时，虔爱者会品味到这种灵性情感。那种使肉身存在通常会延续下去的二元性，被神圣视域达善（*darśana*）所取代，藉此，神及其名字、神及其形象、神及对神的描述，作为彼此并无二致的同一性被经验到。②

依据《圣经》来反对神像崇拜的主张，往往强调所崇拜的形象看似毫无生气、不活动以及无助的外观。我们或许会问，克里希纳作为神像形体，实际上做了什么？外士那瓦会首先回答说，事实上，终极而言是他在做着一切

---

① 在这方面，温达文的六哥斯瓦米尤其强调经典权威性，或许是对察觉到的当时种种不当实践所作的回应。茹帕·哥斯瓦米在其著作《奉爱甘露之洋》（第1篇第2章第101诗节）中警告说，与所有各类权威经典的训喻不相符合的奉爱服务，只不过是公众的灾难，干扰社会秩序。

② 威廉·戴德韦勒解释道，这种词汇及其所指对象之间的同一性“构成该词字面意义几乎不能提供的即时性理解”，由此，只有当这些词汇应用于神时，才有可能认为其字面意义是合理有效的。“我们的世俗经验没有向我们揭示出字义。毕竟，神和神的国度，构成真实而原初的世界，然而我们所处的这个现象世界则是它的仿制品和反射光。不过，神以言语和神像形式，能够在这个世界之内示现他自己。通过将人的心意和感官专注于描述神的言语以及象征神的形象上面，心意和感官逐渐变得纯粹，于是人最终可领悟词汇的本义。”威廉·戴德韦勒：《虔爱者与神像：活在人格的神学中》，第86~87页。

事情，包括给了我们提出这个问题的智力。神像形体是神向受束缚的灵魂给予恩典的诸多渠道之一。正因为如此，它属于化身范畴。通常情况下，化身（神圣降临）从事以下几件事：其一，他们使神易于为受束缚的灵魂所接近（使其有可能超越业报活动的绑缚）；其二，他们行使神圣的正义（特别是惩罚恶徒，由此亦将其从业报活动的束缚中解放出来）；其三，他们重新恢复被湮没的或丧失了的宗教原则，而将自我奉献给神是其中的核心原则。此外，神以其原初的克里希纳形象降临，是为了通过他神圣的名字、形象、品质、娱乐时光和随行人员等，吸引受束缚的灵魂，以唤醒他们先天固有的虔信与奉爱。不仅如此，克里希纳亦作为神像形体接受怀着爱心向他供奉的食物、鲜花、财宝、衣物或祷文，并在享用完后，回馈那些供品的“祭馀”，称为菩莎达（*prasāda*），即仁慈。由此，使克里希纳在《薄伽梵歌》第9章第34节诗所宣说的“将心意专注于他，崇拜他，向他顶礼”这条训令运用到实践中成为可能。

不过，有人也许会争辩说，神像形体在行动或言语方面显然什么都没做。对此，外士那瓦可能会作出如下回应：神的这个最易为受缚灵魂所接近的化身形象，的确看似是最不活跃的。由此，为虔爱者提供了承担积极角色的机会，以其身体、心意和感官从事种种服务。于此主动角色中，人参与到对神热情友好的“严肃游戏”中，让自身愿望服从于神的意志。一直不断地忙于服务是虔爱者的宗旨（而不像传统的一元论学派所主张的不活动），因为正如我们在巴克提的讨论中曾指出的，为使自我彻底满足，服务一定是不含动机的，绵密而不间断的。通过这样始终如一的服务，巴克塔（*bhakta*，虔爱者）越来越多地经验到神的首要性。神是主角，占据主导地位。与之相比，人作为次要的参与者，是配角。

巴克提实践表明，为克里希纳而从事活动的过程中，巴克提本身具有转化内在的特征。如此一来，实践当中所涉及的每一人、事、物的内涵，因参与对克里希纳的服务（*Krishna-sevā*）而被重新定义，具有了非凡意义，不再是寻常事物。[①]在神像崇拜仪式中，崇拜的场所、崇拜中供奉的物

① 正如先前从《莲花往世书》中引用的诗节所表明的，甚至沐浴过神像的水，过后被用作 *caraṇāmṛta*，即“来自神之双足的美妙甘露”。由此可见，这个世界里微不足道的事物，在超验领域，却另有深义，成了最重要、最圣洁的，具有净化力的神圣之物。

品、盛放物品的器皿、所使用的语言、一己的感官和心意——所有这些都被转化而具有灵性属性（*cit-śakti*），以便于崇拜者转化为神的纯粹虔爱者（*śuddha-bhakta*）。随着实践（或演练）日臻完美，崇拜活动本身成为节目表演。而演出场所（克里希纳庙堂）不再是一个普通的地方，而成为布阿佳（Vraja）——克里希纳的非凡之地。在那里，“树木皆是如愿树，地上铺满如意宝珠，水乃玉液琼浆，言语不啻跳跃的音符，一举一动俨然曼妙舞姿”[①]。正是在布阿佳，当人娴熟地参与到神那永远富于变化的、常演常新的爱恋逍遥时，便超越了线性时间的框架。[②]

由以上论述，有人可能会猜想，高迪亚－外士那瓦宗的神像崇拜程序，是高度个人化的事，很少或根本不涉及社团或社会。事实上恰恰相反，这一传统承袭柴坦尼亚所树立的典范。在他看来，会众崇拜具有核心重要性。通过示范哈瑞纳玛－曼陀罗（*harināma mantra*）吟诵，柴坦尼亚及其最亲密的同伴尼提阿南达（Nityānanda）、阿兑塔（Advaita）、嘎达达尔（Gadadhāra）、室利瓦萨（Srivāsa）连同其他人一道，享有“洗劫神爱之宝库，以分发世人”[③]的美誉。柴坦尼亚接受来自低等种姓的合格的巴克塔（*bhaktas*，虔爱者），将对克里希纳（Krishna）的极乐之爱给予他所遇到的人。从前仅为少数人专有的财产，现在世人皆可享用和受益。由此转化整个世界，而非仅仅数位隐居修道者。他因此闻名于世。

神像崇拜实践正在印度以外的庙宇进行着，在对神像崇拜盛行于印度这一文化背景也许不很了解的西方人当中进行着，这可能引发以下思考：传统神学家所阐释的神像崇拜理论，在新形势下的实践中，实际地在扮演着怎样的角色？当然，对这个问题的回答本身构成了又一项研究课题，可能更多地需要以社会学而非神学的视角进行解读。我本人希望，非但从事巴克提的实践者对传统神学知识应像对实践程序一样，有更加透彻的领悟；而且，其他接触到克里希纳－巴克提实践的人，或许也可充分了解克里希纳神像崇拜实

---

① 《梵天本集》第 5 章第 56 诗节。

② 就这一点，高迪亚－外士那瓦神学家们明确阐述了以下复杂理论，即今日印度境内“地上的”布阿佳，与又名为哥楼卡或哥楼卡－温达文的“天上的”布阿佳，是同一、相等的关系。据此，地上布阿佳为具备恰当资格的心灵纯净之人提供了直达天上布阿佳的通道。

③ 《柴坦尼亚生平甘露》初篇第 7 篇第 20 章第 21 诗节。

践背后的神学体系。

希望《服务克里希纳》一书对克里希纳服务仪礼及实践方面，作出颇有见地的呈现。同时，进一步希望本书研究的专题或许可以发展为信仰间对话的主题，不仅在外士那瓦宗与犹太教的实践者之间，而且在前者与基督教、伊斯兰教的实践者之间。因为这两种情形下的对话，都会以不同的方式涉及本书所提出的议题。反过来，诸如此类的讨论，或许可使神像崇拜的比较神学领域产生更多有益的论著（我想，特别是关于正统基督教敬奉圣像传统）。此外，我亦希望《服务克里希纳》一书将有助于外士那瓦社团更好地增进自我理解，以促进自身与其他宗教社团成员之间更有意义的交流。

本书只尝试勾勒出巴克提传统仪礼的某些轮廓，有待于更为资深的学者填充更加丰富和细腻的内容，以使克里希纳－巴克提的神像崇拜仪礼有更为充分的呈现，更易于为读者所理解和接受。

希望对学界有所裨益并作引玉之砖。

Introduction

Within the broad landscape of yoga traditions originating in India, *bhakti-yoga*—the yoga of devotion—stands out as particularly prominent. In the sixteenth century this form of yoga was made popular by a young, charismatic sage named Śrī Caitanya. Traveling throughout India, he encouraged all whom he met—whether learned or unlettered, rich or poor, to practice a simple method of Hare Krishna *mahā*-mantra [①] meditation. In recent years, this practice has been popularized more widely, and even popular musicians have recorded several renditions of the chant, beginning with the Broadway musical entitled *Hair.* [②] Much less known than this form of mantra meditation and less understood by most people are the various meditation centers in which the same chant is performed along with an elaborate program of daily "*sevā* "—service or attendance—to the *arcā-vigraha*, or sacred image, as an integral feature of *vaidhi-bhakti-sādhana*, or the regulated practice of devotional spirituality (*bhakti-yoga*) , also known as Vaiṣṇavism, or the culture of participation in ultimate cosmic order, identified with the name "Vishnu" . As a contribution to the understanding of *bhakti* spirituality, this book is an attempt to present aspects of Gauḍīya-

---

① See Sanskrit & Bengali transliteration pronunciation guides, p. iv.

② Guy L. Beck, "Churning the Global Ocean of Nectar: The Devotional Music of Śrīla Prabhupāda," *Journal of Vaiṣṇava Studies* vol. 6 no. 2 (Spring 1998) : 133-135. The musical started its run on Broadway in New York in April 1968.

Vaiṣṇava theology[1] as it pertains to Traditional Ritual in the Practice of Bhakti Yoga or sacred image service, a way of comprehending divinity in visible form, a form that complements the audible form of divinity, the *harināma*, or divine name, especially as understood by the tradition of Vaiṣṇavism originating in Bengal (northeast India).

A fair amount of literature has appeared in English on the history of Gauḍīya (Bengal) Vaiṣṇavism,[2] focusing on a number of aspects.[3] Yet there has been little attempt to explain to any significant extent the theology of the service of sacred images in the Gauḍīya tradition. Neither do we find any significant attempt to place the theology of image worship next to possible theological objections or reservations to image worship, especially as articulated in the Judeo-Christian traditions. The service of Krishna-images in temples and in homes is becoming increasingly part of the worldwide meditation and yoga landscape. But because the tradition is unfamiliar to many people, they think it is foreign and strange, or they may even think it is threatening and demonic. Hence there is a need of attention to the theology of image service (*mūrti-sevā*) to bring understanding and perhaps appreciation thereof. Due to the need for greater understanding of a

---

① It might be more accurate to speak of a 'matrix of propositions that constitute the world within which [Vaiṣṇavas] conceptualize and practice ritual,' as Richard Davis puts it. Richard H. Davis, *Ritual in an Oscillating Universe: Worshiping Śiva in Medieval India*, (Princeton, New Jersey: Princeton University Press, 1991), 22.

② The term "Vaiṣṇava" is derived from "Viṣṇu" a principle name of Bhagavān, or God. Vaiṣṇavas are generally contrasted with Śaivites, or worshipers of Śiva as the Supreme. Although Gauḍīya Vaiṣṇavas worship Viṣṇu, they understand him to be an expansion of Kṛṣṇa; hence it is Kṛṣṇa, not Viṣṇu as such, who is central to the tradition; alternative designations of the tradition are Bengal Vaiṣṇavism and Caitanyite Vaiṣṇavism.

③ See Rahul Peter Das' chapter "Recent Works On Bengali Vaiṣṇavism," in *Essays on Vaiṣṇavism in Bengal*, (Calcutta: Firma KLM, 1997), for a comprehensive bibliographical survey for Bengali Vaiṣṇavism *in Bengal*. For studies on its presence in the West, especially as ISKCON, see works by Charles R. Brooks, Stillson Judah, Kim Knott, Burke Rochfurt, and Larry Shinn, among others.

tradition that is expanding in different parts of the world, especially due to an expanding worldwide Indian population, this book will be concerned to explore a central theological issue: In what sense, according to Gauḍīya-Vaiṣṇava theology, can an apparently inert material form be seen as divine and therefore venerable, and in what ways is this practice of *arcanam* ① (formal veneration of images) considered a solution to the problem of approaching or being approached by the supreme Being in the Gauḍīya-Vaiṣṇava tradition? The answers to these questions will be located in the interconnection between *avatāra* (divine-descent) theology and devotional praxis, in which the Gauḍīya *vedāntic* doctrine of *acintya-bhedābheda-tattva-vāda*, or inconceivable simultaneous oneness and difference of the one supreme Being in relation to the multiplicity of being, is pivotal.

Since praxis is central to the Gauḍīya-Vaiṣṇnava theology of image worship, I will briefly describe some specific daily ritual procedures in *arcanam*, such as the bathing and dressing of images, the offering of food, the waving of lamps, and the use of *mantras*. But as many of these details will appear similar to those in other image worship practices in South Asia, it will be important to direct attention to particularities of *avatāra*-theology in Gauḍīya-Vaiṣṇavism. These particularities are highlighted in aspects of a certain festival, the *Jagannātha-Rathayātrā*, or public chariot-pulling festival of the image of "the Lord of the Universe," and in scriptural narratives which celebrate the devotional accomplishments of Krishna-devotees.

The method employed in this book will be essentially theological

---

① *arcanam* is pronounced "archanam". There is no apparent etymological connection to the Latin word referring to secrecy or occult knowledge.

explanation[①] and comparison, based on the long-time field work in the temples and holy places in India. I intend to show that image worship in this tradition is sustained in the dynamic relationship between the *bhakta*, or devotee, and Krishna, inasmuch as the presence of the deity is experienced through the practice of *bhakti*. Seen from a 'functional' perspective, as the focus of formal ritual in Gauḍīya-Vaiṣṇavism, the practice of image worship can be understood as a means to bring a sense of direct and immediate experience to the central message of *bhakti*. The word *bhakti* denotes a sustained, transformational, devotional attitude characterized by active service to the supreme divine Being, conceived in Gauḍīya-Vaiṣṇava tradition to be Krishna in his fullest manifestation. This immediacy of *bhakti* is suggested in the expression "Krishna-*sevā*," or "(direct) service to Krishna," in which central importance is placed on the idea that the supreme Being makes himself *accessible* to devotees *through active service* performed according to a prescribed system of veneration—a system of ritual practices that may be best characterized as "sustained (ongoing, uninterrupted) hospitality."

I use the word *functional* with caution, for it may appear to invite readers to entertain a reductionistic perspective of the subject under discussion. However this would be utterly opposed to my purpose. Rather, my underlying aim in this project is to explore the dynamics of interaction between what is understood to be the transcendent realm of Krishna-*bhakti* and the contingent realm of this world in which the practice of Krishna-*bhakti* is necessarily manifested. In this context, attention to image veneration is most fitting,

---

① Paul Griffiths notes that the "doctrinal study of doctrine" is on the wane in the academic study of religion, giving way to analyses of doctrine in terms of social, political, historical, and psychological contexts. In his book *On Being Buddha* Griffiths offers a theory of doctrine "intended to make possible the properly doctrinal study of doctrine." Paul J. Griffiths, *On Being Buddha: Classical Doctrine of Buddhahood*, (Albany, NY: State University of New York Press, 1994), 2. My method here will be not so exacting as his, but perhaps the spirit is similar.

in that the tangible image is understood by the practitioner to demonstrate the ultimate reality of the supreme Being in terms of relationship: *bhagavān*, the supreme Person, is understood as the absolute source of *paramātmā* (the principle of Self animating all beings) and *brahman* (the absolute conceived as non-dual being). Rūpa Gosvāmī, one of the main Gauḍīya-Vaiṣṇava theologians of the 16th century, defines *bhagavān*, the supreme person, as *akhila-rasāmṛta-mūrti*, or "the very form of the nectar of unbounded spiritual relationships."[①] The Sanskrit term *rasa* (liquid, taste, essence), which dominates Indian aesthetic discourse since ancient times, embodies a central concern in Gauḍīya-Vaiṣṇava theology, inasmuch as the ultimate objective of worship is to participate in an eternal relationship with Krishna in terms of a particular modus of loving exchange. It will be necessary therefore to look briefly at *rasa* theology as it relates to image worship, particularly since the latter is generally associated with the less esoteric praxis of *vaidhi-sādhana-bhakti*, where the following of rules and regulations predominates. Image worship as practiced on this level is oriented toward the attainment of increasingly advanced levels of spirituality; hence the practice is sustained and enriched by reference to a body of narratives involving worship of images by *bhaktas* recognized as adepts in the exchange of *rasa* with Krishna and therefore considered to be on the highest levels of spiritual progress.

The structure of this presentation is as follows. After a brief look at Gauḍīya-Vaiṣṇava epistemology, I will make a short presentation of *avatāra*-theology in this tradition, with reference to the Vedāntic formulation of "inconceivable simultaneous oneness and difference." I will then explain basic principles of *bhakti*-theology and the concept of *sādhana* or practice, and how sound and form interrelate to allow a sentient being to become spiritually elevated. The third chapter will focus on *rasa*-theory and the experiences of adepts in relation to images.

---

① *Bhakti-rasāmṛta-sindhu* 1. 1. 1.

The fourth chapter, "Are Vaiṣṇavas Idolators? " aims at comparative theology, whereby image worship in the Krishna-*bhakti* tradition of Gauḍīya-Vaiṣṇavism is juxtaposed with objections to image worship that are voiced in the Abrahamic traditions. Here again, the focus is on the nature of *bhakti*, conceived as the ultimate modus of spirituality, leading toward and bringing about *prema*, or unfettered love for the supreme Being, or Krishna.

Chapter One
Theology of Divine Descent

Of course it is bewildering, O soul of the universe, that You work, though You are inactive, and that You take birth, though You are the vital force and the unborn. You Yourself descend amongst animals, men, sages and aquatics. Verily, this is bewildering.

—Śrīmad-Bhāgavatam 1. 8. 30[①]

I. 1 pramānaḥ—Sources of Knowledge

To understand the theology of image worship in any Indic tradition, and no less the Gauḍīya-Vaiṣṇava tradition, demands entrance into the galaxy

---

① *janma karma ca viśvātmann ajasyākartur ātmanaḥ*
tiryaṅ-nṛṣiṣu yādaḥsu tad atyanta-viḍambanam

All translations from *Śrīmad-Bhāgavatam*, *Bhagavad-gītā*, and *Caitanya-caritāmṛta*, unless noted, are by A. C. Bhaktivedānta Swami Prabhupāda, a member of the disciplic succession of Gauḍīya Vaiṣṇava preceptors descending from Caitanya Mahāprabhu, and Sanskrit scholar, and a prominent 20th century exponent of the Vaishnava bhakti tradition. At times I will offer alternative or more literal translation of a word or phrase if it seems pertinent, or may include in parentheses the Sanskrit word or phrase to which an English word or phrase refers. I also include the transliterated Sanskrit text for each translation in footnotes. The edition of *Śrīmad-Bhāgavatam* (also known as *Bhāgavata Purāṇa*) used by Prabhupāda for translation was: *Śrīmad Bhāgavata Mahāpurāṇam*, ed. Kṛṣṇa-śaṅkara Śāstrī (Ahmedabad, India: Śrī Bhāgavata Vidyāpītha, ND) (present available edition: 1968).

of discourse revolving around the Veda, a group of ancient Sanskrit texts considered within the whole of the tradition to be *apauruṣeya*, without human origin, or divinely revealed. Without dwelling on the complex web of texts which are considered to be elaborations of the original Vedic texts, one may simply note here that within philosophical or theological writings leading to radically differing conclusions, epistemology has been a primary concern, especially in *Vedāntic* discourse, consisting of texts aiming at a systematic explication of the Upaniṣads. ①

The particular strain of theological tradition and reflection we are concerned with received elaborate articulation in the writings of the Six Gosvāmīs. These disciples of Śrī Caitanya Mahāprabhu ② (who himself wrote naught but an eight-verse summary of his teachings) , were commissioned by their master to compile and systematize teachings on *bhakti* spirituality found within existing texts and elaborate on these texts on the basis of their own insights. Of the Six Gosvāmīs ③ Jīva Gosvāmī, in consultation with his colleagues, composed the most comprehensive exposition on Gauḍīya-Vaiṣṇava theology, the *Ṣaḍ-sandarbha*, or 'Six Treatises,' of which the first, *Tattva-sandarbha*, deals exclusively with epistemology.

Near the beginning of this work, in preparation for establishing the centrality of one particular text for Gauḍīya Vaiṣṇavism, Jīva declares his faith in Vedic revelation:

> Human beings are bound to have four defects: they are subject to delusion, they make mistakes, they tend to cheat,

---

① The *Upaniṣads* are a collection of philosophical texts, some said to be composed as early as ca. 800 BCE, ranging up to ca. 200 CE (Holdrege, Barbara A. *Veda And Torah: Transcending the Textuality of Scripture*. Albany, NY: State University of New York Press, 1996. 449n) .

② "Mahāprabhu" is an honorific term, lit. "great master."

③ The other five were Rūpa, Sanātana, Gopāla-Bhaṭṭa, Raghunātha Bhaṭṭa, and Raghunātha Dāsa.

and they have imperfect senses. Thus their direct perception, inference, and so forth are deficient, especially since these means of acquiring knowledge cannot help them gain access to the inconceivable spiritual reality (*alaukikācintya-svabhāva-vastu-sparśāyogyatvāt*). Consequently, for us who are inquisitive about that which is beyond everything, yet the support of everything—which is most inconceivable and wondrous in nature—direct perception, inference, and so on are not suitable means of gaining knowledge. For this purpose the only suitable means is the *Vedas*, the transcendental words that are existing without beginning. They are the source of all mundane and spiritual knowledge and have been passed down in *paramparā* (disciplic succession).[①]

For Jīva Gosvāmī's audience, little endeavor was thought necessary to establish the primacy of the Vedas as infallible sources of truth over against

① Satya Nārāyaṇa Dāsa, *Śrī Tattva-Sandarbha of Śrīla Jīva Gosvāmī Prabhupāda*, (Delhi: Jiva Institute for Vaiṣṇava Studies, 1995), 18, 27.

other sources of knowing.[1] He quickly moves from the original Vedas to a consideration of related texts, the Purāṇas, and through a process of elimination carefully supported by proof texts, Jīva identifies one particular work, the *Bhāgavata-purāṇa*[2] (also known as *Śrīmad-Bhāgavatam*), as the revealed text (*śabda*) which is **most essential, must lucid, most appropriate,**[3] **most authoritative, and accessible to all, including non–**

---

① The primacy of Vedic evidence was accepted by all six of the orthodox Indian medieval schools of philosophy, each of them allowing subordinate, supportive positions to two or more additional types of evidence (*pramāṇas*). Jīva Gosvāmī (and later Baladeva Vidyābhūṣana) accept direct perception (*pratyakṣa*) and inference (*anumāna*) as inclusive of all other standard *pramāṇas*, again, as subordinate and supportive of Veda (*śabda-pramāṇas*) as far as they go to illuminate ordinary existence. One might recall Thomas Aquinas'distinction between knowledge and articles of faith: What cannot be known automatically belongs to the realm of faith, to which belong certain revealed items of doctrine. Yet the Vedas and their corollaries describe experience by persons of super-ordinary existence. Baladeva Vidyābhūṣana, an eighteenth century Gauḍīya commentator (following all the reputed Vaiṣṇava commentators as well as Śankara) designates the Vedas (*śruti*— 'that which is heard') as direct experience (*pratyakṣa*) and the corollaries to the Vedas (*smṛti*— 'that which is remembered') as inferred (*anumāna*) (Narang, 30-42). Guy Beck observes, "To be sure, reason, or rational thinking, in the Western sense has an important and unique place in Indian thought. Yet it runs second place to revelation. The Vedas—revealed texts and thus 'non-rational,' or numinous, from a certain outlook—are the basis of all truth for the Hindu. . . The use of reason in Indian thought (namely, Indian philosophy in the strict sense) is thereby limited to the attempt to reconcile these revelations with human experience and empirical observation." Guy L. Beck, *Sonic Theology: Hinduism and Sacred Sound*, (Delhi: Motilal Banarsidass, 1995), 10-11. Jitendra Mohanty, after presenting his own philosophical analysis of what he sees as weakness in the theory of *śabda-pramāṇatva* (superiority of revealed testimony), concedes, "*Śabda's* claim to be a *pramāṇa* may be weakened by my arguments. . . . but it is restored to its foundational status of defining the parameters of the central core of Indian thinking." Jitendra Nath Mohanty, *Reason and Tradition in Indian Thought: An Essay on the Nature of Indian Philosophical Thinking*, (Oxford: Clarendon Press, 1992), 259.

② Modern scholarship dates this work at ca. 900 CE. The text claims itself to be from the dawn of the Age of Kali, some five thousand years ago. The present redaction may indeed be from the tenth century, with a probability that its oral tradition extends much further back in time.

③ Most appropriate for the present age, the '*kali-yuga*', or era of spiritual darkness.

brāhmaṇas. [1] He also recognizes it as Śrī Vyāsa's [2] own commentary on the *Brahma-sutra.* [3] Thus Jīva declares that his six treatises will essentially be a commentary on the *Śrīmad-Bhāgavatam* whereby he will sometimes, but not always, follow previous commentators. [4] The *Śrīmad-Bhāgavatam*, not unlike other Paurāṇic [5] texts, deals extensively with the concept of *avatāra*, or divine descent, identifying Krishna as *avatārin*, or the source of all *avatāras*.

To facilitate analysis of the contents of the *Bhāgavatam*, Gauḍīya theologians classify the contents in three categories. *Sambandha*, 'relationship,' is concerned with the relation of *īśvara*, or God, to *jagat*, the world; of *īśvara* to *jīva*, the living beings; and of the living beings to the world. *Abhidheya*, 'process,' is concerned with the means by which living beings, on the basis of the knowledge of these relationships, can approach God, which is *prayojana*, the 'purpose' for understanding *sambandha* and practicing *abhidheya.* [6]

In this first chapter of the book dealing with *avatāra* theology we

---

① *brāhmaṇa*: the intellectual class, according to the traditional Indian *varṇa* social system.

② Vyāsa: Kṛṣṇa-Dvaipāyana Vyāsa—the traditionally accepted compiler of the Sanskrit epic *Mahābhārata* and the *Purāṇas.*

③ *Brahma-sūtra*—the most important commentary on the Upaniṣads in the form of extremely dense aphorisms, the standard work upon which all *vedāntic* schools were expected to offer commentary. O. B. L. Kapoor, *The Philosophy and Religion of Śrī Caitanya* (*The Philosophical Background of the Hare Krishna Movement*), (Delhi: Munshiram Manoharlal, 1977), 70.

④ Especially Śrīdhara Svāmī, Rāmānuja, and Madhva.

⑤ Purāṇas are Sanskrit texts which deal largely in narrative form with sacred history on a cosmic scale. Scholars consider them to have been composed from the third or fourth centuries CE up through the fifteenth or sixteenth centuries. Within the tradition they are held to be much older, from shortly after the commencement of the present cosmic era, beginning around 3000 BCE.

⑥ Kapoor, 74-75. *The Philosophy and Religion of Śrī Caitanya* (*The Philosophical background of the Hare Krishna Movement*). Delhi: Munshiram Manoharlal, 1977. 74-75.

are concerned primarily with the principles included in the first category (*sambandha*). The second chapter, concerned with *bhakti*, is the substantial principle of *abhidheya*; and the third chapter will focus on *prayojana*, especially through the principle of *rasa*, the aesthetic active principle in perfected relationship between the devotee and God.

I. 2 Ontology: Vaiṣṇava-vedānta

I. 2. 1 Īśvara—The Controller

The five major traditions of Vaiṣṇava *vedānta*① are all concerned to refute the monistic *vedānta* interpretations of Śaṅkara and his followers by preserving an ontological distinction between living beings and God and thus denying the monistic assertion that multiplicity is *māyā*, or illusion. The central question in Vedānta is, how is the immutable *brahman*, or Absolute Being, related to the contingent world. Madhva (1197-1276) emphasizes the difference between *brahman* and the contingent world with his *dvaita*, or 'dualism' philosophy. Less radically dualistic, yet decidedly rejecting monism, is Rāmānuja (1050? -1137) whose *viśiṣṭādvaita* 'qualified monism' features a concept of the universal 'body of God' to reconcile God/world dichotomy. The Gauḍīyas have attempted to reconcile these two latter positions with their *acintya-bhedābheda* doctrine, the 'inconceivable simultaneous identity and difference' of the supreme Being with the multiplicity of being. O. B. L. Kapoor, paraphrasing Jīva Gosvāmī, states the problem and its solution as conceived by the Gauḍīyas:

---

① Followers of Rāmānuja, Madhva, Nimbarka, Vallabha, and Caitanya. For a survey of the Vedānta systems of each of these, see Manju Dube, *Conceptions of God in Vaiṣṇava Philosophical Systems*, (Varanasi: Sanjay Book Centre, 1984).

The history of philosophy bears evidence that neither immanence nor transcendence can solve the problem of relation between God and the world. The concepts of identity and difference are both inadequate to describe the nature of being. Exclusive emphasis on the one leads to a virtual denial of the world as illusion [monism], while exclusive emphasis upon the other bifurcates the reality into two and creates an unbridgeable gulf between God and the world. Both the concepts, however, seem to be equally necessary. Identity is a necessary demand of reason and difference is an undeniable fact of experience. An ideal synthesis of identity and difference must be the cherished goal of philosophy. But the synthesis, though necessary, is not possible or conceivable. This is the final test of human logic. It fails. But the logic of the infinite succeeds where our human logic fails. In the perfect being there is no conflict between necessity and possibility. Here, what is necessary actually is. ①

The solution as proposed by the Gauḍīyas, recognizing the metaphysical problem of reconciling identity and difference, ② is based on scriptural evidence; it rests on the notion of *acintya-śakti*, or the inconceivable energy of God, an energy by which reconciliation of mutually exclusive concepts is perfectly accomplished in a 'higher synthesis.' The doctrine receives elaboration in the notion of *śakti-parināma*, or 'transformation of energies,' to preserve the immutability of *brahman*: God, the absolute Being, is not himself transformed or altered by multiplicity; rather multiplicity is but transformation of the *energies* of God, which are

---

① Kapoor, 152.

② Dube, 41. We may note that the issue is indeed a metaphysical issue, not simply a "test of human logic" as Kapoor claims, since logic is a mode of functioning of the human mind, over and beyond which lies a metaphysical paradox of a different order than human mental functions.

inseparable from him. ①

This solution is further nuanced by the notion that, depending on perspective, *brahman* ('the greatest') can be conceived in two other equally valid expressions, namely *paramātmā* ('supreme Self') and *bhagavān* ('supreme possessor of opulences') . Although these three perspectives have equal validity in one sense, they can also be graded in terms of advancement of realization. To substantiate this, Jīva Gosvāmī quotes the *Viṣṇu-purāṇa*, another scripture revered by the Vaiṣṇavas:

> The (impersonal) *brahman* is unmanifested; not aging; inconceivable; unborn; without any diminution; indescribable; formless; without hands, feet and the like; it is omnipotent; omnipresent; eternal; the origin of all material elements; causeless; pervading everything, yet nothing is situated in it; that from which everything comes. The demigods [highly evolved souls] see that *brahman* as the supreme abode, the object of meditation for those who aspire after liberation. *Brahman* is the subtle (spiritual effulgence) and abode of Viṣṇu described in the *mantras* of the Vedas. It is *brahman* that is denoted by (the) *bhagavān* (aspect of the Absolute) ,and the supreme Self (*paramātmā*) is the (partial) manifestation of the transcendental form of the imperishable

① It might be interesting to compare this notion of *energies* of God with that of Orthodox Christianity, which asserts that the closest one might come to seeing God directly would be to see the energies of God.

(supreme) Person, *bhagavān*. ①

Bhagavān, or God, is defined as 'the supreme being, who possesses six types of *bhaga*, or opulence, in unlimited magnitude'. ② It is the identification of *bhagavān* as the possessor of all potency which qualifies him as the supreme person, *puruṣottama*, and identifies him as *saguna-īśvara*, ③ or God possessing qualities, superior to *nirguna-brahman*—the unqualified absolute. It is this supreme person who, we shall see, is considered the unique source of all *avatāras*, or divine descents into the world.

I. 2. 2 Jīva—The Living Entity

Quoting *Viṣṇu Purāṇa* again, Jīva Gosvāmī holds that *bhagavān* exhibits his energy in three aspects, namely *svarūpa-śakti* (essential power), *tatastha-śakti* (medial power), and *bahirāṅga-śakti* (extraneous power). ④ *Tatastha-śakti*, literally 'energy situated on the border,' is also known as *jīva-śakti*, or "energy of the living beings"; *bahirāṅga-śakti* is

---

① *yat tad avyaktam ajaram acintyam ajam avyayam*
anirdeśyam arūpañ ca pāṇi-pādādy asaṁyutam
vibhuṁ sarva-gataṁ nityaṁ bhūta-yonim akāraṇam
vyāpy avyāptaṁ yataḥ sarvaṁ tad vai paśyanti sūrayaḥ
tad brahma paramaṁ dhāma tad dhyeyaṁ mokṣa-kāṅkṣibhiḥ
śruti-vākyoditaṁ sūkṣmaṁ tad viṣṇoḥ paramaṁ padam
tad eva bhagavad vācyaṁ svarūpaṁ paramātmanaḥ
vācako bhagavac chabdas tasyādy asyākṣayātmanaḥ
(*Viṣṇu Purāṇa* 6. 5. 66-69, quoted in *Bhagavat-sandarbha* 3. 2. My translation).

② *aiśvaryasya samagrasya vīryasya yaśasaḥ śriyaḥ*
jñāna-vairāgyayoś caiva saṇṇāṁ bhaga itiṅgana (Viṣṇu Purāṇa 6. 5. 47, quoted by Swami Prabhupāda in *The Science of Self Realization*, Chapter 1). The six opulences, according to Viṣṇu Purāṇa, are strength, fame, wealth, knowledge, beauty, and renunciation. See footnote 3 page 126 on six further opulences, or attributes, associated with the accessibility of *bhagavān*.

③ Dube, 5, citing *Viṣṇu Purāṇa* 6. 5. 12-14 (VP. edition not stated).

④ Dube, 44.

identified as the energy of illusion (*māyā-śakti*). As Manju Dube puts it, "Jīva-śakti is responsible for the very being of the individual souls and Māyā-śakti is responsible for the creation, sustenance, and dissolution of the world. Paramātman as their supporter acts as the regulator of the souls and the world."①

In the Vaiṣṇavas'concern to position themselves strongly against the monistic notion that both the world and the living beings are without substance and against the collapsing of individual, personal identity into one conscious Being, they want to preserve the eternal master-servant relationship between God and creatures. Living entities, being products of the medial energy, and being *anu*, or intrinsically minuscule, exist in a relationship of dependence on God, who is *vibhu*, or infinitely great. Although as such they are meant to function in accordance with the *svarūpa-śakti* as eternally liberated souls, out of *avidyā*, ignorance, they subject themselves to the *māyā-śakti*—the potency through which the contingent world is created, maintained, and destroyed, and through which the living entities' seemingly independent desires are facilitated.

Vaiṣṇavism can be contrasted to most forms of Śaivism, which seek to diminish the difference between the *jīva* and Śiva to the point that the individual self may realize a degree of "śiva-ness" (*śivatva*) comparable to Śiva himself.② While in some forms of Śaivism, as in all forms of Vaiṣṇavism, the eternal individuality of each living being (*jīvātmā*) is asserted, in Vaiṣṇavism the *jīva* remains a dependent minuscule portion of *bhagavān*, never an independent entity. As in practically all forms of Indic religious philosphy, Vaiṣṇavism identifies the fundamental problem for the living entity as bondage in the cycle of repeated birth and death (*saṁsāra*). For the Vaiṣṇavas this bondage is due to ignorance of the living entity's real identity in relation to *bhagavān*; the solution to the problem is liberation

---

① Dube, 44.

② Davis, 84, 135.

(*mokṣa* or *mukti*), which can only come about by re-establishing the relation of service by shedding the false conception of oneself as independent doer, controller, or master (*ahaṁkara*). This in turn is afforded by *bhagavān*'s initiative, by making himself accessible to the bound living beings as *avatāras*. Moreover, as the 'knower of the field' (*kṣetra-jña*) or knower of the bodily condition of the living entity, as supreme Self (*paramātmā*), *bhagavān* acts from within the heart of the living entity to guide it out of bondage.

I. 2. 3 Jagat—The World

Through *māyā-śakti*, or the energy of illusion of *bhagavān*, the *jīvātmā* is facilitated to sustain a condition perfectly appropriate for the fulfillment of its desires. The arena of facilitation is *jagat*, 'that which is in flux,' the contingent world of transient names and forms. Each living entity is supplied with a configuration of sensory apparatus, the aggregate of which makes up its physical body, which is subjected to the constraints of matter.

Seen from another perspective, God is revealed through his *māyā-śakti*, that which produces the inanimate world. As God is real, so his energy and hence its manifestation—a transformation of the energy, not of the energetic source—is real. The world, as a transformation of the energy of God, is not God-in-illusory-form; it is not compromised in its status as existent, and hence the experience of the bound living beings—of happiness and distress, of hope and fear, (as also the existence of moral responsibility for action)—is not trivialized. The world is a real effect of the real cause; as such it is one of the unsurpassed attributes of God.[①] In his comparison of the five major Vaiṣṇava theologies, Dube notes,

---

① Sudesh Narang, *The Vaiṣṇava Philosophy According to Baladeva Vidyābhūṣaṇa*, (Delhi: Nag Publishers, 1984), 77.

The reduction of the material world to the Māyā-śakti is an important characteristic of Bengal Vaiṣṇavism. This view strengthens the conception of ultimate Reality as one without a second. The conception of 'acintya bhedābheda' tries to solve the difficulty of reconciling both identity and difference between śakti and śaktimat [the possessor of śakti]. [The] Bengal school does not regard one as real and [the] other as unreal but attributes [to] them a relation which is supralogical and inconceivable. ①

The world facilitates the living entities, but it also facilitates God. The eighteenth century Gauḍīya-Vaiṣṇava commentator Baladeva Vidyābhuṣaṇa (eighteenth century, d. after 1764) gives an analogy from the *Bhāgavatam* (11. 9. 21) to illustrate this:

> Just as a spider creates a web out of itself, maintains it for some time and then reabsorbs it into itself, similarly the Lord creates the universe, maintains it for some time and then reabsorbs it eventually. The sentient part of a spider does not change into web, but it is its non-sentient body from which the web comes out. ②

The spider takes up a position on its creation, its web; similarly the eternal, omnipotent God takes up a position within his creation for the purpose of exhibiting *līlā*, or pastimes, with the aid of his *svarūpa-śakti*. ③ This he does in the form of his various *avatāras*, which appear in various forms at various times within the cosmos.

---

① Dube, 76.

② Narang, 82.

③ *Svarūpa-śakti* is conceived as further divided into a triad of energies, one of which facilitates the pastimes of God free from the danger of blemish which the external energy affords.

I. 3 Cosmology

I. 3. 1 Creation, Maintenance, and Destruction

Cosmic creation and destruction are understood much in the same way as found in the classical Indian *Sāṁkhya* philosophical system. ① Creation is a process of unfolding of several elements and principles—each emerging from the one before it—from which the bodies of living entities are constituted. Cosmic destruction, after set astronomical periods of time, reverses the process of creation. ② Bengal Vaiṣṇavism basically accepts the descriptions of the Purāṇas and Pañcarātra ③ literature of how *bhagavān* participates in this process by a fairly elaborate process of expansion or manifestation in various forms with specific jurisdictions of lordship. All of these are considered manifestations of God conceived as *puruṣa*, the primal Person; hence, because they descend within the world which they bring about, they are known as *puruṣa-avatāras*.

According to the *Bhāgavatam*, a second level of creation, maintenance, and destruction are facilitated by a second type of *avatāra*, the three guṇa-*avatāras* Brahmā, Viṣṇu, and Śiva. At this level, ambiguity enters into the picture in relation to two of these three *avatāras*, Brahmā and Śiva. Whereas Viṣṇu ('he

---

① Narang, 83. There is also therefore much parallelism with Śaiva Siddhānta cosmology, which, like Vaiṣṇavism, rejects monism and considers *māyā* as substantive (*vastutā*), not illusory (Davis, 44).

② This general pattern is also accepted in several other Indian religious and philosophical systems. Davis gives an interesting elaboration of the symmetries of 'emission' and 're absorbtion' which constitute the 'oscillations of the universe' in Śaiva Siddhānta, and how ritual *pūjā* procedures are linked to these conceptions (Davis, 42-74).

③ A branch of Sanskrit literature dealing extensively with the theology and practice of image worship, which emphasizes the concept of *vyuha*, or emanation, of different forms of the deity from one primal form. More discussion of Pañcarātra is to come. See A. K. Majumdar, *Caitanya, His Life and Doctrine: A Study in Vaiṣṇavism*, (Chowpatty, Bombay: Bharatiya Vidya Bhavan, 1969), 296-297, for a brief look at particularities of the Gauḍīya Vaiṣṇava school in relation to Pañcarātra literature.

who enters') is a 'plenary' form of *bhagavān*, and therefore is *Viṣṇu-tattva*, ('of the *Viṣṇu*-suchness' or 'of the *Viṣṇu*-category'), Brahmā is *generally* of the *jīva-tattva*, the category of living entities subject to being fettered within the world; yet occasionally, according to Gauḍīya-Vaiṣṇava commentators, he may be *viṣṇu-tattva*. Śiva is considered by Vaiṣṇava preceptors to occupy his own category, called (not surprisingly) *śiva-tattva*. One text important for the Gauḍīyas, the *Brahmā-saṁhitā*, compares Viṣṇu and Śiva to milk and yogurt, respectively: From milk one can produce yogurt, but yogurt cannot be turned back into milk. There is close affinity, yet milk must be considered superior to yogurt by virtue of being the source of yogurt.

At this level of creation and of increased differentiation of the extraneous potency (*bahiräṅga-śakti*) a slight degree of adverse influence of that energy accrues to Brahmā and Śiva, whereas Viṣṇu, as *bhagavān*, remains fully transcendent and aloof from material blemish. For this reason it is through the agency of Viṣṇu that the delicate balance of the material manifestation is maintained—not only in a physical sense but a moral sense as well. It is as Viṣṇu that *bhagavān* performs the functions expected of majestic ① lordship by overseeing the invisible moral superstructure governed by the principle of *karma*, or (proper and improper) action. And it is *through* Viṣṇu that the numerous *līlā-avatāras* descend, to perform their triple function of blessing the righteous, subduing the unrighteous, and reinstating *dharma*—religious principles—all as elements of their *līlā*, divine pastimes.

After listing the more important of these *līlā-avatāras*, the *Śrīmad-Bhāgavatam* summarizes their essential qualities, then identifies the means by which this subject can be comprehended:

> The Lord, whose activities are always spotless, is the master

---

① I am using John B. Carman's expression from his book *Majesty and Meekness: A Comparative Study of Contrast and Harmony in the Concept of God*, (Grand Rapids, Michigan: Eerdmans Publishing, 1994).

of the six senses and is fully omnipotent with six opulences. He creates the manifested universes, maintains them and annihilates them without being in the least affected. He is within every living being and is always independent. The foolish with a poor fund of knowledge cannot know the transcendental nature of the forms, names and activities of the Lord, who is playing like an actor in a drama. Nor can they express such things, neither in their speculations nor in their words. Only those who render unreserved, uninterrupted, favorable service unto the lotus feet of Lord Krishna, who carries the wheel of the chariot in His hand, [①] can know the creator of the universe in His full glory, power and transcendence. [②]

I. 3. 2 Expansion and Descent: Increasing Availability

As *bhagavān* expands and descends, he becomes in successive categories of expansion increasingly accessible to the *jīvas* who are fettered in the world of *saṁsāra*. *Āgama*, literature [③] describes this increasing accessibility to highlight the importance of the *arcā-vigraha*, also referred to as *arcāvatāra*

---

① 'who holds the wheel of the chariot in his hand' is a reference to Kṛṣṇa's pastime at Kurukṣetra in which he demonstrated his partiality to his devotee at the cost of breaking his promise not to fight in the battle—an incident described in the great epic *Mahābhārata*.

② *sa vā idaṁ viśvam amogha-līlaḥ sṛjaty avaty atti na sajjate 'smin*
bhūteṣu cāntarhita ātma-tantraḥ ṣāḍ-vargikaṁ jīghrati ṣaḍ-guṇeśaḥ
na cāsya kaścin nipuṇena dhātur avaiti jantuḥ kumanīṣa ūtīḥ
nāmāni rūpāṇi mano-vacobhiḥ santanvato naṭa-caryām ivājñaḥ
sa veda dhātuh padavīṁ parasya duranta-vīryasya rathāṅga-pāneḥ
yo ' māyayā santato yānuvṛttyā bhajeta tat-pāda-saroja-gandham (*Śrīmad-Bhāgavatam* 1. 3. 36-38).

③ *Pañcarātra* is one portion of *Āgamas*, a group of texts associated closely with image worship, both in the Śaiva and Vaiṣṇava traditions. The Vaiṣṇava Āgamas are often referred to as *pañcarātra-āgamas*.

—the worshipable physical image. This idea is nicely explained by the Śrī Vaiṣṇava① scholar Srinivasa Chari:

> The *arcāvatāra* which constitutes the foundation for image worship is considered more significant than the other incarnations [sic]② of God. The transcendental form of God (*para-rūpa*) is beyond the approach of human beings since it exists only in the transcendental realm. The *vyūha* forms [quaternary emanations, namely Vāsudeva, Saṅkarṣaṇa, Pradyumna and Aniruddha] too are unapproachable to us. The *vibhava* forms [forms appearing in the world for specific functions or pastimes] have already taken place in the remote past and as such are not available to us at present for direct worship. The presence of God as the indwelling spirit in our heart (*antaryāmin*) though close by is also beyond the scope of worship because the physical sense organs cannot perceive Him. Thus, the Divine Being present in the form of *arcā-vigraha* is always easily available to us for offering worship.③

Chari goes on to explain that later Vaiṣṇava literature speaks of four types of *arcāvatāras* in terms of their apparent origins.④ *Svayamvyakta*, 'self-manifest,' are believed to have appeared by the direct will of *bhagavān*; *daiva*, 'related to a *deva*, or higher mortal,' are said to have appeared on

---

① Śrī Vaiṣṇava: the Vaiṣṇava tradition said to descend from Śrī, or Lakṣmī, of which Rāmānuja is the principal founding teacher.

② 'Incarnation' is the term often used by writers, both Indian and Western, to translate *avatāra*. This is somewhat of a misnomer, although John Carman, well aware of the difference, also uses the term 'incarnation' sometimes in refering to *avatāras*. For his comparison of the two, see Carman, Chapter 10, *passim*, including fn. 9 p. 196, which reviews others' work on this topic.

③ Srinivasa S. M. Chari, *Vaiṣṇavism: Its Philosophy, Theology and Religious Discipline*, (Delhi: Motilal Banarsidass, 1994), 224. See also Carman, 195-96.

④ Chari, 225.

the instigation of one of several cosmic administrative agents [1]; *saiddha*, 'related to a *siddha*, or sage,' appear at the behest of an ascetic by virtue of his highly concentrated will; and *mānuṣa*, 'of a human being,' are images formed and consecrated in accordance with scriptural specifications and procedures, out of one of eight types of material. [2] We might well object that in all cases these images are, at least in some sense, made of ordinary materials such as wood, metal or stone, and hence are clearly perishable. Being of the same substance as all matter, they surely participate in grossness, impurity, and inferiority. Moreover, the images are of particular shape which suggest imperfect human form. Clearly they show none of the characteristics of *puruṣottama*, the 'highest person.' Yet all these apparent disqualifications are, for the Vaiṣṇava, countered by the one basic qualification recognized by the faithful devotee, namely *accessibility*.

John Carman quotes from a commentator who followed Rāmānuja, illustrating the complementarity of *paratva*, or 'supremacy' and *saulabhya*, or 'accessibility' in God:

> How can a lame man climb on an elephant if you tell him to do so? Likewise how can an insignificant soul in this imperfect world... approach the Lord of all...? The answer is surely that the elephant can accommodate itself, kneeling down so that the lame man can mount. God likewise makes Himself very low so that He

---

① "Cosmic administrative agents" are the numerous *devatās* such as Indra, Candra, Agni and Vāruṇa described in Vedic and Paurāṇic literature—powerful *jīvas* granted these positions temporarily as reward for outstanding piety.

② *Śrīmad-Bhāgavatam* 11. 27. 12 states, "The Deity form of the Lord is said to appear in eight varieties—stone, wood, metal, earth, paint, sand, the mind or jewels." Three verses earlier the *Bhāgavatam* offers alternative, aniconic objects as possible representations of *bhagavān*: "A twice-born person should worship Me, his worshipable Lord, without duplicity, offering appropriate paraphernalia in loving devotion to My Deity form or to a form of Me appearing upon the ground, in fire, in the sun, in water or within the worshiper's own heart."

can be worshipped by the soul in this imperfect world. [1]

According to Rāmānuja [2] beauty of bodily form is an attribute of God which demonstrates both his majesty and his accessibility as *avatāra.* [3] As we shall see, this quality will be stressed in the Gauḍīya-Vaiṣṇava theology as one basis for identifying Krishna as *avatārin*, or the source of all *avatāras*, the *puruṣottama* himself.

I. 4 Krishna as the Supremely Attractive Lord

Gauḍīya commentators quote extensively from *Śrīmad-Bhāgavatam* to support the position that Krishna is *svayam bhagavān*, 'God himself,' the source of all *avatāras.* [4] Their concern is to show that although he appears in the world, apparently as an *avatāra* of Viṣṇu, it is he who is the actual source of not only Viṣṇu but also of Nārāyaṇa, the majestic form of *bhagavān* worshipped as supreme in Pañcarātra literature. This is a salient point of distinction between the Śrī Vaiṣṇavas (who mainly follow the *Viṣṇu-purāṇa*) and the Gauḍīya-Vaiṣṇavas, who follow Caitanya's lead in privileging the

---

① Vadakku Tiruvidi Pillai, *Īḍu* 1. 3 intro. , quoted in Carman, *Majesty and Meekness*, 93.

② In the Introduction to his commentary on *Bhagavad-gītā.* Cited in Carman, 91.

③ Carman (p. 91) lists the six attributes of majesty as knowledge, untiring strength, sovereignty, immutability, creative power, and splendor. Rāmānuja's six attributes showing accessibility are compassion, gracious condescension, motherly love, generosity, concern for his creatures' welfare, and tender affection. Apparently 'beauty of bodily form' would be counted as a seventh attribute in each set.

④ An important verse for Jīva Gosvāmī comes from an early portion of the text: "All of the above-mentioned incarnations are either plenary portions or portions of the plenary portions of the Lord, but Lord Śrī Kṛṣṇa is the original Personality of Godhead. All of them appear on planets whenever there is a disturbance created by the atheists. The Lord incarnates to protect the theists (*Śrīmad-Bhāgavatam* 1. 3. 28) .

ete caṁśa-kalāḥ puṁsaḥ kṛṣṇas tu bhagavān svayam
indrāri-vyākulaṁ lokaṁ mṛḍayanti yuge yuge

Śrīmad-Bhāgavatam over other scriptures. But for the Gauḍīyas, the issue is not reducible simply to differing scriptural authority. Rather, they draw a polarity between *aiśvarya*, or lordship, and *mādhurya*, or sweetness—the latter, we may note, having some affinity with, and some significant difference from, Carman's notion of accessibility as articulated by Rāmānuja.

Whereas lordship (*aiśvarya*) is considered a peripheral or accidental quality (*tatastha-lakṣaṇa*) of *bhagavān*, sweetness (*mādhurya*) is referred to as his *svarūpa-lakṣaṇa*, or intrinsic quality. ① However much this argument may appear to defy reason (i. e. denying lordship as a principal feature of God), the Gauḍīyas want to make a statement not only about the nature of God, but also about the nature of the *jīvātmā*, the individual soul: Although the *jīva* is doubtless the eternal subordinate of God, his inclination to serve, and hence his ability to approach God intimately, is afforded *not* by God's lordship as such, but by his beauty and sweetness—by aesthetic qualities. To the Gauḍīyas, Krishna is the supreme being who demonstrates these features. O. B. L. Kapoor, an Indian scholar and practicing Vaiṣṇava, conveys something of this conviction:

> [Krishna] is not the incarnation of Viṣṇu as Śaṁkara and Rāmānuja think, but the hypostasis of Viṣṇu and all other gods. The historical Krishna is the de[s]cent of the eternal Krishna, in whom are embodied supreme puissance, supreme love, and supreme bliss. He is both concrete and expansive. By his infinite nature he encircles the whole universe, but his infinitude is centred in a concrete form. He is all-embracing in the organic unity of his being. His concrete form does not make him limited or restricted in freedom, because the modulations of his being spread everywhere in the infinite expanse of existence. He combines wideness of

① Kapoor, 123.

spirit with intensity of modulations, the eternal peace and calm of perfection with the dynamism of eternally self-revealing and self-fulfilling creative activity, and quickness of movement with intensive harmony and gracefulness. His flute wakes up such modulations in our being that our demands for love, knowledge and peace are all satisfied in an integrative synthesis. It provides freedom, elasticity, harmony and everything that makes for the richest and the most complete spiritual life. [1]

Along with his *mādhurya*, or sweetness, Krishna's 'concreteness' is also central to Gauḍīya-Vaiṣṇavism. [2] It is Krishna who historically [3] appeared in Vṛndāvana, or Vraja, a tract of some 168 square miles of land including the present city of Mathurā, between Delhi and Agra. It was in relation to hundreds of specifically identified places within this holy land that Krishna is remembered for performing his *līlā* in the first eleven years of his childhood and youth with his *parikaras*, or associates. It is the 'concrete,' tangible and specific features of this land which, for devotees, bear witness to the presence of Krishna not only at that time, but in the present—in every stone, tree, and cow of Vraja. And it is the thousands of 'concrete' *arcā* images of Krishna housed in temples, shrines, and religious communities (*āśramas*) which receive the daily devotions of local residents and pilgrims.

I have briefly sketched the theology of the *avatāra* in general terms under

---

① Kapoor, 107.

② This might be equally said for the followers of Vallabhācārya, the "Puṣṭi-mārga," as also of the followers of Nimbarka (Rudra-sampradāya).

③ 'Historically' perhaps not for Western scholarship, but for the Vaiṣṇavas certainly so, if in a sense of historicity which recognizes the possibility of spiritually significant events taking place in historic time which may become obscured to those of fettered perception. For an apropos contemporary Vaiṣṇava discussion on this issue, see Sadāpūta Dāsa, "Rational 'Mythology': Can a rational person accept the stories of the Purāṇas as literally true?" (A lecture presented at the Parliament of the World's Religions, Chicago, 1993) *Back to Godhead* (Jan/Feb 1994).

the category of *sambandha*, 'relationship,' and indicated by it both the significance of the *arcāvatāra* as the object of worship and the significance of Krishna as the most accessible, supreme divinity for the Gauḍīya-Vaiṣṇavas. We must now consider the category of *abhidheya*, 'process,' which is *bhakti*, 'devotional service,' by which *prayojana*, the 'goal,' namely pure love of God, is attained. It is through *bhakti* that the practice of image worship is nourished and sustained.

Chapter Two
Bhakti as Means and End

The manifestation of unadulterated devotional service is exhibited when one's mind is at once attracted to hearing the transcendental name and qualities of the Supreme Personality of Godhead, who is residing in everyone's heart. Just as the water of the Ganges flows naturally down towards the ocean, such devotional ecstasy, uninterrupted by any material condition, flows towards the Supreme Lord.

—Śrīmad-Bhāgavatam3. 29. 11-12①

Ⅱ. 1 Definitions of Bhakti

Ⅱ. 1. 1 Negative Definition of Bhakti

Prompted by their understanding of *Śrīmad-Bhāgavatam* the Gauḍīya-Vaiṣṇava theologians have been concerned to isolate *bhakti* from all practices

① *mad-guṇa-śruti-mātreṇa mayi sarva-guhāśaye*
mano-gatir avicchinnā yathā gaṅgāmbhaso 'mbudhau
lakṣaṇaṁ bhakti-yogasya nirguṇasya hy udāhṛtam
ahaituky avyavahitā yā bhaktiḥ puruṣottame

they consider [1] distinct from *bhakti*, specifically *karma*, *jñāna*, and *yoga*, not to completely reject these latter three, but to highlight *bhakti* as the active, integrative principle through which they come to perfection. [2] *Karma* in this context refers to all efforts made in expectation of gaining material rewards, be they immediately tangible or scripturally promised future rewards (a future auspicious birth, material gains in the next life, etc.). *Jñāna* in this context has to do with the aspiration to gain gnosis, or spiritual knowledge out of a desire for liberation from material, bodily existence. Its perfection consists in the realization of *nirviśeṣa-brahman*, [3] or the non-differentiated, 'impersonal' absolute. *Yoga* as included here refers to the practice of *aṣṭāṅga-yoga*—the classical eight-fold system aimed at realization of *paramātmā*, but which is criticized from the bhakti perspective on the grounds that it tends to distract the practitioner with the acquisition of occult powers which may lead to self-aggrandizement.

These latter three types of practice, profusely extolled throughout Vedic literature, although not held entirely in contempt in the Gauḍīya-Vaiṣṇava school, are regarded with caution as all belonging to the category of 'other desires' (*anyābhilāṣitāḥ*) which serve mainly to perpetuate material existence over against the valued, genuinely spiritual desire of service to *bhagavān*, which is represented by *bhakti*. [4] Only *bhakti* leads one

---

① As Walter G. Neevel Jr. has noted in another context regarding an earlier Vaiṣṇava theologian, Yāmunācārya, the writers we are concerned with would not have seen themselves as *adding anything* to the sources they were drawing from. When I say 'they consider,' it is a bow to modern preconceptions, as Neevel notes, about the importance of individual originality. The Six Gosvāmīs would have considered their task simply "to recover and restate clearly the meaning of [their] sources so as to make it available to [their] contemporaries." Walter G. Neevel, *Yāmuna's Vedānta and Pāñcarātra: Integrating the Classical and the Popular*, (Missoula, Montana: Scholars Press, 1977), 58.

② Kapoor, 182.

③ Kapoor, 177.

④ *anukūlyena kṛṣṇānuśīlanam bhaktir ucyate*: 'that is said to be *bhakti* (which) is conducted for the favoring of Kṛṣṇa.'

to realization of the *bhagavān* feature of the absolute, albeit with possible assistance from the other three in the beginning stages of *bhakti* spiritual practice. ①

This emphasis in the Gauḍīya-Vaiṣṇava conception of *bhakti* places the latter in a position somewhat exclusive from the traditional social structure, the *varṇāśrama* system (which came to be known in the West in its more recent form as the 'caste' system). Whereas *varṇāśrama* caters mainly to the three above mentioned lesser pursuits by focusing on material bodily concerns, Krishna-*bhakti* goes beyond *varṇāśrama* and thereby fulfills its (*varṇāśrama's*) actual purpose. In his *Bhakti-sandarbha*, Jīva Gosvāmī quotes from the *Bhāgavatam*:

> It is therefore concluded that the highest perfection one can achieve by discharging the duties prescribed for one's own occupation according to caste divisions [*varṇa*] and orders of life [*āśrama*] is to please the Personality of Godhead. ②

He then elaborates:

> Pure devotional service [*śuddha-bhakti*] is utterly the best (of spiritual paths). By this verse, therefore, it is said that devotional service is superior to the activities of *varṇāśrama-dharma*. Next he (Sūta Gosvāmī) describes the nature of *bhakti*: Because *bhakti* is naturally and spontaneously blissful, it is unmotivated (*ahaitukī*), that is to say it is without the search for any result other than the service itself; also it is uninterrupted (*apratihatā*), which means because there is an absence of either happiness

---

① Kapoor, 180.

② *Śrīmad-Bhāgavatam* 1. 2. 13, quoted in *Bhakti-sandarbha* 3. 3.

or distress in (reference to) anything (other than devotional service), therefore it cannot be stopped by anything. When *bhakti* is characterized by attraction (*ruci*) (to the Lord), then the practice of *bhakti* (*sādhana-bhakti*), characterized by hearing (about the Lord) and so on, commences. ①

Caitanya and the Six Gosvāmīs do not reject the established social system of class division (unlike some *bhakti* movements, such as that of Kabir ②), yet they subordinate it to the attainment of a higher goal, Krishna-*bhakti*. Since the visible practice of *bhakti* spirituality is significantly related to the temples where images are worshipped, this attitude to *varṇāśrama* becomes important. In accord with the Pañcarātra scriptures which concentrate on the ritual aspect of Vaiṣṇava theology and practice, the Gosvāmīs acknowledge that *bhakti* is for everyone regardless of class membership by birth, in that anyone can become qualified to receive initiation into the practices which constitute the cultivation of *bhakti*—especially the chanting of *mantras*, or mystic utterances, ③ and the worship of divine images (*mūrtis*). Class distinctions are preserved for ordinary social dealings, but they are simultaneously transcended on the higher level of *bhakti*. ④

Bhakti is also contrasted with another categorization of human pursuits, or *puruṣārthas*, namely 'mundane religiosity' (*dharma*); the pursuit of wealth (*artha*); the satisfaction of sense desires (*kāma*); and liberation

---

① *Bhakti-sandarbha* 3. 3. My translation.

② Rabindra Kumar Siddhantashastree, *Vaiṣṇavism Through the Ages*, (Delhi: Munshiram Manoharlal, 1985), 168-71.

③ *mantra*: lit. 'instrument of thought,' a sacred text or speech; 'a sacred formula addressed to any individual deity.' Sir Monier Monier-Williams, *A Sanskrit-English Dictionary*, New Edition, (Oxford: Clarendon Press, 1960).

④ This is discussed also by Bhaktivinoda Thākur in his work *Śrī Caitanya Śikṣāmṛtam*. Kedarnath Datta Bhaktivinoda, *Śrī Chaitanya Shikshamrtam*, trans. (Madras: Sri Gaudiya Math, 1983), 98-99.

(*mokṣa*) —all of which, again, are facilitated by the *varṇāśrama* social structure. Whereas *mokṣa* is seen in almost all formal religious traditions of India as the ultimate human goal (including most Vaiṣṇava systems, which emphasize *bhakti* as the exclusive means to liberation), for the Gauḍīya-Vaiṣṇavas *bhakti* is the goal itself (*sādhya*), and therefore it is inclusive of the four subordinate goals, especially liberation. The importance of all the ordinary human goals is thought to be insignificant in comparison to *śuddha-bhakti*, pure devotion.

Ⅱ. 1. 2 Positive Definition of Bhakti

If *bhakti* is held to be in contradistinction to most ordinary human goals, what is its positive aim? Or if it is inclusive of all other accomplishments, what is its specific characteristic? For the Gauḍīya-Vaiṣṇavas, *bhakti* is devotion specifically to Krishna or one of his many forms, for the exclusive purpose of pleasing him. ① Jīva Gosvāmī substantiates the first aspect of this position with a proof-text from the *Śrīmad-Bhāgavatam* (7. 14. 34):

> O king of the earth, it has been decided by expert, learned scholars that only the Supreme Personality of Godhead, ② Krishna, in whom all that is moving or non-moving within this universe is resting and from whom everything is coming, is the best person to

---

① We may call attention to Krishna Sharma's thesis that the current (at least up to 1987) academic definition of *bhakti* has been unwittingly adopted from the conception of *bhakti* represented in the Gauḍīya school of Vaiṣṇavism. While there may have been some truth to this for some time, I think careful scholarship would show a more nuanced picture today. Krishna Sharma, *Bhakti and the Bhakti Movement: A New Perspective*, (Delhi: Munshiram Manoharlal, 1987), *passim*, esp. Supplement II, 255-279.

② See Graham M. Schweig, "Universal and Confidential Love of God" *Journal of Vaiṣṇava Studies* vol. 6 no. 2 (Spring 1998), 106, for an excellent explanation of Prabhupāda's use of the expression "Supreme Personality of Godhead" to translate the Sanskrit word *bhagavān*. The Sanskrit verse uses the name Hari, an epithet of *bhagavān*.

whom everything must be given. ①

Since it is God in whom "all that is moving or non-moving within this universe is resting and from whom everything is coming," he is compared to the root of a tree which deserves the attentions of watering and nourishment for the benefit of the entire tree; serving him is further compared to human nourishment by the normal process of eating, by which the body's metabolic system assures the proper distribution of energy to all its organs and senses (*Bhāg*. 4. 31. 14). The word *bhakti* comes from the Sanskrit verbal root *bhaj*, 'to divide' or 'to share.' ② Often translated simply as 'devotion,' the Gauḍīya school emphasizes its active quality, as a constant practice of service to the supreme. Since the *svarūpa-lakṣaṇa*, or essential characteristic, of the *jīvātmā* (the individual self) is service, and since the *jīvātmā* has an eternal connection to *bhagavān* (as a ray of sunlight is connected to the sun), the natural object (*viṣaya*) of service and devotion is *bhagavān*.

That *bhakti* has the aim of satisfying *bhagavān* is also indicated in Rūpa Gosvāmī's ③ (1488–156?) definition of the superior (*uttama*) form of *bhakti*. It is *ānukūlyena kṛṣṇānuśīlana*, or the repeated and devoted service to Krishna which is 'according to the current,' i. e. favorable to Krishna. This *svarūpa-lakṣaṇa*, or essential characteristic, of *bhakti*, is a function of the

---

① Quoted in *Bhakti-sandarbha* 286. 44.

② Monier-Williams on verbal root *bhaj*: "to divide, distribute, allot or apportion to, share with, to grant, bestow, furnish, supply; . . . [in this context, from which *bhakti* as 'devotion' is derived:] to serve, honour, revere, love, adore. "*Bhakti*, in this context, he defines as "attachment, devotion, fondness for, devotion to, . . . trust, homage, worship, piety, faith or love or devotion (as a religious principle or means of salvation, together with *karma*, 'works,' and *jñāna*, 'spiritual knowledge.' "

③ Rūpa, one of the Six Gosvāmīs, states this definition as the *svarūpa-lakṣaṇa*, or essential characteristic, of *uttama-bhakti* in his book *Bhakti-rasāmṛta-sindhu*.

svarūpa-śakti, the essential, 'internal' energy[1] of *bhagavān*.

Bhakti is also inherently existing in a dormant condition in the *jīvātmā* (a product of *tatastha-śakti*, or medial potency, as mentioned in Chapter One) who is under the sway of the *bahiraṅga-śakti*, the extraneous potency of *bhagavān*. In other words, the living entity, by virtue of its eternal relation to *bhagavān*, has spontaneous, natural devotion to him;[2] but this devotion has been obscured to a greater or lesser degree by habituation (since time immemorial, from untold previous births) to selfish pursuits inspired by the attractions of the extraneous potency. How one breaks with habit and awakens devotion is ultimately a matter of grace (*kṛpā*, *prasāda*, *vadānyatā*, *anugraha*),[3] received from *bhagavān* by one or more of several means, all based on the ontological relationship of the *jīva* to *bhagavān*.

Krishnadās Kavirāja, one of two principal sixteenth century biographers of Caitanya whose writings are considered canonical by all Gauḍīya-Vaiṣṇavas, claims that the goal of *bhakti*, namely pure love of God, is eternally available within the living being, waiting to be awakened by proper means:

> Pure love for Krishna is eternally established in the hearts of living entities. It is not something to be gained from another source

---

① Sanjukta Gupta explains the general Pañcarātra concept of the *śakti* of *bhagavān* as the aggregate of his six *bhagas*, or glories: "[T] hese six attributes of god [sic], taken together, constitute his Śakti, which may be translated as his power, potency, and potentiality rolled into one. . . . Śakti is god's essential nature, his personality or 'I-ness' (*ahaṁtā*)." Sanjukta Gupta, "The Pāñcarātra Attitude to Mantra," in *Mantra*, ed. Harvey P. Alper, (Albany, NY: State University of New York Press, 1989), 225. Majumdar elaborates on *svarūpa-śakti* in *Caitanya: His Life and Doctrine*, 287-290.

② Bhaktivinoda, 170.

③ *Kṛpā*: lit. 'pity, tenderness, compassion;' *prasāda*: lit. 'graciousness, kindness, kind behaviour, favor, aid, mediation;' *vadānyatā*: lit. 'bounty, liberality, munificence;' *anugraha*: lit. 'favour, kindness, conferring benefits assistance' (Monier-Williams).

(*sādhya*) . When the heart is purified by hearing and chanting, the living entity naturally awakens (C. c. Madhya 22. 107) .

'Hearing' and 'chanting' are types of *sādhana*, or practice which help the *sādhaka*, or practitioner, to awaken the dormant *Krishna-prema*, or unadulterated love for Krishna. The *Bhāgavatam* presents a nine-fold group of interrelated practices conducive to the perfection of *bhakti* which include *śravaṇam*, or hearing topics related to God from qualified sources, and *kīrtanam*, or chanting, speaking about, glorifying God. Also included within these nine is *arcanam*, ① or worshipping God formally, especially by the procedures of *mūrti-sevā*, or service to the divine image. It is this practice with which we are concerned in this book, hence our next topic will be *bhakti* in practice, or *sādhana-bhakti*.

Ⅱ. 2 Vaidhi-sādhana-bhakti—Bhakti as Means

Ⅱ. 2. 1 Regulating the Senses

A contemporary scholar of Gauḍīya-Vaiṣṇavism, Joseph T. O'Connell, gives us a brief explanation of the term *sādhana*:

> . . . [S]*ādhana* is basically a pattern or program of religious practices. The Sanskrit root, *sadh*, means "to accomplish" or "to attain" something. *Sādhana* is the means or the program that one goes through to attain the *sādhya* ("that which is to be attained")

---

① The other six are *smaraṇam*, remembrance of the name, form, qualities and pastimes of God; *pāda-sevaṇam*, literally 'serving the feet,' i. e. rendering menial service to God and his devotees; *vandanam*, offering prayers to God; *dāsyam*, 'servitude,' or participating in the mission of God; *sākhyam*, cultivating intimate friendship with God; and *ātma-nivedanam*, surrendering oneself fully to God.

or the *siddhi* (the "perfection" or the "goal"). In this case, the goal is a yet more perfect experience of *bhakti*, or devotion to the Lord. The *sādhaka* is the person who is striving to attain such perfection.

Sādhana is a program. . . in which the Vaiṣṇava uses not only his or her mind but the physical senses also—eyes, ears, voice—to develop the underlying capacity for devotion into a more perfect culmination of it.[1]

In one of the most important theological writings for the Gauḍīya-Vaiṣṇava community, the *Bhakti-rasāmṛta-sindhu* ('The Ocean of the Nectarean Taste of Devotion'), Rūpa Gosvāmī treats *bhakti* in three categories, the first of which is *sādhana-bhakti*, or devotion in practice.[2] This has two subdivisions, *vaidhi*, or "in reference to regulations," and *rāgānuga*, or "following spontaneously." For the majority of practitioners, the path of following regulations is prescribed, since it is understood that the binding effect[3] of habitual engagement in mundane activities has rendered one more or less incapable of acting on the platform of spontaneous devotion, at least in any sustained way. Following the directions of one's *guru*, or spiritual preceptor, and of *śāstra*, or scripture, the practitioner learns to orient all of his or her physical and mental activities toward the service of God. Krishnadās Kavirāja, after quoting Rūpa Gosvāmī's definition of *uttama-bhakti* (see previous section), elaborates on *anukūlya*, or "favorable" practice, with *sarvendriye*, or "with all one's senses," (whereby in Indian philosophical

---

① Joseph O'Connell, "Sādhana Bhakti," in *Vaiṣṇavism: Contemporary Scholars Discuss the Gauḍīya Tradition*, ed. Steven Rosen, (New York: FOLK Books, 1992), 229-230.

② The other two are *bhāva-bhakti*, spontaneous devotion beyond practice, and *prema-bhakti*, pure ecstatic devotion. We will discuss these later.

③ One might equally speak of the "*blinding* effect" of habitual engagement. Through habitual preoccupation with mundane affairs one becomes unable to perceive one's spiritual identity in relation to God. But the end effect is bondage in material existence (*saṁsāra*).

traditions the mind is considered the interior sense) . He then quotes Rūpa further, who in turn gives reference to *Pañcarātra* scripture:

> *Bhakti* means the service of the supreme Lord of the senses with (one's own) senses. Such service (renders one) free from all material [temporary] designations and (renders the senses) pure. ① (C. c. Madhya 19. 170/BRS 1. 1. 12) .

Krishna is known by the epithet *hṛṣīkeśa*, or "Lord of the senses." The effect of *māyā*, the deluding potential of matter, is to support the bound *jīva's* misconception of his own lordship by facilitating sense activity in relation to sense objects for pleasing results. In the practice of *vaidhi-sādhana*, the practitioner learns to dedicate all activities of the senses to the "Lord of the senses," recognizing *bhagavān's* sensate nature. Thus, for example, one's ability to see is counted as a minute expression of God's unlimited power of sight; similarly the functions of all the other senses are considered testimony to the unlimited sensory power of God, whose desire it is that the *jīva* dedicate its sensory activities to his service as a token of *bhakti*. Dedication of sensory activity to God is rewarded by genuine satisfaction of the senses.

The *Bhagavad-gītā*, revered by most Hindus, especially Vaiṣṇavas of all traditions, ② is generally recognized as a text which emphasizes the importance of *bhakti*. Gauḍīya-Vaiṣṇavas revere it as an essential manual on *bhakti* spoken directly by Krishna to his companion Arjuna. Near the end of the ninth chapter (verse 27) , which deals specifically with *bhakti*, the general concept of dedicating one's activities to God is expressed:

---

① *sarvopādhi-vinirmuktaṁ tat-paratvena nirmalam*
hṛṣīkeṇa hṛṣīkeśa-sevanaṁ bhaktir ucyate (*Caitanya-caritāmṛta*, Madhya-līlā 19. 170, quoting *Bhakti-rasāmṛta-sindhu* 1. 1. 12)

② This is not to say it is exclusively revered, as should be obvious from our frequent mention of other scriptures.

> Whatever you do, whatever you eat, whatever you offer or give away, and whatever austerities you perform—do that, O son of Kuntī [Arjuna], as an offering to Me [Krishna]. ①

This is a generalization of the statement of the previous verse:

> If one offers Me with love and devotion a leaf, a flower, fruit or water, I will accept it. ②

These brief statements indicate the essential theology of sensory engagement as devotional service directed to God—a principle which is extensively elaborated in the *Gītā* itself as also in other scriptures, especially the *Bhāgavatam*. The *Pañcarātra* literature treats this same principle in more technical ways, especially as formalized ritual.

Consolidating and systematizing the numerous injunctions for regulated practice is one of the projects of the Gosvāmīs. Rūpa Gosvāmī offers a list of sixty-four items important for *vaidhi-bhakti-sādhana*, all of which relate directly or indirectly to the worship of God in the *arcā-vigraha*. These injunctions range from basic principles, such as the acceptance of apprenticeship under a properly qualified *guru*, to more specific injunctions, such as the necessity to follow behind processions in which portable *vijaya-mūrtis*, or festival images, are carried. Within this list is found the injunction to worship the image by a daily procedure which is itself elaborated into sixty-four *upacāras*, or items offered, in yet another text, the *Hari-bhakti-*

---

① *yat karoṣi yad aśnāsi yaj juhoṣi dadāsi yat*
yat tapasyasi kaunteya tat kuruṣva mad-arpaṇam

② *patraṁ puṣpaṁ phalaṁ toyaṁ yo me bhaktyā prayacchati*
tad ahaṁ bhakty upahṛtām aśnāmi prayatātmanaḥ (*B. G.* 9. 26)

vilāsa, attributed to Gopāla Bhaṭṭa Gosvāmī.[①]

Ⅱ. 2. 2 Ritual Service Aimed at Devotion

It may be helpful to consider briefly some of the contents of the practice of image worship in the Gauḍīya-Vaiṣṇava tradition. It should be noted that the basic structure and considerable content of this practice is similar to that of other Vaiṣṇava traditions. It has not gone unnoticed by scholars that there is considerable similarity in ritual procedures among Indic traditions; so for example the Śaiva-siddhānta tradition of south India[②] and even "heterodox" traditions, especially Jainism and Buddhism[③] may have almost identical sequences of offering items to the respective object of worship.[④]

Since the *Śrīmad-Bhāgavatam* holds central scriptural authority for the Gauḍīya-Vaiṣṇavas, and since its specific description of image worship

---

① Sanātana Gosvāmī seems to have been involved in its compilation to some extent. See Sushil Kumar De, *Early History of the Vaiṣṇava Faith and Movement in Bengal*, (Calcutta: Firma KLM, 1986), 125-45.

② Davis, *passim.*

③ See Lawrence Babb, *Absent Lord: Ascetics and Kings in a Jain Ritual Culture*, (Berkeley: University of California Press, 1996) for an exploration of Jaina worship and some comparison to Buddhist, Śaiva, and Vaiṣṇava worship.

④ This might suggest similarities in theologies among Indic traditions on levels deeper than their declared differences—a topic for another paper! One useful theoretical distinction in regard to food offering and acceptance (an important aspect of most Indic worship) has been pointed out by Paul Toomey (pp. 5-8): Whereas one group of anthropologists accounts for food offering and receiving ritual in terms of "ranked relationship between worshipper and deity, enacted transactionally," for other anthropologists (including Toomey) who seem to give more recognition to the dynamics of *bhakti*, a "notion that *prasad* [offered food] is a unique cultural idea" is upheld. He goes on to compare *prasad* to the Christian Eucharist. Paul M. Toomey, *Food from the Mouth of Krishna: Feasts and Festivals in a North Indian Pilgrimage Center*, (Delhi: Hindustan Publishing, 1994), 5-8.

Another general approach to this topic could be to consider worship as offering hospitality, a common theme in many Asian forms of worship.

procedure is quite brief and relatively undetailed, we can take advantage of it to become acquainted with the basic elements of worship.

In the twenty-seventh chapter of the eleventh book of this work, Krishna himself is quoted as he outlines the process for his dear friend Uddhava:

> Now please listen faithfully as I explain exactly how a person who has achieved twice-born status (*dvijatvam prāpya*)[1] through the relevant Vedic prescriptions should worship me [in the *arcā-mūrti*] with devotion (*māṁ bhaktyā*).[2]

The *Hari-bhakti-vilāsa* deals at length with the qualifications one needs to achieve "twice-born"[3] status. A person must receive proper initiation from a qualified *guru* and be trained in *sad-ācāra*—proper Vaiṣṇava behavior—before he or she can worship the *arcā-mūrti* directly.[4] Such a *dvija* is then expected to follow a strict daily regimen of actions in relation to the service of God, who may be represented in a small image enshrined in one's own home, or in a *mandira*, or temple, of lesser or greater size. The day begins at the *brahma-muhūrta*, or one-and-a-half hours before sunrise, when one rises to

---

① The expression "twice-born" is a standard literal translation of *dvija*, a reference to a member of the three upper classes who receive initiation (*upanayanam*) into the study of Vedic literature, considered as a second birth from the "mother" of the Veda. It is not to be confused with the western expression associated with evangelical Christianity.

② *yadā sva-nigamenoktam dvijatvaṁ prāpya pūruṣaḥ*
yathā yajeta māṁ bhaktyā śraddhayā tan nibodha me (*Śrīmad-Bhāgavatam* 11. 27. 8, trans. of all 11th Book verses by H. D. Goswami)

③ The *Pañcarātra* system opens up the possibility for persons of all classes to practice *arcanam* by developing the appropriate qualifications of behavior.

④ Kṛṣṇa-kṣetra Dāsa, ed., *Pañcarātra-pradīpa*: *Illumination of Pañcarātra*. Supplement to Volume One, Daily Service. GBC Deity Worship Group, (Mayapur, India: ISKCON-GBC Press, 1995), 11. "Proper Vaiṣṇava behavior" especially refers to the observance of strictures regarding diet (vegetarian), sexual behavior (cohabitation only within marriage, for the purpose of procreation), and complete avoidance of intoxication and gambling.

immediately prepare oneself physically and mentally for approaching God.

> The worshiper should first purify his body by cleansing his teeth and bathing. Then he should perform a second cleansing by applying marks to the body with earth and chanting both Vedic and tantric *mantras* (*Bhāg*. 11. 27. 10). [1]

These and related activities make up *abhigamana*, or acts preparatory to approaching God for worship. *Abhigamana* is one of five divisions (*pañcāṅga*) of *pūjā*, or worship with paraphernalia, found in Pañcarātra literature dealing with the procedures of daily image worship. [2] The second of these is *upādāna*, or gathering items for worship, including collecting offerable flowers and foodstuffs and preparing these and other items for offering, by purification procedures and, in the case of food, proper cooking.

---

① *pūrvaṁ snānaṁ prakurvīta dhauta-danto 'nga-śuddhaye*
ubhayair api snānaṁ mantrair mṛd-grahanādinā (*Śrīmad-Bhāgavatam* 11. 27. 10).

Despite elaborate (mainly western) theorizing over brahminical preoccupation with purity, the explanation for this concern within the tradition is rather straightforward, summed up in our Western adage, "cleanliness is next to godliness." To approach God, who is supremely pure, calls for purity; but purity (especially of the heart, or consciousness) is ultimately bestowed by God. Yet one can, it would be argued, practice acts enjoined directly or indirectly by God which are conducive to purity, beginning with simplest of these, bathing. Perhaps in no other religious tradition of the world does one find such elaborate and detailed specifications for ablution than in brahmanical texts of India, so it is obviously important. Vaiṣṇavas would argue that its importance cannot be reduced to only a concern to maintain social boundaries; rather the contrary: it is the bound souls' disinterest in purity—especially internal purity—which perpetuates its exclusion from direct association with God.

② Chari, 311-16.

> One should worship me in my forms, etc., (*pratimādiṣu*)[1] by offering the most excellent paraphernalia (*dravyaiḥ prasiddhaiḥ*). But a devotee completely freed from material desire may worship me with whatever he is able to obtain, and may even worship me within his heart with mental paraphernalia (*hṛdi-bhāvena*).[2]

The third division is *yoga*, linking oneself (especially internally), or identifying oneself as a servant of God. Ritually this includes a process called *bhūta-śuddhi*, purification of the elements;[3] a brief[4] meditation (*dhyāna*) on the particular form of God one is worshipping (following scriptural descriptions); and *mānasa-pūjā*, or a mental rehearsal[5] of the procedures of worship. Krishna's description of meditation on his form in this section of

---

① *pratimā*: lit. 'an image, likeness, symbol; picture, statue, figure; reflection;' *ādi*, lit. 'having as beginning,' i. e. 'and so on,' here suggests that the God can also be worshipped in various aniconic substances or elements, as was mentioned previously (see footnote 2 page 125).

② *dravyaiḥ prasiddhair mad-yāgaḥ pratimādiṣv amāyinaḥ*
bhaktasya ca yathā-labdhair hṛdi bhāvena caiva hi (*Śrīmad-Bhāgavatam* 11. 27. 15).
We may note tangentially the distinction recognized here between persons of lesser and greater qualifications to worship. The greater the internal qualification, the lighter the injunctive stricture on high-quality offerings. The *Hari-bhakti-vilāsa* elaborates extensively on things fit and unfit for offering, perhaps giving most detail in the matter of offerable and unofferable flowers, for which an entire chapter (out of twenty) is dedicated.

③ *Āgama* texts describe an elaborate procedure of mentally 'deconstructing' one's material body and then 'reconstructing' it with purified material elements. Gauḍīya-Vaiṣṇavas simplify this to the point of a simple meditation on oneself as eternal servant of God, free from all social class (*varṇa*) and life-stage (*āśrama*) designations.

④ In the context of worship under regulations it would generally be brief. The more advanced practitioner might extend the period of meditation as he or she sees fit. The same applies to *mānasa-pūjā*, the next step in *yoga*. The term *yoga* is commonly associated with the classical Yoga system associated with Patāñjalī. However the term has a wide range of meanings depending on context.

⑤ *Manasa-pūjā* involves mentally offering each of the items, just as one will offer them physically after concluding the *manasa-pūjā*, however within the mind there is possibility to embellish the procedure, especially with greater (visualized) opulence than might be possible in the physical worship.

the *Bhāgavatam* is as follows:

> The worshiper should meditate upon my subtle form—which is situated within the worshiper's own body, now purified by air and fire—as the source of all living entities. This form of the Lord is experienced by self-realized sages in the last part of the vibration of the sacred syllable *oṁ*.

With the next step, *avāhana*, or 'calling God down,' the worship proper can begin:

> The devotee conceives of the supreme Self (*paramātmā*), whose presence surcharges the devotee's body, in the form corresponding to his realization. Thus the devotee worships the Lord to his full capacity and becomes fully absorbed in him. By touching the various limbs of the image and chanting appropriate *mantras*, the devotee should invite the *paramātmā* to join the image, and then the devotee should worship (*prapūjayet*) me [in that image]. ①

The fourth of the five aspects of worship, *ijyā*, is the offering of several articles and services in a specific order and with appropriate *mantras*, or sacred verbal expressions. ② As mentioned earlier, sixty-four of these articles

---

① *piṇḍe vāyv-agni-saṁśuddhe hṛt-padma-sthāṁ parāṁ mama*
aṇvīṁ jīva-kalāṁ dhyāyen nādānte siddha-bhāvitām
tayātma-bhūtayā piṇḍe vyāpte sampūjya tan-mayaḥ
āvāhyārcādiṣu sthāpya nyastāṅgaṁ māṁ prapūjayet

Śrīmad-Bhāgavatam 11. 27. 23-24. Verse 24 suggests worship of a temporary, as opposed to a permanent *mūrti*. Vaiṣṇavas mainly worship permanently consecrated images, although the *Śrīmad-Bhāgavatam* seems to give the option of temporary worship as well.

② I will discuss *mantra*-utterance in the context of *arcanam* in Section Ⅱ. 3. 2.

and services, or *upacāras*, are delineated in *Hari-bhakti-vilasa*, all of which together constitute a full day's worship from early morning until late evening, including activities of waking, bathing, dressing, decorating, offering food, entertaining, and putting God to rest. In offering these services, God is treated as either the honored guest in one's home or the lordly monarch in his own palace. In both cases, within *vaidhi-sādhana* (regulated practice) the emphasis will be on careful attention to rules; however, individuals worshipping a home image are less likely to perform such elaborate service daily; more likely all the sixty-four (or more) [1] would be offered in a large temple, with greater attention to punctuality, and not all by one person. Rather, several *pūjārīs*, or ritual specialists, would offer the appropriate services for different times in the course of a day. This temple *nitya-sevā*, or daily program of service, is carried out seven days per week throughout the year; a home image might be worshipped very simply on most days of the week, with a more elaborate service performed once per week or once per fortnight.

Ijyā, the offering of items and services, concludes in a festive mood:

> Singing along with others, chanting loudly and dancing, acting out my transcendental pastimes, and hearing and telling stories about me, the devotee should for some time absorb himself in such festivity. [2]

Although the subject of this chapter of *Bhāgavatam* is *arcanam*, the formal worship of the *arcā-mūrti* as one of nine practices of *bhakti*, this

---

① I am told that the commentator to *Hari-bhakti-vilāsa* points out that service is potentially unlimited, the specifically prescribed items being listed as sixty-four. Hence within the scope of worship under regulations room for spontaneity is suggested.

② *upagāyan gṛṇan nṛtyan karmāṇy abhinayan mama*
mat-kathāḥ śrāvayan śṛṇvan muhūrtaṁ kṣaṇiko bhavet (*Śrīmad-Bhāgavatam* 11. 27. 44).

injunction to sing, chant, and hear in relation to God is also present as both an aspect of *arcanam* and as the substance of the first two most important categories of devotion, *śravaṇam* and *kīrtanam* (hearing and chanting), as we discussed in Section Ⅱ. 1. 2. It is also related to the last of the five divisions of *arcanam*, namely *svādhyāya*, literally "self-study." *Svādhyāya* refers to reading, recitation, and study of sacred texts, alone rather than with others. *Svādhyāya* is the reflective aspect of the practice of *arcanam* which facilitates the cultivation of spirituality and aids the practitioner in avoiding the dangers of routinization, or preoccupation with the details of rules at the expense of the essential purpose of the rules, namely to develop one's natural devotion to God through an attitude of service. Since the texts studied (especially the *Bhāgavatam* and the *Caitanya-caritāmṛta* for the Gauḍīya-Vaiṣṇavas) emphasize other types of service related to the service of the *arcā-mūrti*, the study and recitation of scripture as an aspect of *arcanam* points to the necessity of participating in these other types of service. These revolve around such activities as *Vaiṣṇava-sevā*, or service to Vaiṣṇavas; *nāma-sevā*, or service to the divine names of God (again, through recitation and singing); *ātīthi-sevā*, or reception and service to guests; *prasāda-sevā*, or distributing and eating sanctified food; and *dhāma-sevā*, or service to sacred places associated with God. By careful practice of these *sevās*, the practitioner is expected to progress from a less mature stage of consciousness (characterized by neglect of other *jīvas* on the plea of attentiveness to the *arcā-mūrti*) to a more mature stage of awareness and behavior. This essential aspect of *arcanam* is thus attentive to scriptural warnings such as the following, (attributed to Kapila, counted in the *Bhāgavatam* as an *avatāra* of *bhagavān*):

> One who offers me respect but is envious of the bodies of others and is therefore a separatist (*bhinna-darśī*) never attains peace of mind, because of his inimical behavior toward other living entities. O sinless one, even if one worships with proper rituals and

paraphernalia, a person who is disrespectful of living entities (being not aware of my presence in them) never pleases me by the worship of my image in the temple. ①

Ⅱ. 3 Bhakti as Goal

Ⅱ. 3. 1 Leading Into Līlā: Reciprocation

Having outlined the practices of *vaidhi-sādhana*, or practice according to regulations, we can step back to view the entire progression of devotional practice as it is conceived in Gauḍīya-Vaiṣṇava theology, specifically as articulated by Rūpa Gosvāmī in *Bhakti-rasāmṛta-sindhu*. ② He identifies an eight-fold progression, beginning with initial faith (*śraddhā*) leading to association with other practitioners (*sadhu-saṅga*) with whom one undertakes regulated practice (*bhajana-kriyā*). Substantial progress is then experienced as the cessation of unholy practices (*anartha-nivṛttiḥ*), at which time one becomes firm in conviction (*niṣṭhā*) regarding the efficaciousness of the practice of *bhakti*, and thus one becomes steady in the practice.

In the next stage, one begins to experience *ruci*, or a genuine "taste" or inclination for *bhakti*, especially an inclination for *śravaṇam*, devotional hearing about God. Out of *ruci* develops *āsakti*, or a strong, unshakable attachment to God, out of which develops *bhāva*, or "transcendent

---

① *dviṣataḥ para-kāye māṁ mānino bhinna-darśinaḥ*
bhūteṣu baddha-vairasya na manaḥ śantim ṛcchati
aham uccāvacair dravyaiḥ kriyayotpannayānaghe
naiva tuṣtye 'rcito 'rcāyāṁ bhūta-grāmāvamāninaḥ.
Śrīmad-Bhāgavatam 3. 29. 23-24.

② *Bhakti-rasāmṛta-sindhu* 1. 4. 15-16.

emotion. "As this experience of emotion intensifies and deepens, it allows *prema*, or supreme love of God (that which, as we noted earlier, is considered dormantly present in all living entities) to manifest in the heart.

A similar progression was elaborated some five centuries earlier by the Śrī-Vaiṣṇava Rāmānuja in his *Vedārthasaṁgraha*. In the conclusion of his account of the unfolding of *bhakti*, he stresses the experience of God's grace and the experience of *bhakti* as a goal in itself:

> The supreme person, who is overflowing with compassion, being pleased with such love, showers his grace on the aspirant, which destroys all his inner darkness. *Bhakti* develops in such a devotee towards the highest person, which is valued for its own sake, which is uninterrupted, which is an absolute delight in itself and which is meditation that has taken on the character of the most vivid and immediate vision. Through such *bhakti* is the Supreme attained. ①

Thus *bhakti* is conceived as both a means and an end. It is the means of attaining the supreme person, but once the goal is attained *bhakti* is not given up, for it is the very principle of exchange which constitutes the relationship of *bhagavān* and the *jīva*. Viewed from this perspective, *bhakti* is recognized to be the fundamental modality of transcendent living which alone insures unmediated experience of God's presence. The *Nārada-bhakti-sūtras*, in the typically terse style of the *sūtra*-genre of Sanskrit literature, state, "When one attains this love in *bhakti*, one sees only God, one hears only

---

① Klaus K. Klostermaier, *Mythologies and Philosophies of Salvation in the Theistic Traditions of India*, Canadian Corporation for Studies in Religion, (Waterloo, Ontario: Wilfred Laurier University Press, 1984), 105. Translation of *Vedārthasaṁgraha* by S. S. Raghavachar.

God, one knows only God."[1] It is at this stage that the *accessibility* of God is experienced fully, so that his majestic quality fades to insignificance, giving way to a sense of intimacy. This topic will be treated in more detail in a later section. For now we need simply to note the Vaiṣṇava claim that it is when *bhakti* fully develops and is comprehended as an end in itself that the qualification is reached whereby the presence of God can be properly appreciated and fully experienced—whether as *avatāra* appearing for a particular function, or as *antaryāmin* (the "dweller in the heart"), or as *arcāvatāra* (the consecrated image).

Ⅱ. 3. 2 Sound and Form as Media of Exchange

The stage of *śuddha-bhakti*, or pure devotion, is also the stage at which one is said to comprehend "non-material"[2] sound and form. Classical *advaita* (monistic) *vedānta* sees all sound and form as manifestations of *māyā* (illusion) and *saṁsāra* (the phenomenal world), to be meditated upon by various techniques called *upāsanās*, or "means of approach," in order to ultimately go beyond sound and form. Since sound and form are the objects of the senses, whose activities (*karma*) must cease in order to allow one to gain gnosis (*jñāna*), an aspirant of gnosis must withdraw attention

---

① *Nārada-bhakti-sūtras*, Sūtra 55. *tat prāpya tad-evāvalokayati tad-eva śṛṇoti tad-eva cintayati.* Graham Schweig, trans., "The Bhakti Sūtras of Nārada: The Concise Teachings of Nārada on the Nature and Experience of Devotion." in *Journal of Vaiṣṇava Studies* vol. 6 no. 1 (Winter 1998), 148.

② William H. Deadwyler, "The Devotee and the Deity: Living a Personalistic Theology," in *Gods of Flesh, Gods of Stone: The Embodiment of Divinity in India.* Joanne Punzo Waghorne and Norman Cutler, eds. (New York: Columbia University Press, 1996), 79. Deadwyler faults the *advaita* philosophy for assuming an equation 'form=material', noting that 'formless' must also be a material idea, interdependent with the idea of 'form.' 'Spiritual form', or 'non-material form' is for the *bhakta* not an oxymoron, for *saguṇa-brahman*, the Absolute with qualities, is not, as *advaita* doctrine has it, in any way inferior to *nirguṇa-brahman*, the Absolute conceived without qualities (which the Vaiṣṇavas interpret as "without *material* qualities").

from them. Since such cessation of sense activity is extremely difficult, the *upāsanās* are offered as transitional practices to perfection.

In contrast to *advaita-vedānta*, and like other theistic schools of India, Vaiṣṇavism gives central ontological significance to divine sound and form, as direct revelations from God. Perhaps more than other schools of Vaiṣṇavism, the Gauḍīya-Vaiṣṇavas emphasize the notion of revealed *nāma*, or divine name, as a type of "*avatāra*" by which God becomes most accessible, especially in this present age. ① Krishnadās Kavirāja quotes Śrī Caitanya as saying,

> In this Age of Kali, the holy name of the Lord, the Hare Krishna mahā-mantra, is the incarnation [*avatāra*] of Lord Krishna. Simply by chanting the holy name, one associates with the Lord directly. Anyone who does this is certainly delivered. ②

He goes on to contrast ordinary and divine name, form, and personality:

> The Lord's holy name, his form and his personality are all one and the same. There is no difference (*bheda nāhi*) [no non-

---

① Paurāṇic literature divides cosmic time into repeating cycles of four *yugas*, according to which we are presently (and for the next 428, 000 years) in the Kali-yuga, a time of degradation in which most of us have little or no inclination or capacity for spiritual cultivation. For Gauḍīya-Vaiṣṇavas chanting the Hare Kṛṣṇa *mahā-mantra* (*harināma-kīrtana*) is central to the practice of *bhakti* especially in the form of loud chanting in groups (*harināma-saṁkīrtana*) . (Beck, in *Vaiṣṇavism*, 275) .

② *kali-kale nāma-rūpe kṛṣṇa-avatāra /nāma haite haya sarva-jagat-nistāra.* (*Caitanya-caritāmṛta*, Ādi-līlā 17. 22)

identity] between them. Since all of them are absolute, [1] they are transcendentally blissful. There is no difference [distinction, basis for distinction] between Krishna's body and himself or between his name and himself. As far as the conditioned soul [*jīva*] is concerned, these are all [categorically] different from each other. One's name is different from one's body, from one's original form and so on. [2]

And then he applies this distinction to the problem of approaching the unlimited supreme with *prakṛta-indriya*, limited material senses (quoting from *Bhakti-rasāmṛta-sindhu* of Rūpa Gosvāmī):

Therefore material senses cannot appreciate Krishna's holy name, form, qualities and pastimes. Yet simply when one eagerly renders service by using one's tongue (*jihva*) [to chant the Lord's holy name and taste the remnants of the Lord's food] and other senses, [because the senses become purified] Krishna himself manifests in the world. [3]

Thus Krishna's descent as *avatāra*, to be comprehended, demands

---

① "Since all of them are absolute" is not, strictly speaking, in the verse, but is explanatory as a gloss on *bheda nāhi* (having no distinction). "Absolute" is often used by Prabhupāda as an English equivalent of "non-dual" (*advaya*), perhaps also to be understood as "irreducible".

② *'nāma', 'vigraha', 'svarūpa' — tina eka-rūpa /tine 'bheda' nāhi, — tina 'cid-ānanda-rūpa'*

deha-dehīra, nāma-nāmīra kṛṣṇe nāhi 'bheda' /jīvera dharma—nāma-deha-svarūpe 'vibheda'

(*Caitanya-caritāmṛta* Madhya-līlā 17. 131-32). I have added words in brackets which I think aid the understanding of this translation.

③ *ataḥ śrī-kṛṣṇa-nāmādi na bhaved grāhyam indriyaiḥ*

sevonmukhe hi jihvādau svayam eva sphuraty adaḥ (quoted in *Caitanya-caritāmṛta* Madhya-līlā 17. 136)

response from the *jīva* by activation of the sense organs. To the argument of the *advaitin* (monist) that this means undertaking *karma*, by which the *jīva* becomes further implicated in illusory existence, Vaiṣṇavas would answer that this type of sense activity, even if appearing to be *karma*, is in fact *bhakti*, which has the effect of freeing one from bondage. It is stated in the *Bhagavad-gītā* (9. 28) immediately following the statement I have previously quoted (see Section Ⅱ. 2. 1):

> In this way [by dedicating activities to me, the Lord] you will be freed from bondage to work (*karma-bandha*) and its auspicious and inauspicious results. With your mind fixed on me in this principle of renunciation, you will be liberated and come to me.

As we have discussed previously, in *bhakti* the senses are employed in service to the "God of the senses," and this becomes the basis of reciprocation with God. By God's grace through the medium of sacred sound in particular, the impure *jīva* can, in a sense, retrace back to the position of purity in which communion with God is possible. Central among the sense organs to be employed in this process of return is the tongue, with its double function of articulating language and tasting edibles.

Pañcarātra literature developed an elaborate theology of sacred language interrelating it with cosmogonic and salvific activities of God.[①] This involved a relationship between sound and form much as formulated in earlier speculations. Sanjukta Gupta explains:

> Already, in the early *Upaniṣads*, the world is said to consist

---

① Gupta, 225. Prior to and contemporary with Pañcarātra literature was already considerable linguistic speculation within other schools, especially by the Mimāṁsakas and the Grammarians. But already in the Ṛg Veda hymns there is discussion of divine speech, or Vāc.

of names (*nāma*) and forms (*rūpa*). In systematic philosophy, this same relation becomes that between word (*śabda*) and referent (*artha*). In Pāñcarātra theology, as in all tantric theology, this relation is applied to mantras and their deities: a *mantra* designates a deity. ①

The relation between *mantra*, or potent utterance, and the divinity it designates came to be understood increasingly in terms of *bhakti* in later Pañcarātra literature and practice, wherein the *mantra* is a manifestation of the *anugraha*, or favor of God. In earlier Pañcarātra texts the faithful utterance of the *mantra* received from one's *guru* was understood more as a means to gain power and identity with the referent deity of the *mantra*. The emphasis was on personal effort and meditation, following yogic tradition. In the later formulations *mantras* become embodiments of God's favor, means of attaining communion with God by his grace, which is an emotional experience rather than a meditative one. The earlier and later conceptions were quite disparate, yet a reconciliation was found in the practice of Pañcarātric *upāsanā*, or meditation combined with worship, in which equal importance was placed on the use of *mantra* and the worship of a physical image. ②

The Gauḍīya-Vaiṣṇavas give central importance to *mantra* recitation as the means by which the tongue's ability to articulate language is engaged for God's service. While there are several *mantras* from both Vedic and Pāñcaratric sources used in the daily worship of images, the Gauḍīya-Vaiṣṇava tradition, following the teaching and example of Caitanya, has put greatest emphasis on the so-called *mahā-mantra*, or primary *mantra*. This *mantra* uses three divine names (*hare*, *krishna*, and *rāma*) repeated in different combinations, all in the vocative grammatical case (unlike

---

① Gupta, 230.

② Gupta, 231.

most *mantras* which refer to the divinity worshipped in the dative case). [①] There is considerable literature within the Gauḍīya-Vaiṣṇava corpus dealing with the significance, way of practice, obstacles to avoid in the practice, and transformative results of the devotional chanting of the *mahā-mantra*, including Krishnadās Kavirāja's biography of Caitanya, the *Caitanya-caritāmṛta*. There he describes how Caitanya demonstrated the integration of image worship and the chanting of the *hare krishna mahā-mantra* during the latter part of his life (until 1533) when he resided as a renunciant (*sannyāsī*) in Jagannātha Pūrī, on the central east coast of India. The followers of Caitanya enjoyed a daily festival in the massive temple of Jagannātha, the "Lord of the universe," with Caitanya leading them in loud chanting of the *mahā-mantra* and exuberant dancing before the smiling images of Jagannātha and his associates.

This ancient temple [②] is the shrine of four large wooden images collectively known as Jagannātha, but individually as Jagannātha, Subhadrā, Baladeva, and Sudārśaṇa—considered by the Gauḍīya-Vaiṣṇavas to be special forms of Krishna, Krishna's sister Subhadrā, their older brother Baladeva or Balarāma, and Krishna's fiery disc weapon. Here Caitanya demonstrated *harināma-saṁkīrtana*, or the congregational glorification of God by his divine names, indicating that this is the most simple and

---

① This is the well known *hare krishna hare krishna krishna krishna hare hare*, *hare rāma hare rāma rāma rāma hare hare*. "*hare*" is the vocative for both "*harī*" and "*harā*", the former a name for *bhagavān*, the latter a name for the feminine *śakti* of *bhagavān*.

② The present temple was probably constructed in the twelth century CE., however any number of speculations abound regarding its origins along with the origins and significance of the cult of Jagannatha. Legends regarding both the images and the temple abound in Pauraṇic and other literature. These images are striking for their unusual, semi-iconic appearance, explained as being the result of royal devotional impatience to see the carving work in progress, thus breaking a promise to leave the artist undisturbed. God then communicates that this 'unfinished' form is in fact complete, his desire all along being to receive worship in this particular form. Gopinath Mohapatra, *Jagannātha in History & Religious Traditions of Orissa*, Orissan Studies Project No. 13, (Calcutta: Punthi Pustak, 1982), 45, 380-82).

efficacious means of approaching and pleasing God. For Caitanya's followers it became clear that all the regulations governing ritual worship of God were to be subordinated to a primary rule with two aspects, namely to "always remember the Lord and never forget him."① They were also convinced by Caitanya's ecstatic② behavior that the temple images were to be worshipped as direct manifestations of God. The *Caitanya-caritāmṛta* reports incidents in which the devotees experienced some reciprocation with the images, confirming for them the reality of divine presence in these forms.

An important way in which the followers of Caitanya would experience the presence of the deity in Jagannātha was through the tasting of his *prasāda*, or remnants of food ritually offered to him. One of the special features of this particular temple even today is the centuries-old tradition

---

① *smartavyaḥ satatam viṣṇor vismartavyaḥ na jātucit.* (*Padma-purāṇa*, quoted in *Caitanya-caritāmṛta* Madhya 22. 113)

② About the word "ecstasy" I have noted elsewhere: "To explore the relationship between devotional ecstasy and yogic 'enstasy' it behooves us to consider also the relationship of the former with shamanic ecstasy. Mircea Eliade, in his discussions on the relation of shamanism and Yoga, compares the ecstasy of the shaman with the 'enstasy' of the *yogin*. While the former is characterized by a 'desperate effort to attain the *condition of the spirit* to accomplish ecstatic flight,' the latter is characterized by 'perfect autonomy,' or withdrawal within to a state of liberation, as a *jivan-mukta*, or a soul liberated in this life. See Mircea Eliade, *Yoga: Immortality and Freedom*, (Princeton, NJ: Princeton University Press, 1969), 339-340. As one might expect, a sharp contrast between shamanic ecstasy and devotional ecstasy also exists, as June McDaniel has noted in her book *The Madness of the Saints: Ecstatic Religion in Bengal*, (Chicago: University of Chicago Press, 1997). Referring to Mircea Eliade's etymology of ecstasy, namely 'to stand outside' or 'to be outside,' she emphasizes that devotional ecstasy is 'a radical alteration of perception, emotion, or personality which brings the person closer to what he regards as the sacred. . . The ecstatic often passes through a stage of disintegration, but ultimately experiences an integration that brings parts of the self, or the self and the Divine, into a closer relationship or union' (McDaniel, 2). Whereas ecstasy of the shaman 'manifests the separation of the soul' and thus 'anticipates the experience of death,' that of the *bhakta* involves a supra-consciousness in which all the senses are surcharged or infused with awareness of the worshipable object, God." Kenneth R. Valpey, "Arcana: Der Yoga der Gauḍīya Vaiṣṇavas," *Tattva-viveka* (German) Nummer 5 (Oktober 1996), 8-9.

of offering enormous quantities of cooked food prepared by *brāhmaṇas* according to exacting regulations and following recipes said to be unchanged since the temple's beginning. The daily *saṁkīrtana* festivals of Caitanya would always culminate in a communal feast consisting of such offerings, in which Caitanya would encourage his followers to eat "up to the neck" (*ākaṇṭha*). ① Thus in the Gauḍīya-Vaiṣṇava tradition the second function of the tongue, namely tasting, is considered an essential—indeed joyful—means of practicing *bhakti*, through food exchange. As noted earlier, in the *Bhagavad-gītā* God promises to accept offerings of food which are given with devotion. Although no physical transformation may be evident, the devotees are confident that the accepted offering has been relished by God, and that what remains on the offering plates has become infused by his sanctifying glance to make its eating a transformative, liberating experience. The *Bhagavad-gītā* (3. 13) also speaks of this:

> The devotees of the Lord are released from all kinds of sins because they eat food which is offered first for sacrifice. Others, who prepare food for personal sense enjoyment, verily eat only sin. ②

Food exchange among the practitioners completes the exchange between one practitioner and God. In his book *Upadeśāmṛta* ("Nectar of Instruction"), Rūpa Gosvāmī includes the giving and receiving of food among six forms of loving exchange among devotees of God. ③

The climax of these interactions with Jagannātha as demonstrated by

---

① *Caitanya-caritāmṛta* Madhya-līlā 14. 23-46

② *yajña-śiṣṭāśinaḥ santo mucyante sarva-kilbiñaiḥ*
bhuñjate te tv aghaṁ pāpā ye pacanty ātma-kāraṇāt (*Bhagavad-gītā* 3. 13).

③ The other four are giving and receiving gifts, and speaking and enquiring confidentially. (*Nectar of Instruction* [*Upadeśāmṛta*] 4).

Caitanya were experienced during the annual *Rathayātrā*, when the four images were taken on procession in three towering wooden carriages along the main road of the city.[①] This festival, which even today draws three-to five-hundred thousand pilgrims, took on an esoteric significance for Caitanya and his followers, the explanation of which brings us back to our earlier mention of Vraja, the land identified as Krishna's childhood residence and place of intimate *līlā* with his friends and family members. In Caitanya's ecstatic identification of himself as Krishna's consort Rādhā, his effort to draw the carriage of Jagannātha becomes a re-enactment of Rādhā's effort to bring Krishna back to Vraja some years after his departure to Mathurā, as described in the *Śrīmad-Bhāgavatam.*

In the detailed account of this event in *Caitanya-caritāmṛta*, the occasional inability of the devotees to keep Jagannātha's carriage moving is interpreted as Jagannātha's refusal to move until coaxed by Caitanya, who miraculously[②] brings the massive vehicle into motion single-handedly. For the Gauḍīya-Vaiṣṇavas, this event demonstrates the primacy of *rasa*, or aesthetic-emotional mode of reciprocation, as the substance which sustains the relationship between God and his devotee. Whereas *arcanam* as a practice of *bhakti* is governed largely by rules related to exoteric behavior, the goal (*prayojana*) toward which this behavior is aimed is an essential component

---

① From this event has come the English word juggernaut. Webster defines it thus: "1. Any large, overpowering, destructive object; 2. Anything requiring blind devotion or cruel sacrifice; 3. an idol of Krishna at Puri in Orissa, annually drawn on a huge cart under whose wheels devotees are said to have thrown themselves to be crushed."

② The concept of miracles in relation to images is explored in Richard Davis's collection of articles, *Images, Miracles, and Authority in Asian Religious Traditions* (Boulder, CO: Westview Press, 1998). One article by Robert Brown discusses "expected miracles" which is suggestive of what may have taken place in the account of Caitanya in the Rathayātrā festival. For our purposes in this book we may tentatively accept the Oxford Unabridged Dictionary definition of Miracle: "A marvellous event occurring within human experience which cannot have been brought about by human power or by the operation of any natural agency, and must therefore be ascribed to the special intervention of the Deity or of some supernatural being."

of our understanding of image worship in the Gauḍīya-Vaiṣṇava tradition. This is the topic of the next chapter, in which aspects of image worship more specific to the Gauḍīya tradition should become more evident.

Chapter Three

Bhakti-Rasa: The Aesthetics of Devotion

When You go off to the forest during the day, a tiny fraction of a second becomes like a millennium for us because we cannot see You. And even when we can eagerly look upon Your beautiful face, so lovely with its adornment of curly locks, our pleasure is hindered by our eyelids, which were fashioned by the foolish creator.

—Śrīmad-Bhāgavatam10. 31. 15 ①

Ⅲ. 1 Krishna-śakti Revisited

We have been discussing the mode of *bhakti* known as *arcanam* as the formal offering of worship by the *bhakta*, or devotee, to *bhagavān*, the supreme person. In the Gauḍīya-Vaiṣṇava tradition, however, Krishna is not worshipped alone, but rather with Rādhā, who is considered to be *pūrṇa-śakti*, or the full complementary embodiment of the "energy" of Krishna, who is *pūrṇa-śaktimān*, the full possessor of infinite divine energies. Kapoor explains Rādhā this way:

---

① *aṭati yad bhavān ahni kānanaṁ /truṭi yugāyate tvām apaśyatām kuṭila-kuntalaṁ śrī-mukhaṁ ca te /jaḍa udīkṣatāṁ pakṣma-kṛd dṛśām*

Śrī Krishna is the ultimate source of the infinite [in number] partial manifestations of the divine personality, and Rādhā is the ultimate source of the endless divine energies of Śrī Krishna. The relationship between Krishna and Rādhā is that of inconceivable identity and difference. They are, in essence, one and the same entity, which assumes two different forms to enjoy the bliss of divine sports. Rādhā is one with Krishna, as she is identical with the highest development of the Hlādinī-śakti [energy of bliss] of Krishna. But she is different from him, because she is the predominated moiety [*prakṛti*], while Śrī Krishna is the predominating moiety [*puruṣa*] of the absolute. It is on account of this distinction that Śrī Krishna in his intrinsic selfhood appears in the form of a male, while Rādhā appears in the form of a female. The relationship between them must not, however, be likened to the physical relationship between a male and a female on the mundane plane. The body of Rādhā, like that of Krishna, is made of bliss [*ānanda*] and consciousness [*cit*] and the love between the two is spiritual. ①

As Krishna expands into various *avatāras* (which are generally "male"), *Rādhā* expands into countless female assistants, as *gopīs*, or milkmaids, who

---

① Kapoor, 98. Another explanation of Rādhā's identity given by A. K. Majumdar may be helpful: "Rādhā is Kṛṣṇa's *hlādinī-śakti*, but she is neither a part nor even the representation of the *śakti*; she is the *śakti* herself in its fullest amplitude. Rādhā is the *pūrṇa-śaktī*. . . Rādhā is the realization of the principal emotion being the concretized form of the ideal *hlādinī-śakti* (the energy of bliss), indeed its substratum (*sāra*), in whom the cognizable properties or qualities or attributes or accidents of things have been conceived as inhering in or affecting the essential nature underlying the phenomenon of *mādhurya-rasa*. . . . In the *rasa-maṇḍala* [*rasa*-dance arena]. . . the dance of duality ends in ultimate unity. . . From this unity of Rādhā-Kṛṣṇa emerges the ultimate *rasa*: *raso vai sa*. . . 'He indeed is *rasa*' [*Taittirīya-upaniṣad*]. By himself, Kṛṣṇa is *advaya-jñāna-tattva* [the truth of non-dual gnosis], with Rādhā He is *advaya-rasa-tattva* [the truth of non-dual taste, or feeling]."

assist Rādhā in pleasing Krishna in the land of Vraja by participating in his amorous pastimes (*līlā*). But there are other types of assistants to Krishna in Vraja who, though not seen as expansions of Rādhā, are nevertheless manifestations of Krishna's *hlādinī-śakti* inasmuch as they eternally associate with him for the sole purpose of assisting in his pastimes. These devotees may act as friends and relatives of Krishna, but also as animals (especially cows, monkeys, peacocks and parrots), or even as inanimate plants and trees—each effectively contributing to the ever-increasing pleasure of God.

Each of the associates of Krishna relate to him exclusively in terms of *bhakti*, in accordance with his or her particular *rasa*, or relationship of taste or feeling with him. Just how Krishna is identified as the reservoir of types of relationships is illustrated in a famous passage in the Śrīmad-Bhāgavatam, which describes Krishna after he has left Vṛndāvana to confront and finally kill Kaṁsa, the demonic king of Mathurā:

> The various groups of people in the arena regarded Krishna in different ways when He entered it with His elder brother. The wrestlers saw Krishna as a lightning bolt, the men of Mathurā as the best of males, the women as Cupid in person, the cowherd men as their relative, the impious rulers as a chastiser, his parents as their child, the King of the Bhojas as death, the unintelligent as the Supreme Lord's universal form, the yogīs as the Absolute Truth and the Vṛṣṇis [Krishna's clan] as their supreme worshipable deity. ①
> (*Bhāg*. 10. 43. 17).

One of the early commentators on the *Bhāgavatam*, Śrīdhara Svāmī (14th

---

① *mallānām aśanir nṛṇāṁ nara-varaḥ strīṇāṁ smaro mūrtimān*
gopānāṁ sva-jano 'satāṁ kṣiti-bhujāṁ śāstā sva-pitroḥ śiśuḥ
mṛtyur bhoja-pater virāḍ aviduṣāṁ tattvaṁ paraṁ yogināṁ
vṛṣṇīnāṁ para-devateti vidito raṅgaṁ gataḥ sāgrajaḥ

to 15th centuries), identifies ten *rasas* or types of relationship represented in this passage. Later, Rūpa Gosvāmī systematized the Gauḍīya-Vaiṣṇava *rasa*-theology in his *Bhakti-rasāmṛta-sindhu* and *Ujjvala-nilāmaṇī*, listing twelve *rasas*, of which seven are minor and five are major.① Central to his *rasa*-doctrine is that Krishna is *akhila-rasāmṛta-mūrti*, the very embodiment of the nectar of all *rasa*. Of all possible divinities or semi-divinities② one might choose to evaluate, none match Krishna for his capacity to elicit the emotions of *rasa* to such extent, depth, and sublimity. More importantly, none but Krishna exhibits the *mādhurya-rasa* (conjugal attraction) in any way comparable to him, for this is the *ādi-rasa*, the original or most fundamental *rasa*, to which the other *rasas* are related, or from which they derive their

---

① The seven minor *rasas* are: anger (*raudra*); wonder (*adbhūta*); humor (*hasya*); chivalry (*vīrya*); pity or mercy (*dayā*); fear (*bhayanaka*); horror or ghastliness (*bibhatsa*). The five major *rasas* are: peacefulness (*śānta*); servitude (*dāsya*); friendship (*śakhya*); parenthood (*vatsalya*); and conjugal attraction (*mādhurya* or *śringāra*). Rūpa is noted for systematically combining traditional Indian aesthetics with theology, though before him and before Caitanya some thought and writing went in this direction. Klaus Klostermaier writes: "References to the ontology of beauty, the grounding of feeling in an ultimate reality, were not absent in the literature that developed the *rasa*-theory. To that extent Caitanya's religion of feeling had strong roots in contemporary culture. Equally, the celebration of love between man and woman, based on the attraction of the body as much as on the merging of the souls, its projection unto the divine couple of Rādhā and Krishna, all this was present before Caitanya appeared on the scene. "Klaus K. Klostermaier, "A Universe of Feelings," in *Shri Krishna Caitanya and the Bhakti Religion*, Studia Irenica 33, Edmund Weber and Tilak Raj Chopra, eds. (Frankfurt am Main: Peter Lang, 1988), 115.

② *Devas* or *devatās*, numbering up to thirty-three million in Vedic /Paurāṇic literature, are classified in Gauḍīya-Vaiṣṇava theology as *jīva-tattva*, or of the same ontological status as human beings, animals, and plants. By piety they have gained status which is "divine" only insofar as it is markedly above human qualifications. However such status is temporary, and like any *jīvātmā*, the *devatās* are subject to death.

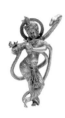

significance.[1] But Krishna's pre-eminence is as it should be, recalling that Krishna is not just one among the many *avatāras*, but the very reservoir of all *avatāras*, or *avatārin*. Even that he is the source of the created universe is secondary[2] to the fact that he is the source of the "universe of feelings," as Klaus Klostermaier expresses it,[3] a universe which has as its purpose the perpetuation of a symphony of *rasa* in which every living being participates in eternity with the Personality of *rasa*. It is *rasa* which distinguishes Krishna from and above even Viṣṇu:

> Even though there is no difference between the true natures of the Lord of Śrī [Viṣṇu] and Krishna (according to established dogma), the true nature of Krishna is made more excellent by *rasa*. This is the position of *rasa* (*BRS* 1. 2. 59).[4]

Because *rasa* necessarily involves relationship, the devotee of Krishna wants to worship him not as *advaya-jñāna-tattva*, the "truth of non-dual gnosis," but rather as *advaya-rasa-tattva*, the "truth of non-dual feeling."For the Gauḍīya-Vaiṣṇavas especially this means to worship Krishna together with Rādhā.

The worship of male divinities together with their female counterparts or

---

[1] Indian aestheticians traditionally argued for either peacefulness (*śānta-rasa*) or pity / compassion (*dayā* or *karuṇā*) as the axial emotion. Gauḍīya Vaiṣṇava focus on *mādhurya-rasa* is concomitant with the doctrine that in relation to Kṛṣṇa it comprehends the most perfect expression of love, the inverse of worldly conjugality which is characterized by lust.

[2] The subordinate value placed on the material creation is further underlined by identifying Kṛṣṇa as the source of the *puruṣa-avatāras*—the forms of Viṣṇu considered the creators of the external world

[3] Klostermaier, "A Universe of Feelings", 113.

[4] Neal Delmonico, "Rādhā: The Quintessential Gopī," *Journal of Vaiṣṇava Studies* vol. 5 no. 4 (Fall 1997), 117.

consorts has a long history in India.[①] In the Śrī-Vaiṣṇava tradition of south India, following Pañcarātra texts, Krishna is worshipped mainly as Viṣṇu or Nārāyaṇa together with his consort Lakṣmī or Śrī. The relationship between Lakṣmī and Viṣṇu is considered to be that of a married couple, or *svakīya-rasa*, in contrast to the relationship between Rādhā and Krishna, which *seems* to be one of paramourship, or *parakīya-rasa*. In the realm of image worship this became a problematic issue in the eighteenth century for the Gauḍīya-Vaiṣṇavas, whose practice of Rādhā-Krishna worship was severely criticized by another Vaiṣṇava group known as Rāmānandīs.[②] When the issue came to a head in Galta, Rajasthan, a debate was staged between the Gauḍīya-Vaiṣṇava scholar Baladeva Vidyābhuṣaṇa and Rāmānandī pundits. The latter had no objection to worshipping Krishna alone, but to worship him together with Rādhā was, they insisted, to condone irreligious behavior. Gauḍīya Vaiṣṇava tradition tells us that the Rāmānandi pundits had to accept defeat by Baladeva, who quoted from his own commentary on the *Brahma-sūtras*.[③] There he argued that the propriety of Rādhā's relationship with Krishna is not an issue, since they are eternally related ontologically as *śakti* and *śaktimān*—as energy and energetic source. If anyone is sanctioned to

---

① See David R. Kinsley, *Hindu Goddesses: Visions of the Divine Feminine in the Hindu Religious Tradition*, (Berkeley: University of California Press, 1988) for an overview of goddesses in relation to gods in Hinduism.

② Rāmānandīs are a north Indian branch of the Śrī-Vaiṣṇavas of south India descending from the fourteenth-century reformer Rāmānanda. See Dayānanda Dāsa, "Baladeva Vidyābhūṣaṇa: The Gauḍīya Vedāntist," *Back to Godhead* (January-February, 1991), 32.

③ Dāsa, Dayananda, 32 (Pt. Ⅱ). Their source for this tradition is a Bengali work, *Śrī Śrī Gauḍīya Vaiṣṇava Abhidhāna*, Śrī Haridās Dās, Haribol Kutir, Śrī Dhāma Navadvīpa, 1955. It would of course be interesting to know what the Rāmānandī tradition has to say about the incident. Practically nothing is written about the history of Rādhā's appearance next to Kṛṣṇa in Gauḍīya-Vaiṣṇava temples (or of other sects, especially the followers of Nimbarka). S. K. De notes that there is no mention of Rādhā in the *Hari-bhakti-vilāsa* of Gopāla Bhaṭṭa Gosvāmī. The ritual worship of Rādhā with Kṛṣṇa apparently developed after the sixteenth century. De, 508.

associate with Krishna, it is Rādhā, for she is the divine heroine of a divine *drama*, the ultimate model of devotion to God, and hence the embodiment of perfect chastity. That Rādhā and Krishna's relationship *appears* to be illicit simply heightens the romantic element of the drama, inviting the worshiper to abandon the distractions of this world to enter into the transcendent realm of rich and exciting transcendent *rasa*. [1]

Ⅲ. 2 Vraja, Land of Sweetness

In section I. 4 I have briefly mentioned Vraja, the land of Krishna's childhood and youth, as the arena where Krishna's concreteness together with his essential feature of sweetness are demonstrated. Sweetness and concreteness combine in Vraja to make Krishna—or more precisely the divine couple Rādhā-Krishna—the accessible recipient of informal devotion, in contrast to the more formal worship afforded to the Lord of the universe, Viṣṇu or Nārāyaṇa (and his feminine counterpart, Lakṣmī or Śrī). If Krishna is the embodiment of *rasa*, he is also the embodiment of *līlā*, the full meaning of which is demonstrated most fully by Krishna in Vraja. David Kinsley remarks,

> In Vṛndāvana [Vraja] Krishna is removed from the ordinary world and the necessity of acting according to pragmatic considerations. In Vṛndāvana he need not play a role but is free to express his essential nature in every action. In the cowherd village,

---

[1] Scholars argue that the doctrine of unmarried love between Kṛṣṇa and the *gopīs* did not prevail until some time after the Six Gosvāmīs. Jīva Gosvāmī presents a case for married love (*svakīya-rasa*) between them, based on inferences from scripture, and also from *rasa-śāstra*, or standard texts of aesthetics, which he says disapprove of illicit conjugal affairs. (De, 348-349). See also Jan Brzezinski, "Does Kṛṣṇa Marry the Gopīs in the End?" *Journal of Vaiṣṇava Studies* vol. 5 no. 4 (Fall 1997).

removed from the world of his mission as an *avatāra*, there are no inhibitions to acting freely. Vṛndāvana is a playground, a magic place, where Krishna can revel freely and continually as a playful child. ①

Certainly there is an element of aimlessness in Krishna's Vraja pastimes, in the sense that they are not part of the realm of mundane necessity or pragmatic purpose. ② But in Gauḍīya-Vaiṣṇava theology, for all the apparent lack of purpose there is a deeper purpose in this play, which is to draw the bound *jīvas* out of their stupefaction typified by striving for worldly accomplishment. According to the *Bhāgavatam*, the basis of increasing worldly inebriation is aspiration after aristocratic birth (*janma*), wealth (*aiśvarya*), learning (*śruta*), and bodily beauty (*śrī*). To remove these aspirations by the spell of his own transcendent charms, Krishna displays his beautiful form (*mādhurya-rūpa*) in Vraja, the particular place which is so enchanting because it is itself a display of Krishna's beauty and charm. In facetious words Rūpa Gosvāmī warns his readers,

> My dear friend, if you are indeed attached to your worldly friends, do not look at the smiling face of Lord Govinda [Krishna] as He stands on the bank of the Yamunā [River] at Keśīghāṭa [a particular place for bathing, in Vṛndāvana]. Casting sidelong glances, He places His flute to His lips, which seem like newly blossomed twigs. His transcendental body, bending in three

---

① David R. Kinsley, *The Sword and the Flute: Kālī and Kṛṣṇa—Dark Visions of the Terrible and the Sublime in Hindu Mythology*, (Berkeley: University of California Press, 1975), 76.

② A useful exploration of the varied meanings of the word *līlā* and a related term *krīḍā* in Vaiṣṇavism is offered by Clifford Hospital in his article "Līlā in Early Vaiṣṇava Thought," in *Gods at Play: Līlā in South Asia*, William S. Sax, ed. (New York: Oxford University Press, 1995).

places, appears very bright in the moonlight. ①

Thus Krishna's beauty in Vraja poses a threat to one's status quo of mundane preoccupations, which cannot be mixed with Krishna-*bhakti-rasa*. If one wants to perpetuate those preoccupations (and thus the sufferings of *saṁsāra*—repeated birth, death, old age and disease), one should stay clear of Vraja. Vraja is a dramatic stage which, if one enters, one will become transformed by, as one is transported to the spiritual realm of perpetual, unpredictable love. John Stratton Hawley highlights this quality of Vraja, contrasting it with other holy places of pilgrimage in India, known as *tīrthas*, or "places of crossing over":

> As a song often sung in the *rāsa līlā* [folk dramas staged around Vraja] says, its [Vṛndāvana's] streets swirl with the floods of love: no order there. And once the unwary traveler is caught in the tide, there is no hope of escape. Safe passage is hardly what one expects at Vrindavan. One comes not to cross [as at a *tīrtha*] but to drown, to drown in love's uncharted sea, and to find in that drowning a tranquillity unknown on dry land. ②

Krishna-*bhaktas* aspire to "drown in love's uncharted sea" by residing, at least for some time, in Vraja. Rūpa Gosvāmī counts living in Vraja as one of five main principles among the sixty-four practices of *vaidhi-sādhana-bhakti*. By residing there, the benefits from observing so many regulations

---

① *smerāṁ bhaṅgī-traya-paricitāṁ sāci-vistīrṇa-dṛṣṭiṁ*
vaṁśī-nyastādhara-kiśalayām ujjvalāṁ candrakeṇa
govindākhyāṁ hari-tanum itaḥ keśī-tīrthopakaṇṭhe
mā prekṣiṣṭhās tava yadi sakhe bandhu-saṅge'sti raṅgaḥ (*Bhakti-rasāmṛta-sindhu* 1. 2. 239, quoted in *Caitanya-caritāmṛta* Ādi-līlā 5. 224).

② John Stratton Hawley, *At Play with Krishna: Pilgrimage Dramas from Brindavan*. (Princeton, NJ: Princeton University Press, 1981), 51.

of service will be multiplied by the attractive force of Krishna's felt presence not only in an image housed in a temple, but in the countless places of Vraja associated with his pastimes. And equally or even more important, one will be blessed by Rādhā, known in Vraja as "Vṛndāvaneśvarī," the presiding goddess of Vṛndāvana, to participate in the divine play, in service to the all-attractive Krishna.

But most persons will not have opportunity to reside in Vraja; for them pilgrimage to and around Vraja is the means of entering into the transcendent realm of Vraja, to be transformed at least for some time into a participant in Krishna's *līlā*. Since the sixteenth century Vraja has been a center of pilgrimage with presently more visitors per year than the Taj Mahal. ① People come there as lone travelers, as families, and in organized groups numbering hundreds and even thousands, to circumambulate (*parikramaṇa*) the town of Vṛndāvana (a four-mile walk), or Govardhana Hill ② (a fourteen-mile walk), or the whole of Vraja (some two-hundred-mile-walk, camping en route). Nowhere on these routes can one go without encountering temples of Krishna, each in a particular place associated with a particular *līlā* of Krishna as described either in canonical scripture or from local tradition. As one progresses (if done "properly," then barefoot, out of respect for the sacred land), one "has *darśana*," or receives a blessed viewing, of one after another of the images of Krishna. And as one thus gains the vision of Krishna, nurtured by the devotional hearing of his *līlā*, the mundane self-

---

① David L. Haberman, *Acting as a Way of Salvation: A Study of Rāgānugā Bhakti Sādhana*, (New York: Oxford University Press, 1988), 193 (fn. 55).

② Govardhana is a very sacred hill in Vraja, said to have been lifted and held like an umbrella by Kṛṣṇa for seven days and nights to protect the residents of Vṛndāvana from the wrath of Indra and his pouring rain.

conceptions [1] (or rather misconceptions) by which one lives in alienation from God become undermined. The senses become "Krishna-ized," or immersed in the experience of Krishna's presence in all the objects of the senses, and it becomes possible to comprehend the transcendent nature of Krishna's name, form, qualities, pastimes, and abode. On this platform of consciousness, the limitations of time and space give way to the ocean of *bhāva*, or transcendent emotion.

Ⅲ. 3 Complementary Paths to Perfection: Bhāgavata-mārga and Pāñcarātrika-mārga

Gauḍīya-Vaiṣṇavas worship images of Rādhā-Krishna, but they do so thinking of themselves as servants of Śrī Caitanya, whom they identify as none other than the "combined form" of Rādhā and Krishna. As accessible as Krishna makes himself, most of the bound *jīvas* of this age of Kali, a cosmic period of spiritual degeneracy, fail to appreciate him and direct their devotion to him. Therefore, Krishnadās Kavirāja tells us, Krishna makes a

① As Steven Gelberg points out, anthropologist Victor Turner calls our attention to the common theme in pilgrimage experience in terms of social marginality, liminality, and consequent experience of *communitas*. Gelberg notes, "Pilgrimage to Vrindaban (and, more so, residence there) is nothing if not a radically liminal experience. More than a vacation from society, it is a vacation from the world itself." Steven J. Gelberg, "Vrindaban as Locus of Mystical Experience," *Journal of Vaiṣṇava Studies* vol. 1 No. 1 (Fall 1992), 23. David Haberman critiques Turner's ideas on pilgrimage in his book *Journey Through the Twelve Forests: An Encounter with Krishna*, (New York: Oxford University Press, 1994), 69-71, with respect specifically to Vraja-pilgrimage. See also A. W. Entwistle, *Braj, Centre of Krishna Pilgrimage*, (Groningen: Egbert Forsten, 1987), 105-107, on special features of Vraja pilgrimage and resistance to generalized anthropological theorizing. Another interesting if rather "monistic" exploration of pilgrimage in the Indian context is that of E. Valentine Daniel in *Fluid Signs: Being a Person the Tamil Way*, (Berkeley: University of California Press, 1984), Chapter 7. Daniel analyzes it (after undertaking a pilgrimage himself) in terms of Charles S. Peirce's phenomenological categories of "Firstness," "Secondness," and "Thirdness" of experience.

special descent, to make even easier for the *jīvas* the means to approach him. This time, as Śrī Krishna Caitanya Mahāprabhu, he descends "playing the part" of his own *bhakta* in order to demonstrate in all detail the mood and behavior of a Krishna-devotee.

> The loving affairs of Śrī Rādhā and Krishna are transcendental manifestations of the Lord's internal pleasure-giving potency. Although Rādhā and Krishna are one in their identity, they separated themselves eternally. Now these two transcendental identities have again united, in the form of Caitanya. I bow down to him, who has manifested himself with the sentiment and complexion of Śrīmatī Rādhārāṇi although He is Krishna himself. (C. c. ṇdi 1. 5) ①

Thus in Gauḍīya-Vaiṣṇava practice of image worship, at least since the last two centuries or longer, ② Caitanya's image has been generally also worshipped along with images of Rādhā and Krishna. But just as often his image will be seen together with that of his closest associate Śrī Nityānanda Prabhu, identified as Balarāma, ③ Krishna's brother in Vṛndāvana-*līlā*. Iconographically, both figures are seen generally with raised arms in

---

① *rādhā kṛṣṇa-praṇaya-vikṛtir hlādinī śaktir asmād*
ekātmānāv api bhuvi purā deha-bhedaṁ gatau tau
caitanyākhyaṁ prakaṭam adhunā tad-dvayaṁ caikyam āptaṁ
rādhā-bhāva-dyuti-suvalitaṁ naumi kṛṣṇa-svarūpam (*Caitanya-caritāmṛta* Ādi-līlā 1. 5)

② As with the history of the worship of images of Rādhā, the history of worship of images of Caitanya is difficult to trace. S. K. De (pp. 227-230) considers the theology of Caitanya/Rādhā-Kṛṣṇa identity a later development, after the writings of the Six Gosvāmīs. However it would not have been very long after, as Kṛṣṇadās Kavirāja, who articulates this doctrine quite extensively in his *Caitanya-caritāmṛta*, apparently had some association with them.

③ *Caitanya-caritāmṛta*, Ādi-līlā 5, *passim.*

dancing pose. The two together are remembered for their missionary spirit of travel and vigorous preaching of Krishna-*bhakti* as portrayed in *Śrīmad-Bhāgavatam*, for their emphasis on *harināma-saṁkīrtana*, or congregational chanting of Krishna's names, and for their ideal example as servants of Krishna's devotees.

In Gauḍīya-Vaiṣṇava theology Caitanya and Nityānanda exemplify that aspect of Krishna-*bhakti* spirituality which emphasizes these last three practices—the study and teaching of *Śrīmad-Bhāgavatam* and related scriptures, the congregational chanting of Krishna's names, and service to Vaiṣṇavas. These practices make up what came to be known as the *bhāgavata-mārga*, literally the "path of the servants of *bhagavān*".[1] Associated with this "path" is also an emphasis on practice of *bhakti* which is inspired by and follows the example of direct associates of Krishna, *rāgānugā-bhakti-sādhana*. Here the emphasis is on spontaneous devotion as opposed to the following of scripturally imposed regulations, but it is nevertheless *sādhana*, or practice. Hence some elements of regulation persist beyond the rule-governed practice of *vaidhi-bhakti-sādhana*.

Complementary to the *bhāgavata-mārga* is the *pañcarātrika-mārga*, characterized by the features of *vaidhi-bhakti-sādhana* which I have already

---

① Historians trace the existence of two more or less distinct cults of Vaiṣṇavism back to early centuries of the Christian era or earlier, one called *Bhāgavatas* and the other called *Pāñcaratras*. According to one scholar, "The main difference between the *Bhāgavatas and the Pañcarātras* seems to lie in the fact that whereas the *Bhāgavata* devotees of Nārāyaṇa had accepted the brāhmaṇical social order, the *Pañcarātras* were indifferent to and were perhaps against it." See Suvira Jaiswal, *The Origin and Development of Vaiṣṇavism: Vaiṣṇavism from 200 BC to AD 500*, (Delhi: Munshiram Manoharlal, 1981), 46. However, in Śaṅkara's commentary on the *Brahmasūtras* he refers to the followers of Pañcarātra texts as Bhāgavatas. See Swami Gambhirananda, trans., *Brahma-Sūtra-Bhāṣya of Śrī Śaṅkarācārya*, (Calcutta: Advaita Ashrama, 1965), Sūtra Ⅱ. ii. 42, 440. In any case, the terms *bhāgavata-mārga* and *pañcarātra-mārga* used here take on a different emphases. As far as my research goes (querying per E-mail a group of scholars of philosophy of Bhakti Yoga), this present usage became especially emphasized by Bhaktisiddhānta Sarasvatī, the prominent Vaiṣṇava scholar of the early part of the twentieth century.

discussed in Chapter Two, especially the practice of regulated worship of the *arcā-vigraha*. Just how these two "paths" are complementary to each other is best understood through devotional narratives such as are found in the *Caitanya-caritāmṛta*, in which incidents involving *bhaktas* recognized as spiritually elevated souls and *mūrtis* of Krishna are described. Also, for the Gauḍīya-Vaiṣṇavas who read or hear these accounts which often contain an element of the "miraculous," these are confirmations of the efficacy of faithful practices of *bhakti* and the reality of God's reciprocating presence in worshipped images.

One example of these narratives may serve to illustrate this sense of complementarity between these two "paths." This story centers around Mādhavendra Purī (ca. 1420–1490), an ascetic highly revered by the Gauḍīya-Vaiṣṇavas as the *guru* of Caitanya's *guru*. Having been ordered in a dream by his Krishna deity in Vraja (named Gopāla) to obtain sandalwood ① in Jagannātha Pūrī, Mādhavendra set out alone to make the long journey. On the way, near his destination, he stopped in Remuṇā where he visited the temple of Gopīnātha (another name of Krishna). While there, it occurred to him that he could do some research on behalf of Gopāla:

> Mādhavendra Purī thought, "I shall inquire from the priest what foods are offered to Gopīnātha so that by making arrangements in our kitchen, we can offer similar foods to Śrī Gopāla." When the brāhmaṇa priest was questioned about this matter, he explained in detail what kinds of food were offered to the Deity of Gopīnātha. The brāhmaṇa priest said,
>
> "In the evening the Deity is offered sweet rice in twelve earthen pots. Because the taste is as good as nectar [*amṛta*], it is named *amṛta-keli*. This sweet rice is celebrated throughout the world

① Sandalwood, when ground to a paste, has a cooling effect when smeared on the body. It is one of the standard items offered to respected persons and images in India.

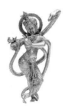

as *gopīnātha-kṣīra.* [1] It is not offered anywhere else in the world."

While Mādhavendra Purī was talking with the brāhmaṇa priest, the sweet rice was placed before the Deity as an offering. Hearing this, Mādhavendra Purī thought as follows.

"If, without my asking, a little sweet rice is given to me, I can then taste it and make a similar preparation to offer my Lord Gopāla."

Mādhavendra Purī became greatly ashamed (*lajjā pāñā*) when he desired to taste the sweet rice, and he immediately began to think of Lord Viṣṇu. While he was thus thinking of Lord Viṣṇu, the offering was completed, and the *ārati* ceremony [2] began. After the *ārati* was finished, Mādhavendra Purī offered his obeisances to the deity and then left the temple. He did not say anything more to anyone.

Mādhavendra Purī avoided begging. He was completely unattached and indifferent to material things. If, without his begging, someone offered him some food, he would eat; otherwise he would fast. A *paramahaṁsa* [3] like Mādhavendra Purī is always satisfied in the loving service of the Lord. Material hunger

---

[1] *Kṣīra* is milk or condensed milk. "Sweetrice" is a favorite sweet preparation consisting of rice cooked slowly in boiled down milk, with sugar. More precisely it would be called *kṣīrānna* (milk and grain/rice), but it is commonly called simply *kṣīra.*

[2] *ārati* or *ārātrika* is a short ceremony of offering various items to the image by waving them in circles while standing and ringing a bell. The main items offered are a lamp (burning camphor or cotton wicks soaked in clarified butter or oil) and a conch shell filled with water. In most temples this ceremony will occur five to eight times in the course of the day, after food has been offered. It is a public event, whereby viewers will either observe silently while offering prayers, or they will sing songs considered appropriate for the particular deity. For an interesting Christian perspective on this ceremony, see Fr. Prasannabhai, "Jesus the Arati Personified—the Eucharist as our Mahā-ārati," *Vidyajyoti Journal of Theological Reflection* no. 60 (1997), 192-199.

[3] *Paramahaṁsa*= "great, swanlike person," an appellative for spiritually advanced ascetics.

and thirst cannot impede his activities. When he desired to taste a little sweet rice offered to the Deity, he considered that he had committed an offense by desiring to eat what was being offered to the Deity. Mādhavendra Purī left the temple and sat down in the village marketplace, which was vacant. Sitting there, he began to chant. In the meantime, the temple priest laid the Deity down to rest. ① Finishing his daily duties, the priest went to take rest. In a dream he saw the Gopīnātha deity come to talk to him, and he [the Lord] spoke as follows.

"O priest, please get up and open the door of the temple. I have kept one pot of sweet rice for the *sannyāsī* (Mādhavendra Purī). This pot of sweet rice is just behind my cloth curtain. You did not see it because of my tricks. A *sannyāsī* named Mādhavendra Purī is sitting in the vacant marketplace. Please take this pot of sweet rice from behind me and deliver it to him."

Awaking from the dream, the priest immediately rose from bed and took a bath before entering the deity's room. He then opened the temple door. According to the deity's directions, the priest found the pot of sweet rice behind the cloth curtain. He removed the pot and mopped up the place where it had been kept. He then went out of the temple. Closing the door of the temple, he went to the village with the pot of sweet rice. He called out in every stall in search of Mādhavendra Purī. Holding the pot of sweet rice, the priest called,

"Will he whose name is Mādhavendra Purī please come and take this pot! Gopīnātha has stolen this pot of sweet rice for you! Please come and take this pot of sweet rice and enjoy the *prasāda*

① *Śayaṇa-sevā*, "resting service": Images are placed in small beds in the evening, unless they are too large and heavy, in which case an *utsava-mūrti*, a smaller, usually metal, version of the main image will be placed in a bed, representing the main image.

> with great happiness! You are the most fortunate person within these three worlds! "[1]
>
> Hearing this invitation, Mādhavendra Purī came out and identified himself. The priest then delivered the pot of sweet rice and offered his obeisances, falling flat before him. When the story about the pot of sweet rice was explained to him in detail, Śrī Mādhavendra Purī at once became absorbed in ecstatic love of Krishna.[2] Upon seeing the ecstatic loving symptoms manifest in Mādhavendra Purī, the priest was struck with wonder. He could understand why Krishna had become so much obliged to him (Mādhavendra), and he saw that Krishna's action was befitting. The priest offered obeisances to Mādhavendra Purī and returned to the temple. Then, in ecstasy, Mādhavendra Purī ate the sweet rice offered to him by Krishna. (C. c. Madhya 4. 115-139)

The narration concludes with the ascetic hastening on his journey to avoid attention from crowds of pious local citizens the next morning.

In this account, a temple priest, attentive to the regulative (*vaidhi-sādhana*) worship of the temple image, wins Krishna's grace in the form of insight into the intimate dealings between God and his spiritually advanced devotee. The ascetic Mādhavendra, with his elevated devotional sensibilities, feels shame for even thinking to taste a food offering to the deity while God was receiving it, even though his thought was not really inappropriate (since his idea was to taste it *after* the completion of the offering). Krishna, usually a seemingly passive recipient of worship and offerings in his *arcā-mūrti*, on this occasion suddenly becomes an active agent "by a trick" (*māyayā*) to assure his devotee that his thought was

---

① "Three worlds" refers to a common Indic cosmogonic conception of earthly, celestial, and intermediary cosmic regions.

② "Absorbed in ecstatic love," *prema-āviṣṭa*: literally "saturated with love."

not offensive. The all-knowing God Gopīnātha (who subsequently becomes famous as Kṣīra-cora-Gopīnātha," "the Lord who stole sweet-rice"), recognizing that Mādhavendra's desire to taste the offering was motivated exclusively by the desire to improve service to himself (Krishna) in his form as Gopāla, turns the situation into an opportunity to act as the servant of his devotee. He breaks the rules, so to speak, as a "thief" to prove that his devotee has not broken any rules but rather has proven the purpose of the rule (that one should not think of enjoying anything unless it has been offered to God for his pleasure). Simultaneously Krishna acts as *guru* to his priest-servant by pointing out to him the elevated spiritual status of Mādhavendra.[①] Finally, the narrator has us understand that the priest is not unable to comprehend the import of what has transpired; rather, his faithful and humble[②] attention to his duties (including details such as bathing before approaching the deity, even in an extraordinary circumstance) qualifies him for such a blessing.

Aside from showing how the "path of devotion" and the "path of rules" are complementary in the context of *arcanam*, this narrative is typical of many which serve to demonstrate to the devotees the active presence of God in his *arcā-mūrti*. As in this account, in others God sometimes "breaks the rules" of ordinary laws of nature, not so much to demonstrate his power, but rather the opposite—to demonstrate his accessibility and readiness to

① It is also significant that as this particular narrative continues, Mādhavendra simply proceeds on his mission to obtain sandalwood for his deity Gopāla. Although it is understood that he has already reached spiritual perfection (he is referred to as a *paramahaṁsa sannyāsī*), and that perfection is further confirmed by the incident with Gopinātha, he does not therefore retire into inactivity to be aloof from the world. Whereas classical *sannyāsī* followers of the *advaita* school are generally known to renounce all endeavors in an effort to terminate karmic reaction, the Vaiṣṇava *sannyāsīs* remain always active, taking liberation as the departure point to eternal service to God. Even in liberated status, a Vaiṣṇava will observe some regulations in worship for the purpose of teaching persons less advanced.

② The priest's humility is implied by his not showing any pride for having been the recipient of special attentions by God in the form of a dream.

become servant to his servant (thereby breaking the "rule" that he is always the master).

Ⅲ. 4 Nuanced Presence in Narrative

As accessible as God becomes in his *arcā-mūrti*, *rasa* can nuance the sense of presence with the opposite sense—of absence: Among the five major *rasas* mentioned earlier, since the time of Mādhavendra Purī[1] Gauḍīya-Vaiṣṇavas single out *mādhurya-rasa*, the mood of conjugal love, as the modus of love for God *par excellence*. The Gauḍīya poets and theologians have been attentive to yet one particular aspect of *mādhurya-rasa*, namely the sense of separation from the beloved (*vipralambha*, or *viraha*[2]), or the sense of the beloved's absence. Again, it is Mādhavendra Pūrī whom Gauḍīya-Vaiṣṇavas celebrate for offering one brief but seminal prayer to Krishna in this mood. He is therefore credited with sowing the seed of Krishna-*prema* in its most exalted expression, which later, in the form of Caitanya Mahāprabhu, became a great tree.

> O my Lord! O most merciful master! O master of Mathurā! When shall I see You again? Because of my not seeing You, my agitated heart has become unsteady. O most beloved one (*dayita*),

---

① Friedhelm Hardy suggests 1420–1490 as plausible dates for Mādhavendra Purī. See Hardy's article, pp. 23-41, for a careful analysis of the verse quoted below. Friedhelm Hardy, "Mādhavendra Purī: A Link Between Bengal Vaiṣṇavism and South Indian *Bhakti*," *Journal of the Royal Asiatic Society of Great Britain and Ireland* (1974).

② *Vipralambha*: lit., "deception, disappointment; separation of lovers; disunion, disjunction." *Viraha*: lit., "abandonment, desertion, parting, separation (esp. of lovers), absence from, lack, want" (Monier-Williams).

what shall I do now? [1]

Mādhavendra Pūrī served his Gopāla deity, feeling in him the presence of Krishna enough to consider a dream as his direct message, convincing him to undertake a difficult and dangerous journey on God's behalf; and yet in this final prayer he expresses his feeling of separation from God. God is present, but in some sense he is not sufficiently present.

Similarly Gopāla Bhaṭṭa Gosvāmī, the south Indian *brāhmaṇa* who compiled the book of Vaiṣṇava ritual *Hari-bhakti-vilāsa*, longed for the direct sight of Krishna even as Krishna was present before him in the form of *Śālagrāma-śīlas* (sacred stones considered direct manifestations of Nārāyaṇa, or Viṣṇu). In his case God satisfied his desire as the "self-

---

① *ayi dīna-dayārdra nātha he/mathurā-nātha kadāvalokyase*
hṛdayaṁ tvad-aloka-kātaraṁ/dayita bhrāmyati kiṁ karomy aham (*Caitanya-caritāmṛta* Āntya-līlā 8. 35).

manifest" image Rādhāramaṇa ('he who gives pleasure to Rādhā') .[①]

Another type of nuancing of the God's presence in the *arcā-mūrti* involves the highlighting of Caitanya's identity as Krishna. Essentially the theme presented in these narratives is that the image (of Krishna) is no doubt directly God (*sākṣāt bhagavān*) , but in some sense Caitanya Mahāprabhu is even "more so," or more importantly so. I want to briefly recount two such narratives before ending this section on *prayojana*, the goal of *bhakti* and hence *arcanam*.

The first of these (again involving food offerings and pranks, but with a different turn) occurs when Caitanya is a small child (known at that time as "Nimai") in the home of his parents in Navadvīpa (in present-day West Bengal) . A *brāhmaṇa* mendicant guest receives conscientious hospitality by Nimai's parents, only to have their efforts utterly spoiled twice in the same evening by their naughty child: Each time the *brāhmaṇa* is about to

① This story begins with Caitanya meeting the young Gopāla Bhaṭṭa during his travels in south India. Becoming Caitanya's follower, he undertook to fulfill his guru's instructions to make the long and arduous trek to the source of the Kali Gandaki River in the Himālayas, on the border of present-day Nepal and Tibet; from there he should bring back several *śālagrāma* stones—round black stones revered by aiṣṇavas as images of Viṣṇu—to join the other Gosvāmīs in Vṛndāvana and practice the daily rituals of worship prescribed for such aniconic forms. This Gopāla Bhaṭṭa did for several years, waiting for the fulfillment of Caitanya's promise to him that eventually he would receive his (Caitanya's) *darśana* until one morning in the Spring of 1542. The night before, Gopāla Bhaṭṭa is said to have lost consciousness while lamenting his unworthiness to see Kṛṣṇa directly, despite all his efforts to worship him with devotion and proper rituals. The next morning he awoke, to notice the lid of the basket in which he kept the *śālagrāmas* hanging overnight askew, and thought that a snake might have entered the basket. Failing to nudge the lid closed with a stick he opened it to find, in place of the stones, a beautiful eleven and one-eighth inch tall image of Kṛṣṇa in his famous triple-bent pose playing a flute and with the distinct marks of one of the *śālagrāma* stones embedded in his shoulder—a *svayam-vyakta*, or 'self-manifest' image. This is the only *arcā-mūrti* of Kṛṣṇa among those of the Six Gosvāmīs which has not been removed from Vṛndāvana to other towns outside Vraja (mainly eventually to Jaipur, Rājasthān) out of fear of Muslim attack. Rādhāramaṇa's worship continues today (in a temple built in 1826) , much according to the same standards established by Gopāla Bhaṭṭa Gosvāmī (Entwistle, 79, 185-186, 413) .

complete the worship of his deity of Krishna with an offering of rice, Nimai pleases himself by barging in the room and stuffing the rice in his mouth. The profusely apologetic parents convince him to make a third offering (fearing a *brāhmaṇas* potent curse). By the time the *brāhmaṇa* completes the third offering the household is sleeping soundly—except of course Nimai, who repeats his prank for a third time. This time, Krishnadās informs us, Nimai manifests his real identity as Krishna before the good gentleman, letting him know that he is the very one to whom he has been offering such devotion in the form of the *Śālagrāma-śīla*. ①

The second narrative involves Caitanya's first visit to the temple of Jagannatha.

After taking to the renounced order (*sannyāsa*) as a young man, on his widowed mother's behest he had agreed to make the town of Jagannātha Pūrī his headquarters, from where she could receive news of him. Arriving in Pūrī ahead of his friends, he goes immediately to the temple to receive God's *darśana* (sight, vision).

An ordinary temple-visitor, after prostrating him or herself, ② rises to stand before the deity with folded hands, offering prayers or simply looking attentively at the form and noting the particular dress and ornamentation of the day. Or the devotee might then bring an offering forward, such as fruit, flowers or sweets, to be offered by a priest to God with appropriate *mantra* after purifying the items by sprinkling water. He or she might then join with others in singing songs of praise to God, or sit for some time in the temple simply to be in the their 'Lord''s presence.

But on this occasion, we are told, as soon as Śrī Caitanya sees 'his Lord' he swoons, remaining unconscious while priests and others wonder

---

① This narrative is found in the Bengali work *Caitanya-bhāgavata* of Vṛndāvanadāsa, *Ādi-khaṇḍa*, fifth chapter.

② Women, according to some scriptural injunctions, should offer obeisance by kneeling, with the head touching the floor.

what to do. Finally Sarvabhauma Bhaṭṭācārya, the senior-most court pundit of the king, has the unknown mendicant brought to his home, sensing that this is no ordinary *sannyāsī*. After some hours Caitanya returns to waking consciousness, and after some time agrees to accept instruction in Vedānta philosophy from Sarvabhauma. Instruction lasts for seven days, during which the young *sannyāsī* remains silent, until Sarvabhauma coaxes his pupil to indicate what he had learned. Caitanya responds candidly (*Caitanya-caritāmṛta* Madhya-līlā 6. 130-132):

> I can understand the meaning of each aphorism [of the *Brahma-sūtra*] very clearly, but your explanations have simply agitated My mind. The meaning of the aphorisms contain clear purports in themselves, but other purports you presented simply covered the meaning of the *sūtras* like a cloud. You do not explain the direct meaning of the *Vedānta-sūtras*. Indeed, it appears that your business is to cover their real meaning. (*Caitanya-caritāmṛta* Madhya-līlā 6. 130-132)

Caitanya then proceeds to expound on Vedānta, refuting the monist interpretation which he had just heard from his teacher. He concludes by giving a learned analysis of a famous verse from the *Bhāgavatam*, the "ātmārāma-verse":

> All different varieties of *ātmārāmas* [those who take pleasure in *ātmā*, or spirit self], especially those established on the path of self-realization, though freed from all kinds of material bondage, desire to render unalloyed devotional service unto the supreme Lord. This means that the Lord possesses transcendental qualities

and therefore can attract everyone, including liberated souls. ①

Sarvabhauma becomes humbled, suspecting that his student could be none other than God himself to be able to display such profound knowledge. As Sarvabhauma prostrates himself, begging forgiveness, Caitanya appears to him as the supreme God, first as the majestic God Viṣṇu and then as the accessible Krishna, to receive his prayers.

The account ends, once again, with the theme of food exchange: The next day Sarvabhauma demonstrates his newfound faith in Caitanya and spontaneous devotion by happily eating some of Jagannātha's remnants received from Caitanya in the early morning upon rising from bed, before making any preliminary brahminical purificatory observances. Krishnadās Kavirāja concludes:

> From that day on, Sārvabhauma Bhaṭṭācārya did not know anything but the lotus feet of Caitanya Mahāprabhu, and from that day he could explain the revealed scriptures only in accordance with the process of devotional service. ②

Again, this narrative brings the *arcā-mūrti*, in this case Jagannātha, into juxtaposition with, we might say, the "hero" of the entire work, such that Jagannātha's divinity is shown to be fully comprehended only through the mercy of God himself.

God appears in two forms here—as the served (*sevya*) and the servitor (*sevaka*), namely Caitanya Mahāprabhu. When Sarvabhauma Bhaṭṭācārya is brought to understand the ontological position of Krishna as *bhagavān*—

---

① *ātmārāmāś ca munayo/nirgranthā apy urukrame*
kurvanty ahaitukīṁ bhaktiṁ/ittham-bhūta-guno hariḥ (*Śrīmad-Bhāgavatam* 1. 7. 10, quoted in *Caitanya-caritāmṛta* Madhya-līlā 6. 186)

② *Caitanya-caritāmṛta* Madhya-līlā 6. 237.

superior to the non-personal conception of the Absolute *brahman*—then he is able to grasp that Caitanya is that very Krishna himself. And at that point it becomes possible for him to fully comprehend the identity of the *arcā-mūrti* Jagannātha by properly honoring the *prasāda* (offered food) of the deity.

God makes himself accessible through his image, but only fully so via his *śuddha-bhakta*, or pure devotee.

In these three chapters I have sketched the Gauḍīya-Vaiṣṇava theology of image worship in terms of Caitanya's three-part classification of the subject matter of Vedic literature, namely *sambandha*, or "relationship," *abhidheya*, or "process," and *prayojana*, or "final goal." My final step in conveying how the apparently material images worshipped in the Gauḍīya-Vaiṣṇava tradition are understood to be worshipable will be to look at this theology from the perspective of one Western religious tradition, that of Judaism.

Chapter Four
Arcanam Versus Idolatry

My dear Lord, You are not a statue; You are directly the son of Mahārāja Nanda (Krishna). Now, for the sake of the old brāhmaṇa, You can do something You have never done before.

—Caitanya-caritāmṛta Madhya-līlā 5. 97[①]

One of the salient self-defining characteristics of the major Middle Eastern monotheistic religious traditions Judaism, Christianity and Islam, has been pointed concern to reject idolatry,[②] the improper worship of God, or the worship of any being other than God. Attention to idolatry by delineating what it is and the necessity to avoid it becomes for these traditions an essential element in the conceptualization of "monotheism": Where God is properly worshiped, there must be absence of idolatry, and where there is idolatry, there must be failure to properly worship the "one true God". This attitude was strongly represented by nineteenth-century Protestant

---

① *pratimā naha tumi—sākṣāt vrajendra-nandana/vipra lāgi'kara tumi akārya-karaṇa*

② An excellent survey of the geneology of the term "religion" and the taxonomy of religions is Jonathan Z. Smith's article "Religion, Religions, Religious," in which the category of "idolatry" is also traced. Jonathan Z. Smith, "Religion, Religions, Religious" in *Critical Terms for Religious Studies*, Mark C. Taylor, ed. (Chicago: University of Chicago Press, 1998).

Christian missionaries in India, who conceived their purpose largely in terms of the eradication of what they perceived as idolatry from the subcontinent.① For them, the ubiquitous worship of sacred images in temples was the very epitome of all that was wrong about the religion of the "Hindoos," to be condemned and eradicated by all means. Of course, these condemnatory efforts were conducted with little or no effort to understand the practices or the theological reflections associated with the practices. What was there to "understand" of practices based simply on superstition and vicious habit? So went the reasoning.

Arguably, as we enter the third millenium, attitudes among religionists (at least within some circles) and scholars of religion have significantly changed,② making much greater possibility for dialogue to occur, founded on mutual respect between and among persons of differing religious traditions, than was possible in nineteenth century India. Whether as a result of this new situation or a cause of it,③ the term "idolatry" is much less likely to be employed in contemporary discussion about non-Western religions. And yet the term has not disappeared, since it does have far-reaching significance in Western monotheistic religion. It may therefore be valuable to explore this notion in the spirit of dialogue, allowing the concept to pose questions and challenges to the practice of image worship in the tradition of this

---

① In this regard see Frederique Marglin, "Jagannātha Purī," in *Vaiṣṇavism: Contemporary Scholars Discuss the Gauḍīya Tradition*, Steven J. Rosen, ed., (New York: FOLK Books, 1992), 214-15, for mention of interesting dealings of the British regarding the Jagannātha temple in the early nineteenth century.

② This change in attitude among Christians would, I suspect, be easily documented by a survey of missionary literature and literature written for the training of missionaries in the last two centuries, with attention to frequency of use of the term 'idolatry.' See footnote 2 page 185 on the history of scholarship and the category 'idolatry.'

③ Mark C. Taylor provides a helpful overview of the inter-relatedness of religion and modernity in his Introduction to *Critical Terms for Religious Studies*, (Chicago: University of Chicago Press, 1998).

study in order to better understand the practice.[①] As a reflective exercise, theologizing is often a border-defining engagement, in response to challenges from opposing positions. If followers of Gauḍīya-Vaiṣṇavism are charged with idolatry, one might then ask, "How will they respond theologically to the challenge? "

The short answer will be, I would suggest, that as with any religious practice, so the practice of image worship within this tradition is prone to degeneration when improperly practiced. Then it may become something akin to the Judeo-Christian notion of "idolatry. "A second short response is that "idolatry" is a highly pejorative term for a wide range of notions or practices which are more or less disapproved within a wide range of Near Eastern religious traditions. So for our subject of study to take the defense against all these notions may not be a very practical or fruitful venture. Rather, what may be most fruitful for understanding the tradition is to try to locate areas of resonance and areas of discord as they reveal themselves by investigating the notion of idolatry as it is understood in some systematic, analytical articulation out of the oldest of the Middle Eastern traditions, Judaism.

This will be afforded by considering five different ways in which the concept of idolatry has been articulated in Jewish tradition as expressed in biblical texts and elaborated on in rabbinical writings—especially of Maimonides. *Betrayal*, *representation*, *myth*, *error*, and *false practice*

---

① My main inspiration for a kind of reflective dialogical mode of encounter between religious traditions comes from Francis X. Clooney, S. J. , and his two important books *Theology After Vedānta* (Albany: State University of New York Press, 1993) and *Seeing Through Texts* (Albany: State University of New York Press, 1996) . My small project here makes no claim to approach the quality of his comparative work, nor the refinement of the spirit of it, but seeks to follow the example of starting from one's own tradition, moving out to encounter the other tradition, and returning to reflect on one's own tradition from a fresh perspective.

are five comprehensive elements of the concept of idolatry ① which I will examine with respect to our topic, not as an exhaustive or exacting exercise in comparative theology, but as a means of calling attention to features of Gauḍīya-Vaiṣṇava doctrine which invite investigation if one is to understand the conceptual fabric surrounding image worship.

Ⅳ. 1 Idolatry and Betrayal

According to Mosche Halbertal and Avishai Margalit, the sense of idolatry as *betrayal* is the one most developed within the Hebrew Bible proper. Within that text, or collection of texts, the notion of idolatry is based heavily on the understanding that there is a unique relationship between God and the people of Israel, a relationship portrayed in the language of human family structures of obligation in monogamous marriage.

> Exemplar of monogamy, God has married only Israel and has taken only the Israelites out of Egypt. The biographical conception of the sin thus also defines those to whom the sin does not apply: It does not apply to those who do not share the history that created the exclusive obligation. The ban on idolatry is not universal because it

---

① The book *Idolatry*, by Moshe Halbertal and Avishai Margalit is an analytical study of the concept of idolatry in the Jewish tradition, from which I am extracting the main five categories for attention here. Each of these divisions will be useful in looking at Gauḍīya-Vaiṣṇava theology of image worship. However, just as the scope of the concept of idolatry as understood in Judaism is far-reaching, so it will be necessary to consider to some extent aspects of Gauḍīya-Vaiṣṇavism which have bearing only tangentially to the practice of image worship. Mosche Halbertal and Avishai Margalit, *Idolatry*, Naomi Goldblum, trans. ,(Cambridge, MA: Harvard University Press, 1992).

was shaped by the metaphor of an exclusive relationship. ①

The exclusive nature of this relationship is amplified by the articulation of the consequences of not honoring it: When individuals or the entire nation of Israel ② offer worship to "other gods," or "play the whore" ③ with other political powers (by making treaties, etc.) they are to be seen as adulterous, in a social milieu where adultery is a most heinous crime, punishable even by death. ④ To be unfaithful to God by worshiping other gods is to call upon oneself painful consequences inflicted by God himself. Having either exacted punishment or at least threatened punishment, reconciliation

---

① Halbertal & Margalit, 22-23. However, as Yehezkel Kaufmann notes in *The Religion of Israel*, although Isaiah, like the other prophets, does not consider idolatry a sin for other nations, "he envisages a time when the nations will forsake idolatry and cleave to God of Israel. "And indeed, Kaufmann observes, there is a complete reversal of attitude in Second Temple times from what prevails during the First Temple, from Israel being a "*terra incognita* to the outsider" to it becoming a hub of mission to eradicate idolatry and paganism from the world. Yehezkel Kaufman, *The Religion of Israel*: *From Its Beginnings to the Babylonian Exile*, Moshe Greenberg, trans., (Chicago: University of Chicago Press, 1996), 449, 450.

② Kaufmann argues that "though some sin of idolatry is found among the people, the people as a whole never apostatize," rather, all are considered answerable for the sins of a few. For example, the sin of worshiping the golden calf is considered the sin of the whole people, although only a small minority are said to have been punished for it (p. 230). The novelty of the Sinaitic covenant was its being given to an entire people through one person, the prophet Moses. Hence "[a] ll the laws of the Torah are given to the nation, and the nation as a whole is answerable for their violation" (p. 234). This perspective makes particularly intriguing the fact that the metaphor of adultery is so much used to describe idolatry: Adultery involves a breach of faith between two individuals, but in connection with idolatry the idea is being applied to one individual and a nation. Thus the nation becomes identified as an individual person (and perhaps one step further, personhood becomes redefined as something which exists only as a collectivity).

③ Halbertal & Margalit, 16, quoting Ezekiel 16: 15-26, 28-34.

④ Ibid., 30. The authors note that the biblical equation of idolatry and adultery worked as long as adultery was understood to be such a grave moral offense. In modern society the relatively relaxed attitude toward adultery results in the "fading of the metaphor."

takes place and the exclusive relationship is restored. [1]

The betrayal of God which is idolatry is compounded by the moral depravity which it engenders. In the Book of Wisdom, chapter fourteen contains a listing of various evils of personal conduct which concludes, "For the worship of infamous idols is the reason and source and extremity of all evil" (BoW 14: 27). According to one commentator on these passages from the Book of Wisdom, the essential character of the evil of idolatry expressed here is preoccupation with the "self," as a lifeless being cut off from God (*New Interpreter's Bible* 5). In order to restore the relationship with God, the moral depravity which is both a source and consequence of idolatry must be purged.

Expressions of exclusivity in the relationship between God and his devotee are found in Vaiṣṇava literature, but always in terms of individuals, never a group or nation, and always to emphasize the strong sense of bonding with God which comes from *bhakti*. For example, in the ninth book of the *Śrīmad-Bhāgavatam* Viṣṇu declares:

> The pure devotee is always within the core of My heart, and I am always in the heart of the pure devotee. My devotees do not know anything else but Me, and I do not know anyone else but them. [2]

It is interesting to note that just before this passage, Viṣṇu compares himself to a faithful husband who is brought under the control of a faithful and loving wife, compared in turn to the *sādhu*, or devotee. In this particular passage the devotees are portrayed as being not attracted to anyone

---

[1] Ibid., 18-20. As the authors explain, the reconciliation between God and Israel involves extensions and transmutations of the marriage-adultery metaphor.

[2] *sādhavo hṛdayaṁ mahyaṁ sādhūnāṁ hṛdayaṁ tv aham*
mad-anyat te na jānanti nāhaṁ tebhyo manāg api (*Śrīmad-Bhāgavatam* 9. 4. 68).

or anything other than God, who reciprocates their devotion with his own feeling of exclusive devotion to them. Thus exclusivity is portrayed in terms of an *undisturbed* human relationship, not as one threatened by betrayal or adultery. If there is a threat of betrayal, it could very well be God, rather than the devotee, who might commit it, considering his ontological identity as the supremely independent being, free of all obligations. Śrī Caitanya expresses his non-conditional commitment to God who is depicted to be in the mood of a paramour to whom the lover has no obligations:

> I know no one but Krishna as my Lord, and He shall remain so, even if He handles me roughly by His embrace, or makes me broken hearted by not being present before me. He is completely free to do anything and everything, for He is always my worshipable Lord unconditionally (*Śikṣāṣṭakam* 8).[①]

The *bhakta*, in contrast to the seeker of benefits in this or the next world (*karmin*), the seeker of gnosis (*jñānin*), and the seeker of mystic perfection (*yogin*), makes no demands on God who, although free of all obligation, never acts neglectfully of his devotee. A famous incident portrayed in the *Mahābhārata* during the great war of Kurukṣetra is seen by Krishna-devotees as evidence that Krishna is not whimsical in his commitment to his devotees and that he holds a relationship (in this case friendship) with his devotee to be more important than to maintain his own reputation as a

---

① *āśliṣya vā pāda-ratāṁ pinaṣṭu mām adarśanān marma-hatāṁ karotu vā*
yathā tathā vā vidadhātu lampaṭo mat-prāṇa-nāthas tu sa eva nāparaḥ (*Caitanya-caritāmṛta Āntya-līlā 20. 47*).

keeper of promises. ①

The faithful devotees of Krishna (or Viṣṇu, or Nārāyaṇa) may not have a problem as potential adulterers, but what about worshipers of other gods, according to the Vaiṣṇavas? The *Bhagavad-gītā* provides the basic concepts related to this issue. Although Krishna is never a "jealous God," ② he does express his displeasure at non-conformity to his will. Most especially this is expressed in two passages—one describing his theophany in the eleventh chapter (in which he is seen by Arjuna as a terrible cosmic figure literally devouring all beings except the faithful Pāṇḍava brothers), and the other in Krishna's description of *asura-bhāva*, the demonic quality, where he warns:

> Those who are envious (*dviṣataḥ*) and mischievous (*krūrān*), who are the lowest among men (*nara-adhamān*), I perpetually cast into material existence, into various demonic species of life. Attaining repeated birth amongst such species, such persons can never approach me. They sink down to the most abominable type of

---

① Kṛṣṇa had made a promise not to personally take up arms in the fratricidal war at Kurukṣetra, a fact which Bhīṣma took to advantage in fighting against Arjuna. With Arjuna's life in danger Kṛṣṇa is moved to fiercely counterattack Bhīṣma (thus satisfying Bhīṣma's desire to see his worshipable Lord display his anger against him, so the *Bhāgavatam* explains). This incident prompts the eighteenth century Gauḍīya-Vaiṣṇava writer Viśvanātha Cakravartī to note that when, in the *Bhagavad-gītā*, Kṛṣṇa orders Arjuna to "declare it boldly that my devotee never perishes," he is anticipating his loss of reputation as a promise-keeper: If Kṛṣṇa himself were to make this declaration, he might not be believed, but since Arjuna will presumably make the declaration, it will be taken seriously.

② There is an account in the *Caitanya-caritāmṛta* regarding Caitanya and his relationship to Advaitācārya which suggests jealousy on the part of Caitanya: Advaitācārya intentionally arouses Caitanya's anger by seemingly propogating monist ideas as a ploy to get Caitanya, who was much junior in age to Advaitācārya, to give up offering him respect as a senior. According to Kṛṣṇadāsa Kavirāja, Advaitācārya saw Caitanya as the supreme Lord, and was therefore embarrassed to receive respect from him (*Caitanya-caritāmṛta* Ādi-līlā 17. 66-69).

existence. [①]

Devotees of other gods (*anya-devatā-bhaktāḥ*) are mentioned in the ninth chapter of the *Gītā* (9. 23). Such persons, Krishna assures, are in fact worshiping him, but in the wrong way. In general the problem with such worship is simply perpetuation of bound existence, sometimes temporarily pleasing, but otherwise leading to repeated birth and death. *Bhagavad-gītā* declares that one is in any case rewarded appropriately for one's misinformed endeavors. Worshipers "go to" (*yānti*) whomever is the object of their worship.

Wrong worship of the wrong form of God can have more severe consequences. An interesting narrative in the fifth book of the *Śrīmad-Bhāgavatam* suggests what could happen if one would attempt to propitiate Goddess Bhadra-Kālī by attempting to offer to her, as a human sacrifice, a devotee of Viṣṇu:

> All the rogues and thieves who had made arrangements for the worship of goddess Kālī were low minded and bound to the modes of passion and ignorance. [②] They were overpowered by the desire to become very rich; therefore they had the audacity to disobey the

---

① *tān ahaṁ dviṣataḥ krūrān saṁsāreṣu narādhamān*
kṣipāmy ajasram aśubhān āsurīṣv eva yoniṣu
āsurīṁ yonim āpannā mūḍhā janmani janmani
mām aprāpyaiva kaunteya tato yānty adhamāṁ gatim (*Bhagavad-gītā* 16. 19-20).

Such condemnation is understood to be possible for an extremely long period, not as absolutely permanent. Eventually all beings may attain beatitude, especially via the mercy of a devotee of God. See for example *Śrīmad-Bhāgavatam* 4. 28. 53-55, 64. Also, throughout the time of the bound soul's existence in the cycle of birth and death, God accompanies as *paramātmā*, or *antaryāmin*, "the indwelling controller."

② The Sānkhya system of classical Indian philosophy analyzes the world in terms of three modalities, *sattva* (illumination or goodness), *rajas* (passion), and *tamas* (darkness, inertia, ignorance). According to disposition persons are understood to be oriented in all their activities and outlook by these modalities or humors.

> injunctions of the Vedas, so much so that they were prepared to kill Jaḍa Bharata, a self-realized soul (*brahma-bhūta*) born in a brāhmaṇa family. . . . there was no reason to kill Jaḍa Bharata, and Goddess Kālī could not bear this. She could immediately understand that these sinful dacoits were about to kill a great devotee of the Lord. Suddenly the image of Kālī burst asunder, and the goddess Kālī personally emerged from it in a body burning with an intense and intolerable effulgence.[1]

The account concludes with a turning of the tables as Bhadra-Kālī renders divine justice by killing the would-be sacrificers of the sage. Thus we find in this passage of *Śrīmad-Bhāgavatam* a rough parallel (in tone if not in content) to some biblical expressions of disapproval of idolatry, except that for biblical authors idolatry was not only depraved but was also foolish for the reason that idols were considered utterly impotent and lifeless. I will discuss further improper worship in the Gauḍīya tradition in section IV. 3. and IV. 4.

IV. 2 Idolatry and Representation

I have selected Judaism as the tradition to represent the Western monotheistic critique of image worship partly because of its very influential thinker Moses Maimonides (1135–1204 CE). Although his view on representation is not necessarily that of biblical Judaism, it does represent an important position in metaphysics which has fueled *via negativa* theology ever since his writing of *The Guide for the Perplexed.*[2] Maimonides articulated a radical dualism wherein God is so utterly different from the world that

---

[1] *Śrīmad-Bhāgavatam* 5. 9. 17-18.

[2] This is not to say that his was by any means the first expression of *via negativa* theology.

pictorial representation or even verbal representation of him is mistaken and misleading. This position places him at odds with our tradition in question and therefore his view deserves special attention. ① If we consider Judaism more broadly, there is one element of commonality with a number of Indic religious traditions regarding representation of the divine, in that there are proper and improper ways in which God can be represented; but Judaism (as also Islam, and rarely Christian traditions) is striking in its concern to maintain a radical rejection of the representation of God by *pictorial* means as mistaken or inappropriate attempts to portray through similarity. ②

According to Menachem Kellner, Maimonides defines the principles of religion specifically in terms of two principles—the unity of God and the prohibition of idolatry. ③ These two principles imply each other. The unity of God, Maimonides insists, precludes the possibility of divine corporeality, and where there is not a clear understanding of the unity of God, idolatry is at hand. Where corporeality seems to be indicated in scripture, it is due to a misunderstanding of the word *zelem*. In the very beginning of his *Guide for the Perplexed* Maimonides expounds on the meaning of the term *zelem* as being different from the ordinary sense of "form" expressed by the Hebrew word *toar*.

---

① It could be inferred from the various descriptions in biblical literature that the idea of God having an image is not rejected; however it is quite clear that pictorial representation, or visual representation for purposes of worship, is forbidden. For Maimonides, however, "Representation is prohibited as a result of the metaphysical claim that since God has no image, any representation of God, and naturally any worship of such a representation, constitutes the worship of a false god. The problem in this case is that any similarity-based representation is mistaken and causes error in the conception of God for anyone who sees or worships such a representation" (Halbertal & Margalit, 45-46). Citing C. S. Peirce, H. & M. distinguish *similarity-based representation* (one thing represents another based on similarity) from *causal representation* (involving relations other than similarity, like metonymy), and *conventional representation* (one thing represents another by convention, as the word "cup" representing an object we drink from).

② Halbertal & Margalit, 45-46.

③ Menachem Kellner, *Maimonides on Human Perfection*, (Atlanta, Georgia: Scholars Press, 1990), 23.

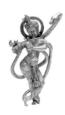

> This term [*toar*] is not at all applicable to God. The term *zelem*, on the other hand, signifies the specific form, viz., that which constitutes the essence of a thing, whereby the thing is what it is; the reality of a thing in so far as it is that particular being. In man the "form" is that constituent which gives him human perception: and on account of this intellectual perception the term *zelem* is employed in the sentences "In the *zelem* of God he created him."[1]

Similarly Maimonides expounds on the homonymous character of several biblical terms which superficially indicate bodily features, such as *panim* (face), *aḥor* (back), and *leb* (heart).[2] In this way Maimonides directs attention to the unity/incorporeality of God whose exclusive right it is to receive worship as he orders. While Maimonides gives credit to the "idolators" for *not* thinking that a stone or metal image is in and of itself the creator of the world, their problem, he claims, is that they "only notice the rites, without comprehending their meaning or the true character of the being which is worshipped," and hence they "renounce their belief in the existence of God."[3]

Thus, according to Maimonides, from superficial (*mistaken*) understanding of scripture one is prompted to make images, initially as intermediaries to God. But pre-occupation with the rites of worship of such images leads to the *error of substitution*. A picture or statue, if worshiped as a representation of God, may easily become the sole focus of the worshiper rather than the Person whom the image represents. From this error, a physical representation can become a fetish, "an object to which people

---

① Moses Maimonides, *The Guide for the Perplexed*, M. Friedlaender, trans., (New York: George Routledge & Sons, 1947), 13.

② Maimonides, 52-54.

③ Maimonides, 52.

attribute powers that it does not have," especially if the representation, by that error, gains "some control over its worshipers." [①] When substitution occurs, the image takes the place of God being worshiped in the eyes of the worshiper. The real object of worship, so Maimonides, loses all importance. In his *Code of Jewish Law* Maimonides concludes his genealogy of idolatry with these words:

> As time gradually passed, the honored and revered Name of God was forgotten by mankind, vanished from their lips and hearts, and was no longer known to them. All the common people and the women and children knew only the figure of wood and stone and the temple edifice in which they had, from their childhood, been trained to prostrate themselves to the figure, worship it, and swear by its name. Even their wise men, such as priests and men of similar standing, also fancied that there was no other god but the stars and spheres, for whose sake and in whose similitude these figures had been made. But the Creator of the universe was known to none, and recognized by none save a few solitary individuals.... (Laws Concerning Idolatry and the Ordinances of the Heathens 1: 2). [②]

If pictorial representation is a *danger* in the biblical traditions, it is, one might say, almost a *necessity* in Hindu theistic traditions, most

① Halbertal and Margalit, 42.

② Isadore Twersky, *A Maimonides Reader*, Library of Jewish Studies, ed. Neal Kozodoy, (West Orange, NJ: Behrman House, 1972), 72-73.

especially Vaiṣṇavism.[1] As we have discussed *avatāra*-theology, it might come as no surprise to us that a descent into the world by *bhagavān* invites pictorial as much as linguistic representation.[2] Since his appearance in the world is as a participant therein, and since his purpose relates specifically to increasing accessibility to bound *jīvas*, God allows, or even invites, pictorial

---

① Peter Bennett has eloquently articulated why idolatry is not an issue in Hinduism in general and devotional traditions in particular. Whereas the binary oppositions of subject and object, and between signifier and signified, dominate western discourse on worship (in models proposed by Sir Edmund Leach, Paul Tillich, Roy Ellen, Victor Turner and others), these oppositions are "in India liable to dissolution according to the notion that the soul (*jīva*), image (*mūrti*) and deity (*deva*) are particularized aspects of divinity. Their differentiation is not reducible to absolute dichotomies. Rather, in many of the devotional traditions, differentiation enables the enlightened soul to realise its innate capacity for experiencing divine bliss (*ānanda*) while enjoying a highly intimate and loving relationship with a personal god of grace." He then points to a western bias "intrinsic to the very idea of the sacred symbol" embedded in dichotomies of human-divine, earth-heaven, profane-sacred, and material-abstract. The symbol thus acts as an "agent of mediation" which may have a special status "by pointing to, and thereby participating in the reality of, that for which it stands." This is where the danger comes, according to E. H. Gombrich (cited by Bennett): We are all "apt to regress at any moment to a primitive state, experiencing the fusion of the image and its model or the name and its bearer. Bennett counters, "But surely in a universe where the apparent gulf separating the two worlds is unreal (and who is to say that such a universe is 'primitive'?) then the reverse might hold true. Enlightenment might only occur when image and prototype, material and abstract, man and divine, signifier and signified, are experienced in their underlying unity. In orthodox western philosophical traditions the holy image is a symbol standing for a higher, intangible reality, while there is always a tendency for the worshiper to see the image as having sacred virtues of its own. Conversely, in Puṣṭi Mārga [the Vaiṣṇava followers of Vallabha, closely akin to Gauḍīya Vaiṣṇavism] I argue that there is a sense in which the material image and supreme divinity are ultimately undifferentiated. To call the image a symbol in a Neoplatonic or Aristotelian sense would be to devalue its inherent sanctity. The symbol is metonymic rather than metaphoric. In a manner of speaking the symbol is that which it symbolizes. The divine image in Puṣṭi Mārga can be quite literally Krishna's own form." Peter Bennet, "Krishna's Own Form: Image Worship and Puṣṭi Mārga," *Journal of Vaiṣṇava Studies* vol. 1 no. 4 (Summer 1993), 114-116.

② An art-historical perspective shows also a parallel development of literary and pictorial representations of *avatāras*. See T. S. Maxwell, *Gods of Asia: Image, Text, and Meaning*, (Delhi: Oxford University Press, 1997), 10-11.

representation as a natural consequence of his appearance, especially as seen or envisioned by spiritually elevated souls.

Although *bhagavān* makes himself visible to all as *avatāra*, it is the spiritually adept sage (*ṛṣi*) or pure devotee (*śuddha-bhakta*) who can receive the form of God as vision (*darśaṇa*), seeing him as he is, and can then communicate that vision for others to hear, repeat, meditate upon, and then sculpt. The sculpted form, if faithful to the specifications of revealed scripture (*āgama-śāstra*, or *śilpa-śāstra*, understood to be the faithful recordings of such visionaries' descriptions), ① can then be worshiped by prescribed procedures which, if properly practiced, enable the practitioner to gain the same vision of God as the sages or devotees who see him "directly." ②

---

① Guidelines for artists are mainly concerned with proportions, standard attributes, and poses (standing, seated or lying). See Jitendra Nath Banerjea, *The Development of Hindu Iconography*, (Delhi: Munshiram Manoharlal, 1974), especially Chapter Ⅷ, "Canons of Iconometry." Adherence to specifications persists today mainly in south Indian image production. Gauḍīya-Vaiṣṇava practice, at least presently, seems less concerned with adherence to scriptural injunctions, perhaps relying more on directions of one's *guru*. In either case there is submission to tradition, as Heinrich Zimmer notes: "[I]t is not granted to any believer to shape by himself, according to his own ideas, the deity's image he wishes to construct in himself, for only the Divine itself can bear witness to what is Divine. The particular manifestation in which God is to appear is His to decide, and to deviate even in the slightest from the traditional way He is perceived and represented—which lies at the heart of sacred tradition—is a patent absurdity, for this tradition, as its literary form attests, is nothing less than the orally preserved self-revelation of God." Heinrich Zimmer, *Artistic Form and Yoga in the Sacred Images of India*, Gerald Chapple and James B. Lawson, trans., (Princeton, N J: Princeton University Press, 1990), 50. An interesting case of sculpting after a "model" is narrated (in an eighteenth century Bengali work *Bhakti-ratnākāra*) regarding a contemporary of Caitanya, Gauridāsa Paṇḍit: Having beseeched Caitanya (and Nityānanda) not to depart from his home in Bengal for Pūrī, his wish is satisfied when the two agree to "pose" for him long enough for him to sculpt the supposedly first images of them, in wood. He kept these images and worshiped them for the rest of his life; they are the selfsame images, we are told by his descendants, that are being worshiped today in that same town near Navadvīpa.

② See Zimmer, 53-64, discussing "outward sight and inner vision," in which he suggests that Indian iconography is conducive to a meditative type of seeing which naturally leads to "inner vision," aided by properly practiced concentration and chanting of the appropriate *mantra*.

Comprehension of divine form, then, involves revelation, linguistic representation, pictorial representation, and regulated worship of the pictorial representation under a preceptor's guidance. As one progresses through the stages of *bhakti* (as outlined in Section II. 3. 1) in the increasing dedication of one's mind and senses to the service of God, the capacity to see the transcendent form of the divinity becomes fully developed. Seeing becomes *re-cognizing*—in the sense that one cognizes the transcendent form of the supreme Person within one's own heart (*hṛdy-anta-stha*). At that stage, the value of the pictorial image does not become diminished (as in some strict monist [*advaita*] traditions, in which the image is purely instrumental). Rather, because *bhakti* is itself the goal, one finds in the image a genuinely *re-presentational* presence, made even more so by the power of *bhakti* to attract God. Rather than making an "error of substitution," the *bhakta* would claim that he or she is, with purified senses and mind, making a *correction in perception*: The error of *not* perceiving God in the world is *corrected* by the process of *bhakti*, which enables one to receive God's blessings in the form of divine sight. ①

That the form of Krishna has been directly cognized by devotees and sages in the past is central to Gauḍīya-Vaiṣṇava doctrine. Gauḍīya-Vaiṣṇavas especially revere in this context the vision of Brahmā, the demiurge said to be the original progenitor of the universe, described in the Sanskrit poetry of the *Brahmā-saṁhitā*. Brahmā, after practicing lengthy austerities (*tapas*), becomes initiated by Krishna into esoteric knowledge of transcendent existence with a sacred *mantra* consisting of names of God. By properly hearing and then reciting this *mantra*, he becomes enabled to gain the sight of Govinda (another name of Krishna), whom he proceeds to describe in

① For example, the *Bhagavad-gītā* (11. 8) describes Kṛṣṇa bestowing "divine eyesight" (*divyaṁ caksus*) on Arjuna, his devoted friend, allowing him to see his universal form (*viraṭ-rūpa*). Also Kṛṣṇa speaks of "understanding by direct perception" (*pratyakṣavagamam*) in *Bhagavad-gītā* 9. 2.

some detail, listing "physical" characteristics but also emphasizing the non-mundane quality of his form:

> Always playing the flute, his eyes like blooming lotus-petals, his head adorned with a peacock feather, his beautiful form the hue of a blue cloud; with the unique beauty that charms millions of cupids—the Primeval Lord, Govinda, do I adore.
>
> Around his neck is a garland of forest-flowers swinging to and fro, and he is adorned with a peacock feather ornament; his flute held in hands adorned with jewelled bracelets, he who eternally revels in pastimes of love, whose charming threefold curved form, Śyāmasundara, is his eternal feature—the Primeval Lord, Govinda, do I adore.
>
> I worship that primeval Lord Govinda, whose form is all-ecstatic, all-conscious and all-truth, and thus full of the most dazzling splendor; every part of that transcendental form possesses the functions of all his senses, as he eternally sees, maintains and regulates infinite universes, both spiritual and mundane (*Brahma-saṁhitā* 30-32). [1]

The first two of these three verses offer graphic, detailed description in terms of physical attributes, emphasizing Govinda's beauty by which he charms his consorts. The third verse gives a more abstract description, reminding the hearer that although God has tangible features, they are

---

① *veṇuṁ kvaṇantam aravinda-dalāyatākṣaṁ/barhāvataṁsam asitāmbuda-sundarāṅgam*
kandarpa-koṭi-kamanīya-viśeṣa-śobhaṁ/govindam ādi-puruṣaṁ tam ahaṁ bhajāmi
ālola-candraka-lasad-vanamālya-vaṁśī-/ratnāṅgadaṁ praṇaya-keli-kalā-vilāsam
śyāmaṁ tri-bhaṅga-lalitaṁ niyata-prakāśaṁ/govindam ādi-puruṣaṁ tam ahaṁ bhajāmi
aṅgāni yasya sakalendriya-vṛtti-manti/paśyanti pānti kalayanti ciraṁ jaganti
ānanda-cinmaya-sad-ujjvala-vigrahasya/govindam ādi-puruṣaṁ tam ahaṁ bhajāmi
(*Brahma-saṁhitā* 5. 30–32. *trans. by Sagar*, 81–85).

of a higher nature than ordinary physical features. He has a "body," but every "part" of it can function in the same way as any other "part." This latter verse echoes other types of description found in Vedic literature (all of which is understood as revelatory, i. e. "envisioned" by sages or devotees), [1] as for example this description of God from the *Śvetāśvatara Upaniṣad* (8. 13):

> He has no feet or hands, yet He is the swiftest runner and can grasp anything. Though without eyes or ears, He sees and hears. Nobody knows Him, yet He is the knower and the object of knowledge. Sages describe Him as the supreme, original Personality of Godhead. [2]

Such paradoxical language in this last passage, which holds a tension between form and formlessness, [3] leans more toward the sense of dignity and majesty of God than accessibility and intimacy which is preferred in the Gauḍīya-Vaiṣṇava tradition, which seeks to resolve the paradox by making a distinction between "material form" and "spiritual form." The former is

---

① A concise presentation of the vision of the Vedic seers (*ṛṣis*) is offered by Rajendra P. Pandeya in his article "The Vision of the Vedic Seer," in *Hindu Spirituality*, Sivaraman, ed., (New York: Crossroad, 1989).

② *apāṇi-pādo javano grahītā paśyaty acakṣuḥ sa śṛṇoty akarṇaḥ*
sa vetti vedyaṁ na ca tasya vettā tam āhur agryaṁ puruṣaṁ purāṇam
Translation by H. D. Goswami, in the 'Purport' to *Śrīmad-Bhāgavatam* 10. 87. 28, in Bhaktivedānta, *Complete Works*.

③ There is a parallel between this form/formlessness tension and the "finite/infinite" dichotomy which Robert Cummings Neville discusses in his book *The Truth of Broken Symbols*, (Albany: State University of New York Press, 1996). In his theological analysis of symbol, he sees images or symbols as border-limits or boundary-markers between the finite and infinite which mediate between the two (p. 69). When they fail to accurately mark that boundary, symbols become idolatrous: "Religious symbols can be false by being idolatrous, that is, identifying their referent with the meaning of some finite, non-divine, or profane thing and not indicating how the meaning does not apply quite adequately" (p. 20).

characterized by limits of time and space comprehended by the bound *jīva*; the latter is characterized as partaking of the "form of eternal-cognizant-bliss" (*sac-cid-ānanda-vigraha*) which is the essential nature of God.

What Brahmā's verses suggest for the followers of Caitanya is that what is being denied in the *Śvetāśvatara Upaniṣad* is not form or image or body with appendages as such. Rather, form or image in reference to God conceived as having the same sorts of limitations as those we normally experience is denied. In this way God's infinity is preserved without compromising his omnipotence. ① The omnipotence of God is, for Vaiṣṇavas, further demonstrated by his bestowing to pure devotees the power of divine sight and power to communicate that sight to others.

This argument for "spiritual form" and the possibility of comprehending it would not be to Maimonides' liking, no doubt, as he insists that all words used to describe God must be understood as figurative descriptions, and

---

① We might be reminded of Maimonides'view that although the sentence "God is wise" in its literal sense has no cognitive meaning, it is better for didactic purposes to say this than to say its cognitively equally meaningless opposite, "God is not wise." The first statement creates an attitude of respect for the deity, whereas the second statement creates an attitude of disrespect (Halbertal and Margalit, 153-54). One might argue that to claim material forms are forms of God would be an insult to God. Vaiṣṇavas might answer that this would be quite the case, were it so that the forms were merely material. Since it is understood that they have been declared non-material (at least not *merely* material) by scripture (*arcye viṣṇoḥ śīlā-dhīḥ. . . yasya vā narakī saḥ*: "One who thinks the worshipable form of Viṣṇu to be merely stone. . . possesses a hellish mentality" [Padma Purāṇa]), the potential insult is removed. It has also been pointed out by Swami Prabhupāda that Kṛṣṇa identifies the material elements of this world as his "separated nature" (*bhinna-prakṛti*). Although consisting of the external energy (*bahiraṅga-śakti*) of God, material forms are nevertheless *his* energy, transformable at will into internal energy (*antaraṅga-śakti*). Another perspective which touches on the Christian notion of God's humiliation as the Incarnation is the suggestion by John Carman (p. 195) that "The consecrated image is the ultimate in God's 'descent' . . . , coming down to a level even lower than that of God's human worshipers. This 'real presence' of divine mercy manifests God's grace in physical weakness at the mercy of those who handle—or even mishandle—him." From this perspective, if the material form is a minimization of the dignity of God, it is one which he has chosen to accept for the sake of blessing bound souls.

should therefore not be taken as indicating the bodily features or human qualities they suggest. The *Śrīmad-Bhāgavatam* raises this question of language transparency in a different way:

> Śrī Parīkṣit said: O brāhmaṇa, how can the Vedas directly describe the Supreme Absolute Truth, who cannot be described in words? The Vedas are limited to describing the qualities of material nature, but the Supreme is devoid of these qualities (*nirguṇa*), being transcendental to all material manifestations and their causes. [1]

Indeed later in the discussion the Vedic statements are described as tying up "like animals" persons who are inimical to God. The gist of the answer to Parīkṣit's question is that God is fully capable of revealing himself to the person he desires to bless, and that the Vedas themselves are *sometimes* blessed by him to comprehend his pastimes (*līlā*). Again, the Upaniṣads emphasize that it is the prerogative of God to reveal himself to the one he chooses:

> This Supreme Self cannot be reached by argumentation, or by applying one's independent brain power, or by studying many scriptures. Rather, he alone can achieve the Self whom the Self chooses to favor. To that person the Self reveals His own true, personal form. [2]

Bhaktisiddhānta Sarasvatī, the leading scholar of Gauḍīya-Vaiṣṇavism in the early part of the twentieth century, spoke of revelation of the "true Form of God" in terms of receptivity by the "unmixed soul" while defending

---

① *Śrīmad-Bhāgavatam* 10. 87. 1

② *nāyam ātmā pravacanena labhyo na medhayā na bahunā śrutena*
yam evaiṣa vṛṇute tena labhyas tasyaiṣa ātmā vivṛṇute tanūṁ svām.
(Kaṭha Upaniṣad 2. 2. 23 and Muṇḍaka Upaniṣad 3. 2. 3), H. D. Goswami trans.

image worship against the charge of idolatry in an interview with an American scholar, Professor Albert E. Suthers:

> If a pure entity or unmixed soul sees that Eternal Form of God and receives It in his own pure receptacle and then places this Transcendental Form in the world from his heart as illuming the intrinsically and essentially true Form of God, that never deserves to be called an idol. Just as even by coming down to this phenomenal world, God remains untouched by the influence of *māyā* by dint of His inscrutable power, so does His true Form, too, as revealed to the unmixed entity of His devotee, remain above it even though brought down here. . . . The *Śrī-Vigraha* [sacred image] of the Vaiṣṇava philosophy cannot but be the direct indication of the Essential Form of God. By way of an imperfect comparison it may be said to be the proxy of the essential Form of God which is beyond the cognisance of the material eye, just as there are, in art and science, crude representations of invisible matter. ①

The idea of a *proxy* suggested here also indicates representation, but in a different sense from "pictorial" or "linguistic representation." A proxy is a *person* who represents someone else in a particular function, and in this sense acts as substitute, *on the authority of the person represented.* In that Vaiṣṇavism emphasizes worship as personal exchange, one could say that this type of substitution is occurring, except that the representing and represented

---

① Rūpa Vilāsa Dāsa, *A Ray of Vishnu*: *The Biography of a Śaktyāveṣa Āvatāra*, *Śrī Śrīmad Bhaktisiddhānta Sarasvatī Gosvāmī Mahārāja Prabhupāda*, (Washington, Mississippi: New Jaipur Press, 1988), 93. Bhaktisiddhānta Sarasvatī, a native of Bengal, wrote and spoke fluent English. The text quoted is part of a longer conversation (from 1929, in Krishnanagar, W. Bengal) which was transcribed later by a disciple who was thought to have audiographic memory. In any case the transcription was approved by the speaker.

Person are one and the same. This would certainly not be regarded as an *error* on the part of the bound *jīva*, rather Vaiṣṇavas would see it is a *correction* on the part of the omnipotent God for the sake of the bound *jīva*.[1]

It may be worth noting that Maimonides'radical dualism has had its counterbalance within Judaism in the medieval mystical tradition of Kabbalah, which posits two aspects to the deity, the unknowable *Ein Sof* and the revealed ten emanations (*sefirot*). Hasidism, John Carman notes, developed these ideas and affirmed an intimate personal relationship between God and the Hasidic mystic.[2]

IV. 3 Idolatry and Myth

The Jewish notion of idolatry is inseparable from the notion of paganism, according to Yehezkel Kaufmann. And yet, he notes, the Bible is "utterly unaware of the nature and meaning of pagan religion."[3] Whereas the Bible conceives only the "lowest level" of paganism, articulated in its polemic against idolatry as stigmatization of pagan gods as "the handiwork of man," or "wood and stone," (Deut. 4: 28; 28: 36, 64) it does not, he claims, show any knowledge of the mythological features of the gods it condemns. The battle against idolatry waged in the Bible is solely based on

---

[1] Some comparison might be made here to the attitude of the ninth century iconodules who defended icon-veneration against the iconoclasts in the Orthodox Christian tradition. But in making a distinction between *worship* and *veneration* the iconodules put perhaps a different value to the concept of "symbol" than the devotional Indic traditions would do. For the latter, the image is fully worshipable to the same extent that God's name or God's devotees are worshipable, as capable of transmitting God's presence to the devoted soul. One might say that the worshipable image (*arcā-vigraha*) as symbol is not Robert Neville's "broken symbol" so much as a "breaking symbol," that is to say one which is capable of *breaking down* the structure of superficial designations (*upādhis*) by which one's existence in bondage persists.

[2] Carman, 256-258.

[3] Kaufmann, 7-20.

the argument of fetishism and nowhere argues against the existence of the gods being worshipped in the images, nor against the truth of those gods' mythologies. "The Bible nowhere denies the existence of the gods; it ignores them." Kaufmann continues,

> The Bible's ignorance of the meaning of paganism is at once the basic problem and the most important clue to the understanding of biblical religion. It underscores as nothing else can the gulf that separates biblical religion from paganism. A recognition of this gulf is crucial to the understanding of the faith of the Bible. Not only does it underlie the peculiar biblical misrepresentation of paganism, it is the essential fact of the history of Israelite religion. ①

This view, if not typical of scholars on biblical religion, is indicative perhaps of a typical Jewish apologetic expression of the contrast between Jewish monotheism and the supposed "mythological polytheism" of all other religions. Vaiṣṇavism is likely not the only religious tradition in the world which does not conform to Kaufmann's (rather extensive) generalizations of paganism. Nevertheless as a typical expression of possible objection (*pūrvapakṣa*) ② to *arcanam* in the Gauḍīya-Vaiṣṇava tradition we may briefly examine the supposed characteristics of pagan religion and consider how Gauḍīya-Vaiṣṇavism departs from these typifications.

Also, insofar as image worship in Gauḍīya-Vaiṣṇavism involves ritual activity, we do well to examine what Kaufmann (followed by Halbertal and Margalit) presents as contrasts between biblical worship of God and pagan

---

① Kaufmann, 20.

② *Pūrvapakṣa*, lit. "initial claim," is the term commonly used in Indian philosophical dialectics for a portrayal of an idea to be refuted.

worship, bound as it is, in their view, to *myth*, [1] which extends idolatry from mere fetishism to a complete worldview. The first of these contrasts is between limited power of pagan gods and the absolute will of God. Whereas pagan gods are limited by fate and nature, God creates the world "by his word and not by war." [2] Kaufmann writes,

> The mark of monotheism is not the concept of a god who is creator, eternal, benign, or even all-powerful; these notions are found everywhere in the pagan world. It is, rather, the idea of a god who is the source of all being, not subject to cosmic order, and not emergent from a pre-existent realm. . . The High gods of primitive tribes do not embody this idea. [3]

Second, according to this view, the absolute divinity of God determines the nature of ritual as distinct from that related to pagan gods. Whereas the latter rites are characterized by magic, whereby some form of control of the gods is won (they being bound to primordial nature, which one ritually manipulates), biblical ritual functions within the context of covenant: "God consents to do what man asks of him because his will has been fulfilled, and not because he has been compelled, by a magical or ritual technique,

---

① In this context Halbertal and Margalit seem to define myth as "the collective science of a traditional society," whereby the society is "closed," in contrast to the modern "open" society which allows for confrontation among rival theories. "What distinguishes myth from modern theories is not the obvious falseness of myth and the principled correctness of theories, nor even that myth is primitive and theories are developed. The difference between them is social. Myth serves a closed society, and modern scientific theories serve an open society. . . . The transition from myth to logos is thus not the transition from an obvious falsehood to a theory that is correct at first approximation. It is the transition from a closed society to an open society. The difference lies not in what the theory says but in the social context of what is said" (pp. 85-86).

② Halbertal and Margalit, 68-69.

③ Kaufmann, 29.

to act on man's behalf." Kaufmann finds in paganism a "confusion of realms," there being a "common womb" out of which both gods and the world have appeared, and hence there is a removal of "any fixed bounds between [the gods] and the world of men and other creatures."①

Third, the type of mediation between man and the divine is different: In pagan prophecy there is requirement of skill on the part of the prophet or priest, in contrast to biblical prophecy whereby God selects a messenger to communicate *his* will.

Fourth, pagan morality is embedded in nature, in contrast to biblical morality originating in the will of God.② In these writers' view, pagan myth can be further characterized by a multiplicity of independent beings participating in the drama of a sacred story, unlike monotheistic narratives, in which there is no multiplicity of beings "with a will capable of limiting the divine will".③

In light of much of what we have already discussed regarding the ontology-doctrine of Gauḍīya-Vaiṣṇavism, it may be clear that the above characterizations of pagan mythic narrative of gods would not be entirely apt for describing the Vaiṣṇava conception of *bhagavān* and his pastimes (*līlā*) which include cosmic creation, nor of the *bhakti* type of worship directed to

---

① Kaufmann, 35.

② Halbertal and Margalit, 69. The authors cite Yehezkel Kaufman as the source for these distinctions. Along with Ernst Renan and Henri Frankfort, he considers myth "a form of expression unique to paganism." The authors consider whether this is a fair assessment, or whether the Bible is not itself myth, generally concluding that whether or not he has given the best definition of myth, he "has indeed put his finger on an essential difference between the two worlds, and this difference exists even if it is not analogous to the difference between mythological and nonmythological literature" (p. 71). The authors go on to qualify their own view that God of the Bible is characterized more by personhood than absolute will, which involves him in "emotional interdependency" "in a complex relationship with the world and gives the biblical story a mythic dimension even in Kaufmann's own terms. . . . The dependency we have identified is like a person's dependency on his beloved, or upon prior obligations" (p. 73).

③ Halbertal and Margalit, 79.

him. Regarding the position of God, or *bhagavān*, I have already noted (in section I. 2. 3) the example from the *Śrīmad-Bhāgavatam* of a spider and its web as analogous for God and his creation. The topic of God's independence is dealt with exhaustively in the *Śrīmad-Bhāgavatam*, beginning with the opening verse. The four core verses of the entire work, found in the second book, treats of this theme as well. The first of these states,

> Brahmā, it is I, the Personality of Godhead, who was existing before the creation, when there was nothing but Myself. Nor was there the material nature, the cause of this creation. That which you see now is also I, the Personality of Godhead, and after annihilation what remains will also be I, the Personality of Godhead.[1]

In light of the independence of God, Krishna-*bhakti* is contrasted with other types of worship. As mentioned in Section IV. 1, in the *Bhagavad-gītā* Krishna refers to worship of "other gods" as being in fact worship of himself, but performed "in a wrong way" (*avidhi-pūrvakam*).[2] Since the fruits of such indirect worship are limited and temporary, the worshipers have a lack of good judgment (*alpa-medhas*).[3] Whereas such worshipers seek favors of the *devatās* (administrative cosmic beings), thus performing rites which in some sense are meant to compel those beings by manipulative means, Krishna condones only direct approach to the absolute God, which can be accomplished properly only by means of non-manipulative *bhakti*:

> One can understand Me as I am, as the Supreme Personality of

---

① *aham evāsam evāgre nānyad yat sad-asat param*
paścād ahaṁ yad etac ca yo 'vaśiṣyeta so 'smy aham (Śrīmad-Bhāgavatam 2. 9. 33.)

② Bhagavad-gītā 9. 23.

③ Bhagavad-gītā 7. 23.

Godhead, only by devotional service (*bhakti*). And when one is in full consciousness of Me by such devotion (*tattvato jñātvā*), he can enter into the Kingdom of God (*viśate tat-anantaram*). ①

The *Śrīmad-Bhāgavatam* emphasizes that devotion service to God should not be confused with business transactions:

> Otherwise, O my Lord, O supreme instructor of the entire world, You are so kind to Your devotee that You could not induce him to do something unbeneficial for him. On the other hand, one who desires some material benefit in exchange for devotional service cannot be Your pure devotee. Indeed, he is no better than a merchant who wants profit in exchange for service. ②

This notion is not dissimilar from Maimonides' expression of the proper attitude for reading Torah:

> Whoever engages in the study of the Torah in order that he may receive a reward or avoid calamities is not studying the Torah for its own sake. Whoever occupies himself with the Torah, neither out of fear nor for the sake of recompense, but solely out of love for the Lord of the whole earth who enjoined us to do so, is occupied with

---

① *bhaktyā mām abhijānāti yāvān yaś casmi tattvataḥ*
tato māṁ tattvato jñātva viṣate tad-anantaram (*Bhagavad-gītā 18. 55*)

② *nānyathā te 'khila-guro ghaṭeta karuṇātmanaḥ*
yas ta āśiṣa āśāste na sa bhṛtyaḥ sa vai vaṇik (*Śrīmad-Bhāgavatam 7. 10. 4*)

the Torah for its own sake.[1]

According to Vaiṣṇavas, genuine *bhakti* is accomplished by learning from qualified *bhaktas*, referred to in the *Bhagavad-gītā* as literally "seers of thatness," or "seers of the truth" (*tattva-darśinaḥ*) whose powers of spiritual understanding have been awakened by the favor of God:

> That very ancient science of the relationship with the Supreme (*yoga*) is today told by Me [Krishna] to you [Arjuna] because you are My devotee (*bhakta*) as well as My friend (*sakhā*) and can therefore understand the transcendental mystery (*uttamaṁ rahasyam*) of this science.[2]

These "seers of the truth" may not conform to the biblical concept of prophets as messengers chosen by God, but neither are they simply magicians or skilled priests mediating the petitions of favor-seekers. Considerable attention is given to the qualifications of a spiritual preceptor, especially in the *Pañcarātrika* literature which focuses on the ritual aspect of image worship. Most essential of these qualifications is that he must be fixed in knowledge of *brahman*, or the Absolute, as indicated by his freedom from material preoccupations. The *Śrīmad-Bhāgavatam* states,

> Therefore any person who seriously desires real happiness

---

① Twersky, 86-87 (Mishneh Torah 1, Repentance 10. 5). Contemporary Vaiṣṇavas might recognize in such expressions the idea of *bhakti* which they hold to be present to greater or lesser degrees in religious traditions throughout the world. Another potential topic for study of comparative theology would be to cull from Jewish sources such expressions comparable to Vaiṣṇava expressions of *bhakti*. The Song of Songs would be an obvious starting point.

② sa evāyaṁ mayā te 'dya yogaḥ proktaḥ purātanaḥ
bhakto 'si me sakhā ceti rahasyaṁ hy etad uttamam (*Bhagavad-gītā* 4. 3)

must seek a bona fide spiritual master (*guru*) and take shelter of him by initiation (*prapadyeta*). The qualification of the bona fide guru is that he has realized the conclusions of the scriptures by deliberation and is able to convince others of these conclusions. Such great personalities, who have taken shelter of the Supreme Godhead (*brahmany upaśamāśrayam*), leaving aside all material considerations, should be understood to be bona fide spiritual masters. ①

Concerning the moral dimension of interaction between *bhagavān* and other beings, we have already discussed this briefly in relation to the identity of Rādhā, the *pūrṇa-śakti*, or fully representative "consort" of God. Initially moral order is established in the Vedas, which in Vaiṣṇava theology have their origin in the "breathing" of *bhagavān*. Hence he is the author of the moral order as well as its sustainer, especially in his function as the inner controller of the *jīva*, as the "supersoul" (*paramātmā*). But he is also the originator and sustainer of the moral order (*dharma*) through his various *avatāras*. When God comes into conflict with demonic beings as one of his several *avatāras*, he may engage in "battles" with them, but he is never actually threatened by them since they are merely his servants specifically deputed to amuse him as viable fighting partners. ② Thus there is no "multiplicity of independent beings" in these pastimes. Rather than opposing and limiting the divine will, they participate in and enhance it.

---

① *tasmād guruṁ prapadyeta jijñāsuḥ śreya uttamam*
śabde pare ca niṣṇātaṁ brahmaṇy upaśamāśrayam (*Śrīmad-Bhāgavatam* 11. 3. 21).

② This theology of divine fighting entertainment is elaborated in the *Śrīmad-Bhāgavatam*, especially in relation to the conflict between Viṣṇu and the two demons Hiraṇyākṣa and Hiraṇyakaśipu. Such "demons" are essentially devotees who have been temporarily denied the memory of their devotional character in order to facilitate the *līlā* of fighting. They ultimately manifest the will of God, but as do all *jīvas*, they preserve minute independence. They are not simply shadows or reflections with no will of their own.

Finally, as a corollary to God's independence, the creation is, as a manifestation of *bhagavān*'s extraneous energy (*bahiraṅga-śakti*), subordinate to him; he is never under the control of primordial nature. Rather, he enters into the world as *avatāra* for the purpose of expanding his *līlā* and sustaining *dharma*. As for the *arcāvatāra*, the physical image, it is recognized that the image is composed of physical elements, which are subject to decay; however precisely because those elements are subordinate to *bhagavān*, it would be claimed, he can, by his will "enter into" (*pratiṣṭha*) that image to receive the worship of his devotees and reciprocate with them.[1]

The rhetoric which identifies "paganism" with "myth" is problematic in several ways, the analysis of which is not my topic. Suffice to say that to define myth simply as "imagination" and hence as "an untrue story" (as would be likely in a critique of "paganism") would make any use of the term by practitioners of Krishna-*bhakti* unlikely in relation to the revered sacred narratives in their scriptures. These scriptures do contain narratives which are explicitly to be understood in an allegorical sense, but in general there is not the concern to impose the critical eye of historical inquiry into scripture.[2] The interpretation of scripture is always from within a matrix of hermeneutics circumscribed by the tradition of teachers (*guru-paramparā*) for whom the purpose of scripture—the attainment of pure devotion to God (*prema-bhakti*)—is always to be maintained.

---

① The Vaiṣṇava and other Indian traditions deal with the problem of physical decay of images simply by repair or replacement: Through ritual procedure God is invited to reside temporarily in a vessel until repairs are completed, or a new image is prepared. In the case of the wooden images of Jagannātha, an elaborate procedure of "body renewal" (*nava-kalevaram*) takes place every twelve to fourteen years which involves a transfer of "*brahman as wood*" (*dharu-brahman*) from old to new images, after which the old images are ceremonially buied in the temple courtyard.

② This topic is related to the issue of how western scholars might go about studying the practice of image worship in India without improperly imposing western perspectives. See Bennet, *passim*.

IV. 4 Idolatry as Error and as Improper Practice

I have discussed Maimonides'concern about the superficial reading of scripture as leading to the making of images for worship (in Section IV. 2). Such improper action is, for Maimonides, the result of improper belief, consisting essentially of the philosophical, conceptual *error* of conceiving multiplicity and complexity in God. It is hardly to be expected that Maimonides, radical dualist that he is, would be impressed with arguments from the "qualified non-dualist" (*viśiṣṭādvaita-vādin*) or "inconceivable-identity-and-distinctionist" (*acintya-bhedābheda-vādin*) positions which identify the multiplicity of being which is the world more or less with the Being which is God. Since for him "perfection" is the essential nature of God, Maimonides demands utter austerity of pictorial and linguistic expression to preserve it. ①

The Vaiṣṇava *bhakti* theology (and Vaiṣṇava-*vedānta* philosophy) recognizes the necessity of upholding the perfection of God, but it is not troubled by the notion that his perfection would be compromised in the minds of humans by the imperfections of language or form. Rather, it holds to the need for keeping two notions in mind simultaneously—that God maintains aloofness from the world and simultaneous involvement with the world, as suggested in the *Bhagavad-gītā*, where Krishna says,

> By Me, in My unmanifested form (*avyakta-mūrti*), this entire universe is pervaded. All beings are in Me, but I am not in them. And yet everything that is created does not rest in Me. Behold My mystic opulence (*yogam aiśvaram*)! Although I am the maintainer of all living entities and although I am everywhere, I am not a part of this cosmic manifestation, for My Self is the very

① Halbertal and Margalit, 111.

source of creation.[1]

The perfection of God in the Vaiṣṇava *bhakti* tradition is preserved and expanded by encompassing the *apparent* imperfections of contingency: If having form and body is an imperfection, then Krishna confounds that conception with his body (*vigraha*)[2] of *sac-cid-ānanda* (eternity-cognition-bliss). If action in the world demonstrates imperfection, then Krishna confounds that conception by his *līlā*, as the "perfect" master, friend, son, or paramour. And if the attempt to describe God in terms of these features—all considered revelatory—is considered error, then the Krishna-*bhakta* will accept that "error" as the core of profound insight, the truth of the "universe of feeling" which is *bhakti*.[3]

Halbertal and Margalit note the contrast in approach between the philosophers such as Maimonides and the twelfth-century Jewish thinker and poet R. Judah Halevi (ca. 1075-1141). Maimonides'concern for

---

① *mayā tatam idaṁ sarvaṁ jagad avyakta-mūrtinā*
mat-sthāni sarva-bhūtāni na cāhaṁ teṣv avasthitaḥ
na ca mat-sthāni bhūtāni paśya me yogam aiśvaram
bhūta-bhṛn na ca bhūta-stho mamātmā bhūta-bhāvanaḥ (*Bhagavad-gītā* 9. 4-5).

② *Vigraha*: With the verbal root>*kṛ*, to do or make, *vigraha-kṛ* means 'to separate, i. e. individual form or shape, form, figure, the body'' (Monier-Williams). The *Brahmā-saṁhitā* describes Kṛṣṇa as *sac-cid-ānanda-vigraha*, "he whose form is eternal, cognizant and blissful."

③ Daniel Sheridon, writing on the *Śrīmad-Bhāgavatam*, notes a "special genius of India" visible in that work which, he says combines depth of intellectual discourse with heightened emotional resonance and exciting imagery. "The heightened emotion [aroused in the work] becomes essential for the understanding while understanding that does not evoke intense emotional responses can hardly be accepted as authentic insight." Daniel P. Sheridon, *The Advaitic Theism of the Bhāgavata Purāṇa*, (Delhi: Motilal Banarsidass, 1986), viii. Regarding "divine error," the *Śrīmad-Bhāgavatam* stresses repeatedly the failure of the most elevated souls, the associates of Kṛṣṇa in Vṛndāvana, to recognize the divinity of Kṛṣṇa, not because they are foolish, but because they are functioning under the influence of *yogamāyā*—God's energy through which *līlā* becomes possible. *Yogamāyā* is in contradistinction to *mahāmāyā*, God's energy by which the bound soul remains forgetful of its relationship to God.

error is replaced, for Halevi, with a concern for improper worship. The philosopher's concern is the proper *object* of worship (determined by philosophical reasoning); hence there is less concern for the proper *means* of worship. For Halevi it is the opposite. According to him, since for the Rabbinic Jewish tradition the object of worship is determined by tradition (according to the halakhah), the main concern is with establishing a model of proper worship "determined in general by the intention, sincerity, and seriousness of the worshiper." ① Halevi's conclusions in this regard, for better or worse, isolate Judaism over against the other biblical monotheistic traditions, which are all identified with the idolatrous religions due to departure from revelation as transmitted in Judaism. ②

The scriptural and oral tradition of Gauḍīya-Vaiṣṇava image worship has

① Halbertal and Margalit, 189.

② Halbertal and Margalit, 190.

detailed delineations of correct and incorrect worship of the *arcā-vigraha*.[1] As mentioned in Section Ⅱ. 1. 2, *arcanam* is one of nine overlapping categories of devotional practice listed in the *Śrīmad-Bhāgavatam*, all of which, as means of cultivating *bhakti* (as process—*abhidheya*), involve purposeful action with the senses and mind aimed at the satisfaction of God. *Arcanam* is the most formal of these, and thus Rūpa Gosvāmī (quoting Paurāṇic literature), lists not less than sixty-four "offenses" in worship (*sevā-*

---

[1] Many factors may be involved in determining what is correct and incorrect in *arcanam*, such that the proper application of rules becomes an art. Narottama Dās, an important eighteenth century Gauḍīya Vaiṣṇava poet, suggests a system of checks and balances consisting of scripture (*śāstra*), preceptor (*guru*), and association of practitioners (*sadhu*). The devotee's business is to find, using his or her own discriminating power, the proper way to proceed under the direction of these three guides and thus avoid the mistake referred to by Rūpa Gosvāmī as *niyamāgraha*—the imbalanced condition of either following rules for rules' sake or being neglectful of rules out of whimsy. A Vaiṣṇava might agree that the imbalanced situation of *niyamāgraha* would be a condition in which the worship of God becomes improper and therefore "idolatrous". Where this imbalance prevails, worship takes on the coloration of motivations other than service to God. The whole purpose becomes lost when the desire prevails to make God one's own servant rather than to make oneself into a fit servant of God. Therefore in the ongoing effort to find the proper balance regarding the regulations in *vaidhi-bhakti-sādhana*, there is an emphasis on caution whereby the mood of reverence is privileged over the assuming of more intimate moods of service (friendship, parenthood, paramourship). Thus, for example, while worshiping *mūrtis* of Rādhā-Kṛṣṇa, practitioners are advised to do so *as if* worshiping Lakṣmī-Nārāyaṇa. Lakṣmī-Nārāyaṇa are none other than Rādhā-Kṛṣṇa, but they are exhibiting the principle of lordly splendor in married conjugality rather than rustic charm in non-socially sanctioned conjugality. One might ask, why then would one not simply worship forms of Lakṣmī-Nārāyaṇa directly, rather than forms of Rādhā-Kṛṣṇa "as if" they are Lakṣmī-Nārāyaṇa. Gauḍīya Vaiṣṇavas would likely answer that they are followers of Caitanya Mahāprabhu, who specifically advented to teach the worship of Rādhā-Kṛṣṇa as the highest goal. In following Caitanya, they also find the basis of balanced worship in his emphasis on the chanting of the names of God, especially the Hare Kṛṣṇa *mahāmantra*, as the most essential activity in worship. In fact all the procedures of *arcanam* are understood to be secondary and supportive of the central activity of *harināma-saṁkīrtana*, the congregational chanting of the names of God before the *arcā-mūrti*. Caitanya demonstrated this way of worship during his residence in Jagannātha Purī, and his followers continue to observe this practice.

aparādha) [1] to be avoided when practicing *arcanam*. All of these offenses have to do with some lack—lack of purity, of respect, of endeavor, or of faith—which would be interpreted within the tradition as greater or lesser disregard for God's direct presence in the image. Most of the offenses listed are understandable analogously with potentially offensive behavior before a superior person in human society. Thus, for example, one is forbidden to be in an unclean condition in the presence of the deity; one should not display pride before the deity; one should not neglect to offer seasonal fruit to the deity, and so on. It is understood that all offenses can be avoided for the most part by controlling six urges of the senses—the urges of speech, mind, anger, tongue, belly and genitals. Offenses of this type are generally considered relatively serious, but they are easily corrected by sincere observances of prescribed penances. [2]

More serious than the above are *nāma-aparādha*, offenses in belief, attitude, words or practice in regard to the divine names of God, ten of which are delineated in the *Padma-purāṇa*. Since the name of God has an equivalency with God (*abhinnatva*) , negligence in the pronunciation or chanting of the name (*hari-nāma*) reflects on one's behavior in relation to God. Of these, the most serious offenses are three: disrespect (especially verbal, *ninda*) toward *bhaktas*; disobedience to the preceptor (*guru*) under whose guidance one is learning the practice of *bhakti*; and indulging

---

① *Aparādha*, lit. "offense, transgression, fault; mistake" (Monier-Williams) . Gauḍīya Vaiṣṇavas give an etymology which indicates its meaning to be "to be distanced from worship. " See Bhakti Promode Puri Goswami, *The Heart of Krishna*: *Vaishnava Aparadha & the Path of Spiritual Caution*, (San Francisco: Mandala Media, 1995) , 1.

② Both the Rabbinic Jewish and the Vaiṣṇava Hindu practitioners are operating under systems of rules. Yet we must acknowledge a difference in the nature of these rules by virtue of the difference in the type of revelation from which they stem. The Law of Torah, as the substance of the Covenant, differs in character from the rules (*vidhi-niṣedha*) of which we are dealing here, which are composed of "remembrance" (*smṛti*) of sages and saints honored in the tradition. There are quite severe warnings, in some cases, regarding consequences of making certain offenses in *arcanam* or in relation to the *arcā-mūrti*, especially regarding theft of items (such as jewelry) belonging to the deity.

in sinful practices or attitudes (*pāpa-buddhi*) with the idea that the sin will be counteracted by further meditation on the name. It is expected that the beginning practitioner will be subject to committing the *nāma-aparādhas*, for which the solution is to continue the practice of chanting-meditation while simultaneously cultivating a prayerful desire to become free from the offenses.

The most serious type of *aparādha* is *Vaiṣṇava-aparādha*, or the offending of a fellow practitioner of Krishna-*bhakti*, either with one's body, words, or mind. The only means of correcting such an offense is to beg forgiveness from the offended person, as it is warned that even God himself is not in a position to counteract the offense.[1]

We may notice in this progression from lesser to greater seriousness of offense a parallel progression of *proximity* of identity with God. Thus although there is a principle of identity between God and the image of God, a "greater identity" is acknowledged between God and his name, and "greatest identity" is acknowledged between God and his pure devotee.[2] As we may recall, Viṣṇu declares in *Śrīmad-Bhāgavatam* (9. 4. 68) that he considers the devotees to be his very heart. "My devotees do not know anything else but me, and I do not know anyone else but them."

All of the various types of offense mentioned here have to do with lack of respect in one form or another, and all are considered to stem from either simple ignorance of the nature of the object of respect and worship or refusal to appreciate that nature. The *Padma-purāṇa* summarizes the faulty attitude in this way:

> One who thinks the image of Viṣṇu to be made of stone (*śīla-dhīḥ*), who thinks of the spiritual preceptors as an ordinary man

---

① *Śrīmad-Bhāgavatam* 9. 4. 69-71. Puri Goswami Mahārāja, 13-18.

② This "greatest identity" is, however, not to be misconstrued as ontological identity, which would go utterly against the Vaiṣṇava recognition of the *jīva's* eternally distinct identity as servant of God.

(*guruṣu nara-matiḥ*), who thinks the Vaiṣṇava to belong to a certain caste or creed (*jāti-buddhiḥ*) or who thinks of the water which has bathed the image of Viṣṇu or the feet of the Vaiṣṇava, or Ganges water, as ordinary water (*ambu-buddhiḥ*), who considers the name of Viṣṇu or his *mantra*, although they are able to destroy the evil effects of the age of Kali, to be ordinary words (*śabda-sāmānya-buddhiḥ*), and who considers Viṣṇu to be equal (not superior) to his creation (*tad-itara-sama-dhīḥ*) —such a person is surely a resident of hell (*nārakī*) (*Padma-purāṇa*). [①]

A "resident of hell" is understood to be essentially one who is not progressing in the development of devotion to God despite the numerous opportunities afforded to do so by God's grace. As mentioned near the beginning of our discussion on idolatry, God's displeasure in response to repeated disregard of his guidance comes in its severest form as condemning the recalcitrant *jīva* to repeated birth in demonic species (*asura-yonim*). But the teachers of the tradition assure us that rather than punish, God is much more inclined to instruct through qualified practicing preceptors (*ācāryas*), and through *śāstra*, or revealed scripture. The practice of regular submissive

---

① *arcye viṣṇau śilā-dhīr guruṣu nara-matir vaiṣṇave jāti-buddhir*
viṣṇor vā vaiṣṇavānāṁ kali-mala-mathane pāda-tīrthe 'mbu-buddhiḥ
śrī-viṣṇor nāmni mantre sakala-kaluṣa-he śabda-sāmānya-buddhir
viṣṇau sarveśvareśe tad-itara-sama-dhīr yasya vā nārakī saḥ

Another severe warning about thinking of the arcā image as mere material elements comes from Pillai Lokācārya and Maṇavāla Māmunikal (14th century, of the Śrī Vaiṣṇava tradition) in the context of considering the birth or caste of a devotee. Vasudhā Nārāyanan writes that they warn, "[P] lacing importance on the caste of a devotee is as reprehensible as the questioning or analyzing the elements which compose the arcāvatāra. Both are as despicable and as vulgar as regarding the reproductive organ (yoni) of one's own mother as a common sex object." Vasudha Narayanan, "Arcāvatāra: On Earth as He Is in Heaven," in Gods of Flesh, Gods of Stone: The Embodiment of Divinity in India, Joanne Punzo Waghorne and Norman Cutler with Vasudha Narayanan, eds., (New York: Columbia University Press, 1996), 62.

hearing of revealed knowledge from proper sources is, for the Vaiṣṇava, the most essential practice to avoid deviation into improper worship.

In his interview with Bhaktisiddhānta Sarasvatī, Professor Suthers must have been surprised to hear his assertive response to the professor's suggestion that Vaiṣṇavas practice idolatry. Sarasvatī took the aggressive rather than defensive role, charging several classes of religionists, both Western and Indian, of being "idolaters," appropriating the biblical term to designate any person not engaged in the practice of *bhakti*:

> How can those, that have not in their heart Love of God which is the true function of the soul and is the science[①] of the true knowledge of realities, think of the *Śrī-Mūrtis* (*Śrī Vigrahas*) as other than idols? The deliberations of the Vaiṣṇava philosophy are very fine. These have shown by true scientific analysis that they are all, more or less, idolaters who declare themselves as partisans either of the doctrine of no Form of God or that of His material Form. Just as those who attribute God-ship to matter and worship it like the fire worshippers among the uncivilised people or the worshippers of the planets, such as Jupiter, Saturn, etc., of Greece, are crude idolaters, in a similar manner the others, who declare everything beyond matter as formless, and become exponents of the doctrine of non-distinction, are equal or even greater idolaters. The Henotheists or worshippers of one of the Vedic deities or the worshippers of the five deities (called *Panchopasakas*) worship imaginary icons, considering them God.

---

① "Science" is likely Sarasvatī's English rendering of '*vijñāna*', a term with a multiplicity of meanings in Sanskrit related to knowledge, wisdom, understanding, recognition, and discernment. I think here he means something like "properly applied wisdom," which would also suggest the Sanskrit term *prajñā*. "True scientific analysis," two lines later, suggests "analysis on the basis of accepted scriptural authority and accepted theologians."

According to them, God has no *sat-cit-ānanda-vigraha*, and as without some form there can be no subject for contemplation, to make it easy to meditate on Him, some form has got to be imagined. They are all idolaters. So also is the conduct of some of the yogis and others to be regarded as idolatry, who, for purifying their heart or improving the functions of the mind, imagine a God and perform practices of contemplation, etc. , of some imaginary form of His. Those who consider *jīvas* as God are the most blasphemous idolaters, because to imagine any worldly thing or form as God is idolatry.

> There is a world of difference between the worship of *Śrī-Mūrtis* as ordained by the Vaiṣṇava philosophy and the doctrines of God with Form and without Form of the other thinkers. Mahāprabhu Śrī Caitanya Deva has refuted all sorts of idolatry and instructed the service of the *Arcāvatāras* of the All-merciful God of Inscrutable Potency. ①

Thus the claim is that the possession of "Love of God" in the heart is the first qualification for determining what is proper and improper worship, and that "fine deliberations" make further discrimination thereof possible. Of course it is not the purpose of the Vaiṣṇavas to accuse others of being "idolaters," but to question the type of thinking which would condemn the worship of any image by anyone as idolatry, as well as to indicate that the Gauḍīya-Vaiṣṇavas would themselves not endorse all forms of image worship. Exactly to what extent differences in theologies of image worship would be visible in differing methods of worship (for example such as might not be endorsed by Gauḍīya Vaiṣṇavas) is a topic in itself which deserves investigation in another paper.

---

① Rūpa Vilāsa Dāsa, 94.

Conclusion

I have raised the questions at the beginning of this book, "In what sense, according to Gauḍīya-Vaiṣṇava theology, can an apparently inert material form be seen as divine and therefore venerable, and in what ways is this practice of *arcanam* considered a solution to the problem of approaching or being approached by the supreme Being in the Gauḍīya-Vaiṣṇava a tradition?" The question betrays a suspicion about worship in relation to tangible objects, a suspicion which finds its full expression in the biblical prohibition against the making and worship of images of any kind. The biblical prohibition is intrinsic to the biblical conception of monotheism: To worship the one Living God *means* above all, at least in terms of negative injunctions, to *not* worship images, either of the one God or of "other gods." In sharp contrast to the biblical tradition, Vaiṣṇavism in general, and Gauḍīya Vaiṣṇavism as a particular case, strongly encourages or even prescribes the worship of holy images of God, as an integral aspect of proper religious human behavior and spirituality. What is more, Vaiṣṇavas (of all sects) consider themselves to be also monotheistic, although certainly their conception of "monotheism" is radically different from that of Near Eastern religions. One might well conclude that the term "idolatry" in reference to this tradition would not be a very accurate or descriptive term for what is going on. In this book the attempt is to offer an alternative description, allowing the scriptures of the tradition to speak on behalf of those who dedicate themselves to this practice.

Much as Judaism is a religion of scripture, so also is Gauḍīya Vaiṣṇavism a scriptually oriented tradition. [①] I have tried to call attention to some portions of the scriptural basis for the worship of Krishna and show thereby that it is by no means an unreflective practice, or a case of naive confusion of categories. Rather it has reference to a systematic theology which is a solution to the problem of God's supremacy and consequent apparent inaccessibility. This theology takes into account the nature of materially embodied existence on the one side and the omnipotent nature of God on the other.

As the worship of the *arcā-mūrti* is not unreflective or naive, it is also not whimsical or amoral in its practice. Rather the worship of Krishna is strictly regulated by scriptural injunctions, *guru's* instructions, and tradition which aim always to maintain purity and propriety as necessary prerequisites allowing genuine devotional interaction with the Deity to occur. [②]

We can also see that Gauḍīya Vaiṣṇava worship is, in its practice, a solution to human imperfection which affirms the potential for human beings to act and experience on a platform of devotional perfection, allowing one to transcend the limitations imposed by bodily existence. *Bhakti* is the via media of contact by which the *bhakta* is allowed to enter into the "universe of feelings" where Krishna reigns as reservoir of spiritual emotion, or *rasa*. In Gauḍīya Vaiṣṇavism, this takes place specifically at a stage of development of *bhakti* known as *bhāva*. The dualities under which bodily existence is normally conducted are superseded by *darśana*, or divine vision, whereby

① This is not to ignore the vast differences in the way scripture is conceived in both traditions, beginning with the Jewish emphasis on the written text versus the Indic attention to the spoken or chanted text. See Barbara A, Holdrege, *Veda and Torah: Transcending the Textuality of Scripture*, (Albany: State University of New York Press, 1996). There is important similarity simply in that both traditions identify themselves largely in terms of their respective scriptures, which hold positions of some kind of absolute authority.

② The Six Gosvāmīs of Vṛndāvana put particular emphasis on scriptural authority in this regard, possibly in response to perceived improprieties at the time. Rūpa Gosvāmī warns in *Bhakti-rasāmṛta-sindhu* (1. 2. 101) that devotional service which does not conform to the injunctions of all the various canonical scriptures (*śruti-smṛti-purāṇādi pañcarātra-vidhim*) is simple a public calamity (*utpāta eva*), a disturbance of social order.

God and his name, God and his image, as well as God and his description are experienced as non-different from each other. ①

Biblical polemic against image worship often dwelled on the seeming deadness, inactivity, and helplessness of the images worshipped. We might ask, what does Krishna as *arcā-mūrti* actually *do*? Vaiṣṇavas would answer first that in fact it is *he* who is ultimately doing everything, including giving us the mental ability to ask this question. The *arcā-mūrti* is one of several means by which God bestows grace to conditioned souls. As such it belongs to the category of *avatāras*. In general *avatāras*, or divine descents, do several things. First, they make God accessible to bound souls (making it possible for them to transcend the bondage of action [*karma-bandhana*]); second, they execute divine justice (especially punishing the wicked [*duṣkṛti-nāśana*], thereby releasing them also from the bondage of action); third, they re-establish obscured or lost religious principles (*dharma-saṁsthāpana*), the central principle being the necessity to offer oneself to God (*Krishna-samarpanam*). In the original form of Krishna God descends additionally to *attract* bound souls, awakening their innate devotion, through his divine name, form, qualities, pastimes and associates. Also, as *arcā-mūrti* Krishna accepts devotional offerings (of food, flowers, wealth, cloth, or prayers), and reciprocates by bestowing "remnants" (*nirmālya*) of those offerings as his *prasāda*, or mercy. He thus makes possible the practical application of his injunction (*Bhagavad-gītā* 9. 34) to fix one's mind on him, worship him, and offer obeisances to him.

---

① William Deadwyler explains that this identity between word and object "constitutes an immediacy of apprehension for which the term *literal* hardly serves," whereby it becomes possible to consider the literal meaning of terms as valid *only* when they apply to God. "Our worldly experience does not reveal to us the literal meaning. God and the kingdom of God, after all, constitute the real and original world, while this world is its imitation and reflection. Yet God is able to manifest himself within this world in the form of words and images, and by concentrating one's mind and senses on the words that describe God and on the images that depict God, the mind and senses gradually become purified, and then one can at last apprehend the literal meaning" (Deadwyler, 86-87).

Still, one might argue, the *arcā-mūrti* is obviously not *doing* anything in the sense of moving or speaking. Vaiṣṇavas would likely respond that indeed this form of *avatāra*, while the most accessible to bound souls, *seems* to be the least active so that the devotee is given opportunity to take on the active role by rendering all types of services with his or her body, mind and senses. In this active role one is engaging in the "serious play" of being hospitable to God, subordinating one's own desires to his wishes. The aim is to be constantly engaged (rather than to become inactive as classical monistic schools advocated), for, as noted in our discussion of *bhakti*, service must be unmotivated and uninterrupted in order to completely satisfy the self. Through such constant engagement the *bhakta* experiences increasingly the primary agency of God, in relation to whom one is a secondary actor.

In this undertaking of acting on behalf of Krishna, the *practice* of *bhakti* manifests its transformative character, whereby everything *ordinary* which is involved in the practice becomes redefined in terms of service to Krishna (*Krishna-sevā*) thus becoming *extraordinary.*[①] Within *arcanam* ritual, the place of worship, the objects offered in worship, the utensils and language used, one's own senses and mind—all are transformed into spirit (*cit-śakti*) in order to facilitate the transformation of the worshipper into a *śuddha-bhakta*, a pure devotee of God. As practice (or rehearsal) transforms into perfection, action becomes performance, and the place of performance (a Krishna temple) becomes not an ordinary place, but Vraja, the extraordinary land of Krishna where "The trees are wish-fulfilling trees, the land is made of touchstone, the water is nectar, words are musical vibrations, and all movements are dancing."[②] It is in Vraja that the confines

---

① As suggested in a previously quoted verse from *Padma Purāṇa*, even the water which has bathed the image is afterward served as *caraṇāmṛta*, or the "ambrosia from the feet of God". What is insignificant in this world becomes most significant and sanctifying in the transcendent realm.

② *Brahma-saṁhitā 5. 56.*

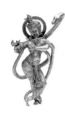

of linear time are overcome [1] as one becomes adept at participating in God's perpetually variegated, ever fresh pastimes of love.

From this presentation one could suspect that the process of *arcanam* in Gauḍīya Vaiṣṇavism is a highly individual enterprise, with little or no reference to a community or society. In fact it is quite the opposite case in the tradition following Caitanya, for whom congregational worship was of central importance. Through the practice of *harināma mantra* chanting Caitanya is credited with having "plundered the storehouse of love of God" [2] together with his most intimate associates Nityānanda, Advaita, Gadadhāra, Srivāsa and others. By accepting as qualified *bhaktas* persons from lower castes, infusing those he met with ecstatic love of Krishna, he is celebrated for having made available to the world what was previously the property of a very few, transforming the world itself rather than merely some isolated individuals.

The fact that this practice of image worship is going on in temples outside India, among westerners perhaps less familiar with the cultural context in which *arcanam* flourishes in India, could provoke the question, what role does this theology of image worship as delineated by the tradition's theologians actually play in the practice as found in these new situations? The answer would of course be a study in itself, with attention perhaps more on sociology than theology. It is my own hope both that persons engaged in the practice will be well informed in the theology of the tradition as much as the practices, and that other persons encountering the practices of Krishna-*bhakti* may become sufficiently informed about the theology behind the practice of worshipping the *arcā-mūrti* of Krishna.

This hope for an informed observance of Krishna-*sevā* as well as an

---

① The Gauḍīya Vaiṣṇava theologians have articulated an elaborate doctrine of equivalency between the earthly Vraja identifiable in present-day India and a celestial Vraja, also known as Goloka or Goloka-Vṛndāvana, whereby the earthly Vraja can yield direct access to the celestial Vraja for one who is properly qualified by a pure heart.

② *Caitanya-caritāmṛta* Ādi-līlā 7. 20-21.

informed practice of Krishna-*sevā* suggests my further hope—that the subject of this book might develop into a topic of interfaith dialogue, not only between practitioners of Vaiṣṇavism and of Judaism, but also between the former and practitioners of Christian and Islamic faiths, both of which have dealt in different ways with the issues raised here. Such discussion, in turn, might generate additional useful work in comparative theology of the worship of images (particularly, I am thinking, in regard to the tradition of icon veneration in Orthodox Christianity) which would be helpful for the Vaiṣṇava communities to promote better self-understanding, out of which more meaningful communication with members of other religious communities could take place.

This thesis is but an attempt to sketch a few contours of a topic which has yet to be filled in with the rich and subtle colors of more qualified devotion and scholarship to make fully accessible the presence which is the *arcanam* process of Krishna-*bhakti*.

It is hope that it will serve a purpose in generating further discussion.

Works Consulted

Babb, Lawrence A. *Absent Lord: Ascetics and Kings in a Jain Ritual Culture.* Berkeley: University of California Press, 1996.

Banerjea, Jitendra Nath. *The Development of Hindu Iconography.* Delhi: Munshiram Manoharlal, 1974.

Beck, Guy L. "Sonic Theology." in *Vaiṣṇavism: Contemporary Scholars Discuss the Gauḍīya Tradition.* Edited by Rosen, Steven. New York: FOLK Books, 1992.

__________. *Sonic Theology: Hinduism and Sacred Sound.* Delhi: Motilal Banarsidass, 1995.

__________. "Churning the Global Ocean of Nectar: The Devotional Music of Srila Prabhupāda." *Journal of Vaiṣṇava Studies* vol. 6 no. 2 (Spring 1998).

Bennet, Peter. "Krishna's Own Form: Image Worship and Puṣṭi Mārga." *Journal of Vaiṣṇava Studies* vol. 1 no. 4 (Summer 1993).

Bhaktivedānta Swami Prabhupāda, A. C. *Bhagavad-gītā As It Is*, Second Edition. Los Angeles: Bhaktivedanta Book Trust, 1990.

__________. Complete Works. Bhaktivedānta Vedabase CD-ROM. Sandy Ridge, NC: The Bhaktivedanta Archives, 1998.

Bhaktivedānta Swami Prabhupāda, trans., & Svāmī, Acyutānanda; Jayaśacinandana. *Songs of the Vaiṣṇava Ācāryas.* Los Angeles: Bhaktivedanta Book Trust, 1979.

Bhaktivinoda, Kedarnath Datta. *Sri Chaitanya Shikshamrtam.* Translation from Bengali. Madras: Śrī Gauḍīya Math, 1983.

Brzezinski, Jan. "Does Krishna Marry the Gopīs in the End?" *Journal of Vaiṣṇava Studies* vol. 5 no. 4 (Fall 1997) .

Carman, John B. *Majesty and Meekness: A Comparative Study of Contrast and Harmony in the Concept of God.* Grand Rapids, Michigan: Eerdmans Publishing, 1994.

Chari, Srinivasa S. M. *Vaiṣṇavism: Its Philosophy, Theology and Religious Discipline.* Delhi: Motilal Banarsidass, 1994.

Clooney, Francis X. , S. J. *Seeing Through Texts: Doing Theology among the Śrī Vaiṣṇavas of South India.* Albany, N. Y: State University of New York Press, 1996.

__________. *Theology After Vedānta: An Experiment in Comparative Theology.* Albany, N. Y: State University of New York Press, 1993.

Daniel, E. Valentine. *Fluid Signs: Being a Person the Tamil Way.* Berkeley: University of California Press, 1984.

Das, Rahul Peter. *Essays on Vaiṣṇavism in Bengal.* Calcutta: Firma KLM, 1997.

Dāsa, Dayānanda, & Dāsī, Nandarāṇī Devī. "Baladeva Vidyābhūṣaṇa: The Gauḍīya Vedāntist. "*Back to Godhead*, (January-February 1991) : 30-34 (Part I) , & (March-April 1991) : 22-26, 32 (Part II) .

Dasa, Hayagriva. *The Hare Krishna Explosion: The Birth of Krishna Consciousness in America (1966-1996)* . Palace Press, 1985.

Dāsa, Krishna-kṣetra, ed. *Pañcarātra-pradīpa: Illumination of Pañcarātra. Supplement to Volume One, Daily Service.* GBC Deity Worship Group. Mayapur, India: ISKCON-GBC Press, 1995.

Dāsa, Rūpa Vilāsa (Robert D. MacNaughton) . *A Ray of Vishnu— The Biography of a Śaktyāveṣa ṇvatāra: Śrī Śrīmad Bhaktisiddhānta Sarasvatī Gosvāmī Mahārāja Prabhupāda.* Washington, Mississippi: New Jaipur Press, 1988.

Dāsa, Śrī Satya Nārāyaṇa, trans. , and Kundalī Dāsa. *Śrī Tattva-Sandarbha* of Śrīla Jīva Gosvāmī Prabhupāda. Delhi: Jiva Institute for Vaiṣṇava Studies, 1995.

Dāsa, Sadāpūta. "Rational 'Mythology' : Can a rational person accept the stories of the Purāṇas as literally true? " (A lecture presented at the Parliament of the World's Religions, Chicago, 1993) *Back to Godhead* (Jan/Feb 1994): 22-31.

Davis, Richard H. *Images, Miracles and Authority in Asian Religious Traditions*. Boulder, CO: Westview Press, 1998.

__________. *Ritual in an Oscillating Universe: Worshiping Śiva in Medieval India*. Princeton, New Jersey: Princeton University Press, 1991.

De, Sushil Kumar. *Early History of the Vaiṣṇava Faith and Movement in Bengal*. Calcutta: Firma KLM, 1986.

Deadwyler, William H. "The Devotee and the Deity: Living a Personalistic Theology. " In *Gods of Flesh, Gods of Stone: The Embodiment of Divinity in India*. Edited by Joanne Punzo Waghorne and Norman Cutler. New York: Columbia University Press, 1996.

Delmonico, Neal. "Rādhā: The Quintessential Gopī. " *Journal of Vaiṣṇava Studies* vol. 5 no. 4 (Fall 1997).

Dube, Manju. *Conceptions of God in Vaiṣṇava Philosophical Systems*. Varanasi: Sanjay Book Centre, 1984.

Eck, Diana. *Darśan: Seeing the Divine Image in India*. Chambersberg, PA: Anima Publications, 1985.

Eliade, Mircea. *Yoga: Immortality and Freedom*. Princeton, NJ: Princeton University Press, 1969.

Entwistle, A. W. *Braj, Centre of Krishna Pilgrimage*. Groningen: Egbert Forsten, 1987.

Gambhirananda, Swami, trans. *Brahma-Sūtra-Bhāṣya of Śrī Śaṅkarācārya*. Calcutta: Advaita Ashrama, 1965.

Gelberg, Steven J. "Vrindaban as Locus of Mystical Experience. "*Journal of Vaiṣṇava Studies* vol. 1 no. 1 (Fall, 1992).

Griffiths, Paul J. *On Being Buddha: The Classical Doctrine of Buddhahood*. Albany, NY: State University of New York Press, 1994.

Gupta, Sanjukta. "The Pāñcarātra Attitude to Mantra. "In *Mantra*, Harvey P. Alper, ed. Albany: State University of New York Press, 1988.

Haberman, David L. *Acting as a Way of Salvation: A Study of Rāgānugā Bhakti Sādhana*. New York: Oxford University Press, 1988.

__________. *Journey Through the Twelve Forests: An Encounter with Krishna*. New York: Oxford University Press, 1994.

Halbertal, Mosche, and Margalit, Avishai. *Idolatry*. Translated by Naomi Goldblum. Cambridge, MA: Harvard University Press, 1992.

Hardy, Friedhelm. "Mādhavendra Purī: A Link Between Bengal Vaiṣṇavism and South Indian *Bhakti*." *Journal of the Royal Asiatic Society of Great Britain and Ireland* (1974).

Hawley, John Stratton (with Shrivatsa Goswami). *At Play with Krishna: Pilgrimage Dramas from Brindavan*. Princeton, New Jersey: Princeton University Press, 1981.

Holdrege, Barbara A. *Veda And Torah: Transcending the Textuality of Scripture*. Albany, NY: State University of New York Press, 1996.

Hospital, Clifford. "Līlā in Early Vaiṣṇava Thought." In *Gods at Play: Līlā in South Asia*. William S. Sax, ed. New York: Oxford University Press, 1995.

Jaiswal, Suvira. *The Origin and Development of Vaiṣṇavism: Vaiṣṇavism from 200 BC to AD 500*. Delhi: Munshiram Manoharlal, 1981.

Judah, J. Stillson. *Hare Krishna and the Counterculture*. A Wiley-Interscience Publication. New York: Wiley, 1974.

Kapoor, O. B. L. *The Philosophy and Religion of Śrī Caitanya (The Philosophical background of the Hare Krishna Movement)*. Delhi: Munshiram Manoharlal, 1977.

Kaufmann, Yehezkel. *The Religion of Israel—From Its Beginnings to the Babylonian Exile*. Translated by Moshe Greenberg. Chicago: University of Chicago Press, 1966.

Keck, Leander E., editor. *The New Interpreter's Bible Commentary*, 10 volumes. Nashville: Abingdon Press, 2015.

Kellner, Menachem. *Maimonides on Humna Perfection*. Atlanta, Georgia: Scholars Press 1990.

Kinsley, David R. *Hindu Goddesses: Visions of the Divine Feminine in the Hindu Religious Tradition*. Berkeley: University of California Press, 1988.

__________. *The Sword and the Flute: Kālī and Krishna, Dark Visions of the Terrible and the Sublime in Hindu Mythology*. Berkeley: University of California Press, 1975.

Klostermaier, Klaus K. *Mythologies and Philosophies of Salvation in the Theistic Traditions of India*. Canadian Corporation for Studies in Religion. Waterloo, Ontario: Wilfred Laurier University Press, 1984.

__________. "A Universe of Feelings." In *Shri Krishna Caitanya and the Bhakti Religion*. Studia Irenica 33. Edited by Edmund Weber/Tilak Raj Copra. Frankfurt am Main: Peter Lang, 1988.

Mahārāj, Tridaṇḍī Swāmī Bhakti Hṛdaya Bon. *Śrī Rūpa Gosvāmī's Bhakti-rasāmṛta-sindhuḥ*. Vol I. Vrindaban, U. P., India: Institute of Oriental Philosophy, 1965.

Maimonides, Moses. *The Guide for the Perplexed*. Translated by M. Friedlaender. New York: George Routledge & Sons, 1947.

Majumdar, A. K. *Caitanya, His Life and Doctrine: A Study in Vaiṣṇavism*. Chowpatty, Bombay: Bharatiya Vidya Bhavan, 1969.

Marglin, Frederique. "Jagannātha Purī." In *Vaiṣṇavism: Contemporary Scholars Discuss the Gauḍīya Tradition*. Edited by Steven J. Rosen. New York: FOLK Books, 1992.

Maxwell, T. S. *Gods of Asia: Image, Text, and Meaning*. Delhi: Oxford University Press, 1997.

McDaniel, June. *The Madness of the Saints: Ecstatic Religion in Bengal*. Chicago: University of Chicago Press, 1989.

Mohanty, Jitendra Nath. *Reason and Tradition in Indian Thought: An Essay on the Nature of Indian Philosophical Thinking*. Oxford: Clarendon Press, 1992.

Mohapatra, Gopinath. *Jagannātha in History & Religious Traditions of Orissa*. Orissan Studies Project No. 13. Calcutta: Punthi Pustak, 1982.

Monier-Williams, Sir Monier. *A Sanskrit-English Dictionary*, New Edition. Oxford: Clarendon Press, 1899 (reprint, 1960).

Narang, Sudesh. *The Vaiṣṇava Philosophy According to Baladeva Vidyābhūṣaṇa*. Delhi: Nag Publishers, 1984.

Narayanan, Vasudha. "Arcāvatāra: On Earth as He Is in Heaven." In *Gods of Flesh, Gods of Stone: The Embodiment of Divinity in India*. Edited by Joanne Punzo Waghorne and Norman Cutler with Vasudha Narayanan. New York: Columbia University Press, 1996.

Neevel, Walter G., Jr. *Yamuna's Vedānta and Pāñcarātra: Integrating the Classical and the Popular*. Harvard Theological Review/Harvard Dissertations in Religion Number 10. Edited by C. Bynum & G. Rupp. Missoula, Montana: Scholars Press, 1977.

Neville, Robert Cummings, *The Truth of Broken Symbols*. Albany, N. Y: State University of New York Press, 1996.

O'Connell, Joseph. "Sādhana Bhakti," In *Vaiṣṇavism: Contemporary Scholars Discuss the Gauḍīya Tradition*. Edited by Rosen, Steven. New York: FOLK Books, 1992.

Pandeya, Rajendra P. "The Vision of the Vedic Seer." in *Hindu Spirituality*. Sivaraman, ed. New York: Crossroad, 1989.

Prasannabhai, Fr. "Jesus the Arati Personified—the Eucharist as our Mahā-ārati." *Vidyajyoti Journal of Theological Reflection* 60 (1997).

Puri Goswami Maharaja, Bhakti Promode. *The Heart of Krishna: Vaishnava Aparadha & the Path of Spiritual Caution*. San Francisco: Mandala Media, 1995.

Sagar, Tridandi Bhiksu Sri Bhakti Ananda, trans. *Śrī Brahma-saṁhitā: Quintessence of Reality the Beautiful*. Navadwip, W. B., India: Śrī Chaitanya Sāraswat Maṭh, 1992.

Schweig, Graham M, trans. "The Bhakti Sūtras of Nārada: The Concise Teachings of Nārada on the Nature and Experience of Devotion." *Journal of Vaiṣṇava Studies* vol 6 no. 1 (Winter 1998).

__________. "Universal and Confidential Love of God: Two Essential

Themes in Prabhupāda's Theology of *Bhakti*." *Journal of Vaiṣṇava Studies* vol. 6 no. 2 (Spring 1998).

Sharma, Krishna. *Bhakti and the Bhakti Movement: A New Perspective—A Study in the History of Ideas*. Delhi: Munshiram Manoharlal, 1987.

Sheridon, Daniel P. *The Advaitic Theism of the Bhāgavata Purāṇa*. Delhi: Motilal Banarsidass, 1986.

Siddhantashastree, Rabindra Kumar. *Vaiṣṇavism Through the Ages*. Delhi: Munshiram Manoharlal, 1985.

Sivaraman, Krishna, ed. *Hindu Spirituality: Vedas through Vedanta*. Volume 6 of World Spirituality: An Encyclopedic History of the Religious Quest. New York: Crossroad, 1989.

Smith, Jonathan Z. "Religion, Religions, Religious."in *Critical Terms for Religious Studies*. Edited by Mark C. Taylor. Chicago: University of Chicago Press, 1998.

Taylor, Mark C., ed. *Critical Terms for Religious Studies*. Chicago: University of Chicago Press, 1998.

The New Interpreter's Bible in Twelve Volumes. vol. 5. Nashville, Abingdon Press, 1997.

Thākur, Srila Sachidānanda Bhakti Vinode, *Shri Chaitanya Shikshāmritam*. Translated by Sri Bijoy Krishna Rarhi. Madras: Sri Gaudiya Math, 1983.

Toomey, Paul M. *Food from the Mouth of Krishna: Feasts and Festivals in a North Indian Pilgrimage Center*. Delhi: Hindustan Publishing Corp., 1994.

Tripurari, Swami B. V. *Aesthetic Vedānta: The Sacred Path of Passionate Love*. Eugene, Oregon: Mandala Publishing Group, 1998.

Twersky, Isadore. *A Maimonides Reader*. Library of Jewish Studies, ed. Neal Kozodoy. West Orange, N. J: Behrman House, 1972.

Valpey, Kenneth R. "Arcana—der Yoga der Gauḍīya Vaiṣṇavas." *Tattva-viveka* 5 (German) (Oktober 1996).

Ward, J. S. Keith. *Images of Eternity: Concepts of God in Five Religious Traditions*. London: Darton, Longman and Todd, 1987.

Zimmer, Heinrich. *Artistic Form and Yoga in the Sacred Images of India*.

trans. Gerald Chapple and James B. Lawson. Princeton, New Jersey: Princeton Unversity Press, 1990.

The following works quoted in the text have been accessed through the Bhaktivedanta Vedabase CD-ROM (see above) :

Brahma-saṁhitā. Translation and purports by Bhaktisiddhānta Sarasvatī Goswami Thākura.

Bhagavad-gītā of Krishna-Dvaipāyana-Vyāsa. Translation and Purports by A. C. Bhaktivedānta Swami Prabhupāda.

Caitanya-caritāmṛta by Krishnadās Kavirāja. Translation and Purports by A. C. Bhaktivedānta Swami Prabhupāda.

Nectar of Devotion, (summary study of *Bhakti-rasāmṛta-sindhu* of Rūpa Gosvāmī) . by A. C. Bhaktivedānta Swami Prabhupāda.

Nectar of Instruction (*Upadeśāmṛta* of Rūpa Gosvāmī) . Translation and Purports by A. C. Bhaktivedānta Swami Prabhupāda.

Śrīmad-Bhāgavatam of Krishna-Dvaipāyana-Vyāsa. Translation and Purports by A. C. Bhaktivedānta Swami Prabhupāda.

The Science of Self-Realization. Lectures and Conversations of A. C. Bhaktivedānta Swami Prabhupāda.

Sanskrit Texts

Śrī Bhakti Sandarbhaḥ of Śrīla Śrī Jīva Gosvāmī Prabhupāda. Edited by Śrī Haridāsa Śāstri. Vṛndāvan, India: Sad-Grantha-Prakāśaka, 1984.

Viṣṇu Purāṇa of Vedavyāsa. Edited by Sītarāmadās Oṁkaranāth. Calcutta: Satya-dharma-pracāra-saṅgaḥ, ND.

Śrīmad Bhāgavata Mahāpurāṇam of Vedavyāsa. Edited by Krishna-śaṅkara Śāstrī. Ahmedabad, India: Bhāgavata Vidyāpītha, 1968.

词表（Vocabulay）

–A–

Abhidheya—process，方法、程序。

abhigamana—acts preparatory to approaching God for worship，为崇拜神像而做的准备活动。

ācārya—qualified practicing preceptors，以身作则的资深导师。

acintya-bhedābheda-tattva-vāda—inconceivable simultaneous oneness and difference of the one supreme Being in relation to the multiplicity of being，不可思议即一即异论，或称不可思议不一不异论。最高存在与多样性的生物之间不可思议地既同一又有差异。

acintya-śakti—inconceivable energy of God，神不可思议的能量。

ādi-rasa—original or most fundamental rasa，最原始的、最基础的茹阿萨。

advaita—monist，不二一元论者。

advaya-jñāna-tattva—truth of non-dual gnosis，非二元灵知的真理。

advaya-rasa-tattva—truth of non-dual feeling，非二元情感的真理。

ahaitukī—unmotivated，不含动机。

amṛta—nectar，甘露。

ānanda—bliss，妙乐，极乐，喜乐。

antaryāmin—dweller in the heart，内心的居住者。

anugraha—favor of God，神的恩典。

anukūlya—favorable，顺意的。

ānukūlyena kṛṣṇānuśīlana—repeated and devoted service to Krishna which is ‘ according to the current,’ i. e. favorable to Krishna，为克里希纳做顺意的、重复不断的、具有献身精神的服务。

apratihatā—uninterrupted，不受打扰的、连续不断的。

Arcanam—formal veneration of divine images，正式的神像崇拜。

Arcāvatāra—the worshipable physical image，可以用来崇拜的物化形象，神像。又作 *arcā-vigraha*。

Arjuna—Krishna's companion，阿周那，或称阿尔诸纳。克里希纳的朋友。

ārati—阿尔提仪式，崇拜神像时的吉祥灯仪。

arcā-vigraha—sacred image，神像。

āśrama—orders of life，人生阶段；religious community，宗教社区。

aṣṭāṅga-yoga—eight-fold system，八部瑜伽，旨在领悟最高我。

asura-bhāva—demonic quality，阿修罗－巴瓦。恶魔品性。

asura-yonim—demonic species，恶魔种族。

ātīthi-sevā—reception and service to guests，接待和服务客人。

āsakti—a strong，unshakable attachment to God，对神的依恋之情，强烈而不可动摇。

ātmā—spirit self，阿特玛。灵性本我。

ātma-nivedanam—surrendering oneself fully to God，完全向神臣服皈依。

avāhana—calling God down，呼唤神降临。

avatāra—divine descent，阿瓦塔、阿凡达。化身、神圣降临。

avatārin—source of all *avatāras*，所有化身的源头，即克里希纳。

avidyā—ignorance，愚昧无知。

avyakta-mūrti—unmanifested form，克里希纳未展示的身相。

–B–

bahirāṅga-śakti—extraneous power，外在能量。

Baladeva—Krishna's elder brother，巴拉提婆，或称巴拉戴瓦、巴拉罗摩、巴拉茹阿玛。克里希纳的哥哥。在佳甘纳特·普瑞供奉着他的特别形象。

Baladeva Vidyābhuṣaṇa—巴拉提婆·维迪亚布善。高迪亚－外士那瓦学者。

Bhadra-Kālī—帕德拉－卡利女神。

bhāgavata—薄伽梵派。

bhāgavata-mārga—薄伽梵派之道，文中简称为“薄伽梵道”。强调三种实践活动，即学习和教授《薄伽梵往世书》及相关经典著作，齐颂克里希纳圣名，为外士那瓦（Vaiṣṇavas，克里希纳的虔爱者）服务。

Bhāgavata-purāṇa—*Śrīmad-Bhāgavatam*，《薄伽梵往世书》，又作《圣典薄伽瓦谭》。

bhagavān—

• the supreme Person，薄伽梵，神，至高无上的人，被认为是最高我与梵的绝对源头。

• supreme possessor of opulences，一切富裕的最高拥有者。

bhakta—devotee，巴克塔。虔信者、虔爱者、奉献者、信徒。

bhakti—devotion or devotional service to bhagavān，巴克提。虔信、虔爱、信爱、奉爱；对薄伽梵的奉爱服务。特指对克里希纳或他众多形象之一的虔信与奉爱。其宗旨只有一个：取悦克里希纳。

Bhakti-rasāmṛta-sindhu—*The Ocean of the Nectarean Taste of Devotion*，《奉爱甘露之洋》，茹帕·哥斯瓦米所著，是高迪亚－外士那瓦社团中最重要的神学著作之一。

bhakti-yoga—yoga of devotion，巴克提瑜伽。虔信瑜伽、虔爱瑜伽、奉爱瑜伽。

bhāva—transcendent emotion，超然的情感。

bheda nāhi—no difference，no non-identity，没有差别，不异。

brahma-bhūta—a self-realized soul，觉悟了自我的灵魂。

brahman—Absolute Being，绝对存在，梵。

brahma-muhūrta—one-and-a-half hours before sunrise，太阳升起前的一个半小时，这时外士那瓦立即起床，从身、心两方面做好准备以接近神，开

始每天的服务。

Brahma-sūtra—the most important commentary on the Upaniṣads，《 梵经》，即《奥义书》最重要的评注。

–C–

Caitanya—Śrī Krishna Caitanya Mahāprabhu，柴坦尼亚，即室利·克里希纳·柴坦尼亚·摩诃帕布（1486—1533），印度圣哲，哈瑞－克里希纳摩诃曼陀罗的倡导者。

Caitanya-caritāmṛta—Krishnadās Kavirāja's biography of Caitanya，《柴坦尼亚查瑞塔密瑞塔》，即《柴坦尼亚生平甘露》，又名《永恒的柴坦尼亚经》。克里希纳达斯·卡维罗阇撰写的柴坦尼亚传记。

cit—consciousness，知觉，意识。

–D–

darśana—sight，divine vision，达善。见、神视。

dāsyam—literally“ servitude ”，or participating in the mission of God，字面意思为“侍奉”，即参与神的使命。

devatās—administrative cosmic beings，负责宇宙事务的诸天神。

dhāma-sevā—service to sacred places associated with God，服务与神有关的圣地。

dharma—religious principles，达摩、法、宗教原则。

dhyāna—meditation，冥想。

dvaita—dualism，二元论。

dvija—twice-born，二次出生；再生者。

–G–

Gauḍīya Vaiṣṇava—高迪亚－外士那瓦。亦称为毗湿奴教派孟加拉支派，或毗湿奴教派柴坦尼亚支派。

Gauḍīya Vaiṣṇavas—高迪亚－外士那瓦们，柴坦尼亚派信徒。

Gopāla—哥帕拉。克里希纳的另一名字。

Gopāla Bhaṭṭa Gosvāmī—哥帕拉·巴塔·哥斯瓦米。南印度婆罗门，著有《哈瑞奉爱之美》，为毗湿奴派仪轨汇编。

gopīs—milkmaids，哥琵。牧牛姑娘。协助茹阿达，在布阿佳，参与克里希纳恋爱的逍遥时光，以此取悦克里希纳。

Gopīnātha—哥琵纳塔。克里希纳又一个名字。意为“牧牛姑娘的主人”。

Govardhana—哥瓦尔丹山。

Govinda—another name of Krishna，哥文达。克里希纳的又一名字。

guṇa-avatāras—three *guṇa-avatāras* Brahmā，Viṣṇu，and Śiva，三个属性（三德）化身——梵天、毗湿奴、湿婆，促成第二级创造、维系和毁灭。

guru—spiritual preceptor，古鲁。上师、精神导师、灵性导师。

guru-paramparā—tradition of teachers，上师传承体系。

–H–

harināma-saṁkīrtana—congregational chanting of Krishna's names，哈瑞纳玛－桑克尔坦。齐颂克里希纳的圣名。

hlādinī-śakti—energy of bliss，克里希纳的喜乐能量。

hṛṣīkeśa—Lord of the senses，瑞希凯施。感官的主人，克里希纳的又一名字。

–I–

ijyā—offering of several articles and services in a specific order and with appropriate *mantras*，以特定的顺序服务并供奉几样物品给神像，同时吟唱恰当的曼陀罗。

Īśvara—controller，伊士瓦尔。主宰者。

–J–

Jagannātha—Lord of the universe，佳甘纳特。宇宙之主。在佳甘纳特－普瑞供奉的佳甘纳特神像，被认为是克里希纳的特别形象。

Jagannātha Pūrī—佳甘纳特－普瑞。

Jagannātha-Rathayātrā—檀车节。公众拖动“宇宙之主”的檀车进行巡游的庆典。

Jīva—individual self，吉瓦。个我、灵魂。

jīvātmā—living entity，生物，生命体。

Jīva Gosvāmī—吉瓦·哥斯瓦米。六哥斯瓦米之一，撰写了高迪亚－外士那瓦最为全面的神学注释《六论》。

jñāna—gnosis，真知，知识。

jñānin—seeker of gnosis，追求真知者、知识思辨者。

–K–

Kali-yuga—era of spiritual darkness，灵性的黑暗时代。据古史文献记载，是一个退化和堕落的年代，大多数人有很少的或根本没有耕耘灵性的倾向和能力。

Kapila—卡皮拉。克里希纳的一个化身。

Karma—羯磨。业、行为活动。

karmin—求福报者、追求今生或来世利益者。

kīrtanam—chanting，speaking about，glorifying God，克尔坦。歌唱、谈论、荣耀神。

Krishna—克里希纳，又译黑天、讫里瑟拿[①]、克释拿、奎师那[②]、克里须那、克里希那。即“薄伽梵”。史有其人，为雅达瓦族之长。[③]其名字在佛教著作中称为“甘诃”，按照发音来说，等于是 Krishna。[④]

Krishna-bhakti—克里希纳－巴克提。对克里希纳的虔敬奉爱。

Krishna-prema—unadulterated love for Krishna，克里希纳－普瑞玛。对克里希纳纯粹的热爱。

Krishna-sevā—service to Krishna，克里希纳－塞瓦。服务克里希纳。

kṛpā—grace，恩典。

Kṣīra-cora-Gopīnātha—the Lord who stole sweet-rice，偷甜奶饭的主。

–L–

Lakṣmī—拉克希米。毗湿奴的配偶。

Līlā—divine pastimes，丽拉。神的娱乐活动、神圣游戏、逍遥时光。

līlā-avatāras—众多的逍遥时光化身。降临世上，执行三重功能。其一，祝福中正之人；其二，降伏邪恶之人；其三，重建宗教原则（*dharma*，达摩，法）。以上三方面均属逍遥时光化身的神圣娱乐活动（*līlā*，丽拉）。

–M–

Mādhavendra Purī—玛达文陀·普瑞（1420—1490）。柴坦尼亚的古鲁的古鲁，一位深得高迪亚－外士那瓦尊崇的苦行者。

---

① ［英］查尔斯·埃利奥特著，李荣熙译：《印度教与佛教史纲》第二卷，高雄：佛光出版社，1991 年，第五篇，《印度教》，各处。

② ［印］摩诃提瓦著，林煌洲译：《印度教导论》，台北：东大图书公司，2002 年，第 41 页。

③ ［印］室利·阿罗频多著，徐梵澄译：《薄伽梵歌论》，北京：商务印书馆，2010 年，第 656 页。

④ ［英］查尔斯·埃利奥特著，李荣熙译：《印度教与佛教史纲》第二卷，高雄：佛光出版社，1991 年，第五篇，《印度教》，第 238 页。

mādhurya—sweetness，甜美。薄伽梵内在固有的品质。

mādhurya-rasa—conjugal attraction，两性间的爱慕，情侣之爱。

mādhurya-rūpa—beautiful form displayed by Krishna in Vraja，克里希纳在布阿佳示现的美丽迷人的形体和相貌。

Madhva—摩陀婆，又译玛达瓦（1197—1276）。吠檀多毗湿奴派哲学家，主张二元论。

Mahābhārata—《摩诃婆罗多》。印度史诗。

mahā-mantra—摩诃－曼陀罗。为高迪亚－外士那瓦所持念的首要真言。（*hare kṛṣṇa hare kṛṣṇa kṛṣṇa kṛṣṇa hare hare*，*hare rāma hare rāma rāma rāma hare hare*. 哈瑞，克里希纳；哈瑞，克里希纳；克里希纳，克里希纳；哈瑞，哈瑞。哈瑞，罗摩；哈瑞，罗摩；罗摩，罗摩，哈瑞，哈瑞）

Mahārāja Nanda—摩诃罗阇・南达。南达王，克里希纳的养父。

mānasa-pūjā—a mental rehearsal of the procedures of worship，对崇拜程序做内心演练。

mantra—mystic utterances，曼陀罗。神圣的真言。

Mathurā—马图拉。位于今德里与阿格拉之间。

māyā—illusion，摩耶。幻象、幻觉。

māyā-śakti—摩耶－沙克提。错觉能量、迷幻能量、幻力，负责世界的创造、维系和毁灭。

māyayā—by a trick，耍个小把戏。

mokṣa/mukti—liberation，解脱。

mūrti-sevā—image service，服务神像。

–N–

nāma—name，名字。

nāma-aparādhas—冒犯克里希纳的圣名。

nāma-sevā—service to the divine names of God through recitation and singing，通过吟诵和歌唱的方式服务神的圣名。

Nārada-bhakti-sūtras—《拿拉达虔信经》。

Nārāyaṇa—那罗衍那。

Navadvīpa—纳瓦兑帕。柴坦尼亚的出生地，位于今西孟加拉境内。

Nimai—尼迈。柴坦尼亚·摩诃帕布儿时的昵称。

nitya-sevā—daily program of service，日常服务程序。

–O–

oṁ—唵，奥姆。吠陀圣音。

–P–

pāda-sevaṇam—rendering menial service to God and his devotees，为神及其虔爱者做谦卑的服务。

Pañcarātra—潘查茹阿陀。五夜派。

pañcarātrika-mārga—五夜派之道，文中简称五夜道。以规范化的练习（外迪－萨达纳－巴克提），尤其是以规范化的神像崇拜实践为特征。

Pāṇḍava brothers—潘达瓦（般度）五兄弟。

Paramahaṁsa—great，swanlike person，an appellative for spiritually advanced ascetics，帕罗摩汉萨。天鹅般的崇高人物。对一位灵性造诣极高的苦行者的称谓。

Paramātmā—supreme Self/supersoul，最高我 / 超灵。至尊人薄伽梵超验形象的局部展示。居于每一生命体之内。

parakīya-rasa—paramourship，情侣关系。

parikramaṇa—circumambulate，绕拜。

prapūjayet—worship，崇拜。

prasāda—remnants of food ritually offered to deity，菩莎达。祭馀，按照仪式程序供奉过神像的食物。

prasāda-sevā—distributing and eating sanctified food，派发和进食供奉过的食物。

prayojana—purpose，宗旨、目的。

pūjā—worship with paraphernalia，普佳。用物品来举行崇拜仪式。

pūjārī—ritual specialist，祭司。祭祀仪式专家。

Purāṇas—《往世书》。梵语文献，主要以叙事的方式记载全宇宙范围内的神圣历史。

pūrṇa-śakti—full complementary embodiment of the "energy" of Krishna，克里希纳"能量"的具体体现和完满化身。

pūrṇa-śaktimān—full possessor of infinite divine energie，无限神圣能量（*pūrṇa-śakti*）的完全拥有者。

puruṣa—the primal Person，菩鲁沙。原初之人、原人、原人神我。

puruṣa-avatāras—菩鲁沙 - 阿凡达（阿瓦塔）。原人的众多化身。

puruṣārthas—不同于巴克提的另一类人生追求，包括世俗的宗教信仰（*dharma*）、追求财富（*artha*）、满足感官欲望（*kāma*）以及解脱（*mokṣa*）。

puruṣottama—the supreme person，至尊人、最高神我。

–R–

Rādhā—茹阿达，即 Śrīmatī Rādhārāṇi，室利妈媞·茹阿达茹阿妮。克里希纳的爱侣。

Rādhāramaṇa—he who gives pleasure to Rādhā，茹阿达罗曼。给予茹阿达快乐的人，指克里希纳。

rāgānuga—following spontaneously，spontaneous devotion，自发的奉爱。

Rāma—罗摩，又译茹阿玛。

Rāmānuja—罗摩奴阇，又译茹阿玛努佳。吠檀多毗湿奴派哲学家。主张限定不二论。

rasa—茹阿萨。与克里希纳之间甜美关系与神圣情感的品味。

Rathayātrā—檀车节。

ṛṣi—spiritually adept sage，瑞希。在灵性方面称得上行家里手的圣人。

ruci—对巴克提的品味或喜好。

rūpa—form，身相。形体。

Rūpa Gosvāmī—茹帕（鲁跋）·哥斯瓦米，室利·柴坦尼亚的弟子，六哥斯瓦米之一。著有《奉爱甘露之洋》，全称为《奉爱服务的纯粹甘露之洋》。

–S–

śabda—revealed text，天启圣典。

sac-cid-ānanda-vigraha—form of eternal-cognizant-bliss，永恒－全知－妙乐的身相。

sad-ācāra—proper Vaiṣṇava behavior，外士那瓦（毗湿奴派信徒）的恰当举止。

sādhana—practice，萨达纳。练习、实践。

sādhana-bhakti—practice of *bhakti*，萨达纳－巴克提。巴克提实践或修习、练习。

sādhaka—practitioner，萨达卡。实践者、练习者、修习者。

sādhu—a devotee of Krishna，萨杜。克里希纳的虔爱者。

sadhu-saṅga—association with other practitioners，和其他修习者交往。

sākhyam—cultivating intimate friendship with God，培养和神之间的亲密关系。

śakti—energy，沙克提。能量。

śaktimān—energetic source，沙克提曼。能量的拥有者和来源。

śakti-parināma—transformation of energies，能量转化。

Śālagrāma-śīlas—圣石。被奉为那罗衍那或毗湿奴直接展示的神圣小石头。

Sambandha—relationship，关系。

saṁsāra—repeated birth，death，old age and disease，反反复复的生、老、病、死。

Śaṅkara—商羯罗。印度中世纪吠檀多不二一元论哲学家。

sannyāsa—renounced order，遁世期，生命的弃绝阶段。

sannyāsī—桑尼亚西。托钵僧。

sarvendriye—with all one's senses，以所有感官。

śāstra—scripture，经典。

Sevā—service or attendance，塞瓦。服务，服侍。

sevaka—servitor，仆人。

sevā-aparādha—offenses in worship，神像崇拜中的冒犯。

sevya—the served，被服务者、主人。

smaraṇam—remembrance of the name，form，qualities and pastimes of God，记忆神的名字、形象、品质和娱乐活动等。

śravaṇam—hearing topics related to God from qualified sources，从有资格的讲授者那里聆听有关神的话题。

śraddhā—faith，信心。

Śrī—室利。幸运女神。那罗衍那的配偶。

Śrīmad-Bhāgavatam—《薄伽梵往世书》，又称《圣典薄伽瓦谭》。

Śrī Nityānanda Prabhu—室利·尼提阿南达帕布。室利·柴坦尼亚的亲密同伴。被确认为是克里希纳在温达文娱乐时光中的哥哥巴拉罗摩。

Śrī Vaiṣṇava—室利毗湿奴派，毗湿奴女神派。毗湿奴派的又一传系。据说传自室利，即拉克希米。罗摩奴阇是这一传承中主要的创始导师。

Śrī-Vigraha—sacred image，神圣形象。

Subhadrā—苏芭朵。克里希纳的妹妹。在佳甘纳特·普瑞供奉着她的特别形象。

Sudārśaṇa—Krishna's fiery disc weapon，苏达尔珊纳，克里希纳炽热的神碟武器。

śuddha-bhakta—pure devotee，殊达－巴克塔。纯粹的虔爱者。

śuddha-bhakti—pure devotional service，殊达－巴克提。纯粹的奉爱服务。其特征是：出于天性，自发而充满喜悦，不含任何动机，不受干扰，永不间断，绵密无漏。

svādhyāya—literally“self-study”，字面意思是“自修”，指独自一人阅读、吟诵以及学习神圣典籍。神像崇拜实践中的一个反思环节。

svakīya-rasa—a married couple，已婚夫妇关系。

svarūpa-śakti—essential power，内在能量。

Śvetāśvatara Upaniṣad—《白骡奥义书》。

svayam bhagavān—God himself，神本人。

Śyāmasundara—夏玛逊达尔。克里希纳又一名字。双臂持笛、三度曲线的唯美形象。

–T–

tantric mantras—坦特罗（谭崔）曼陀罗。

tapas—austerities，苦行。

tatastha-śakti—medial power，亦称为吉瓦－沙克提（*jīva-śakti*），字面意思是“处于边界的能量”，中间能量，生物能量，负责个我灵魂的存在。

tattva-darśinaḥ—seers of thatness or seers of the truth，明心见性者、证悟实相者。

–U–

Uddhava—乌达瓦。克里希纳的亲密朋友

upacāras—items offered，供奉给神像的物品。

Upadeśāmṛta—*Nectar of Instruction*，《教诲的甘露》。茹帕·哥斯瓦米著作。

uttama-bhakti—superior form of *bhakt*，巴克提高级阶段。

–V–

vaidhi—in reference to regulations，按照规范。

vaidhi-sādhana-bhakti—外迪－萨达纳－巴克提。规范练习阶段的奉爱服务。以遵守规范原则为主，神秘性较少。

Vaiṣṇava—外士那瓦。即毗湿奴派信徒，最高神克里希纳的虔信者。

Vaiṣṇavas—外士那瓦们。Vaiṣṇava 的复数形式。

Vaiṣṇava-aparādha—the offending of a fellow practitioner of Krishna-*bhakti*，either with one's body，words，or mind，对外士那瓦的冒犯，即以自己的身体，言语或心意，得罪了一位在练习克里希纳－巴克提的同修。

Vaiṣṇava-sevā—service to Vaiṣṇavas，服务外士那瓦。

Vaiṣṇavism—外士那瓦宗。即毗湿奴派。崇拜毗湿奴，但认为毗湿奴不过是克里希纳的一个扩展。故在其传统中，占中心地位的是克里希纳，而不是毗湿奴。

vandanam—offering prayers to God，向神供奉祷文。

varṇa—caste divisions，瓦尔那。种姓阶层。

varṇāśrama—瓦尔那刷玛。社会四阶层与人生四阶段制度。晚近以种姓制度（cast system）渐为西方人所知。

vedānta—吠檀多。终极韦达经、吠陀的终结、吠檀多派。

vigraha—body，身体。

vijaya-mūrtis—festival images，庆典神像。

viraha/vipralambha—separation from the beloved，与心上人的分离。

Vishnu—毗湿奴、维瑟奴，唐译为毗搜纽或毗奴。①

viśiṣtādvaita—qualified monism，限定不二论。

viśiṣtādvaita-vādin—qualified non-dualist，限定不二论者。

Vraja—布阿佳。克里希纳从小生活的地方（直到 11 岁）。

Vṛndāvana—Krishna's most beloved forest in Vraja，where He enjoys pastimes with the cowherd boys and the young gopis；also，the entire district of Vraja. 克里希纳在布阿佳最喜欢的一处森林，他在那里和牧牛童及牧牛姑娘们享受美妙的逍遥活动；也可指布阿佳全境。

Vṛndāvaneśvarī—presiding goddess of Vṛndāvana，Rādhā，温达文内湿瓦瑞。温达文首席女神茹阿达。

Vṛṣṇis—Krishna's clan，维施尼。克里希纳的族人。

Vyāsa—毗耶娑、维亚萨、毗耶舍。全名为：克利须那・兑帕亚纳・毗

---

① 参见［印］室利・阿罗频多著，徐梵澄译《薄伽梵歌论》，北京：商务印书馆，2010 年，第 660 页。

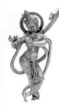

耶娑（Kṛṣṇa-Dvaipāyana Vyāsa），传统上被公认为梵文史诗《摩诃婆罗多》及《往世书》的编纂者。

–Y–

yānti—go to，去到，出生。

yoga—瑜伽。意为“连接”，尤指从内在与自我相连，将自己看成是神的一位仆人。

yogam aiśvaram—mystic opulence，克里希纳玄秘的富裕。

yogin—seeker of mystic perfection，追求完美的神秘主义者、瑜伽行者、瑜伽师。

yugas—古史文献将宇宙时间划分为四个年代的循环周期。每一个年代称为一个 *yuga*，现在正处于 *Kali-yuga*，即，喀历年代（包括未来的 42 万 8 千年在内）。

译后记

这是华培教授第一部以中文出版的著作。此前，他有两篇学术论文被译成中文发表，其一是《权威的经验与经验的权威——论〈薄伽梵歌〉与现代“宗教经验”的对话》[①]，其二是《菩提达摩的〈入道四行观〉与〈薄伽梵歌〉：以印度教毗湿奴派的视角看禅宗》。[②]

华培教授非常喜爱中国。1989 年他第一次踏上中国这片土地，同行的还有正在剑桥大学宗教学系攻读博士学位的托玛斯·赫兹格先生[③]，他们怀着对中国文化的喜爱与欣赏，访问了广州和西安。2007—2011 年，华培教授被聘为香港中文大学文化及宗教研究系的客座教授，期间他开设了“印度的传统与现代”“印度圣地学”及“印度文化中的爱”等课程。

华培教授与大陆学术界的交流始于 2007 年底。其时他正执教香港中文大学印度宗教与文化教席，应赖品超和谭伟伦两位教授之邀，参加了在北京大学哲学系举办的题为“宗教经验与宗教对话”的学术会议。这是北京大学哲学系与香港中文大学文化及宗教研究系联合举办的小型校际交流会。前面提到的《权威的经验与经验的权威——论〈薄伽梵歌〉与现代“宗教经验”的对话》一文，便是他在该会上所作的报告。那以后，他有了更多的机会到

---

① 肯尼斯·华培著，张雪松译：《权威的经验与经验的权威——论〈薄伽梵歌〉与现代“宗教经验”的对话》，收录于赵敦华主编：《哲学门》（总第十八辑），北京：北京大学出版社，2009 年 2 月，第 189~197 页。

② 肯尼斯·华培：《菩提达摩的〈入道四行观〉与〈薄伽梵歌〉：以印度教毗湿奴派的视角看禅宗》，收录于张凤雷主编，王博译，惟善审校：《宗教研究》2015 年（秋），北京：宗教文化出版社，2016 年 11 月，第 173~180 页。

③ 托玛斯·赫兹格先生后来以“古道华”为笔名，著有一本小说，以中文出版。古道华：《新世纪瑜伽：李广施的故事》，太原：北岳文艺出版社，1994 年 5 月。

访中国大陆的高等学府进行讲学。[①] 2012 年 10 月，他在武汉大学哲学学院做了三场分别题为“印度宗教思想的变迁”（上、下）、“宗教比较研究”的讲座。以此为开端，几乎每年华培教授都来中国大陆的高等学府及科研机构进行学术交流。截至 2018 年 3 月，先后有清华大学翻译与跨文化研究中心、中央民族大学世界人类学民族学研究中心等几十家院校和科研机构邀请他前来讲学。[②] 交流的主题涉及语言学、翻译学、人类学、社会学、心理学、动物伦理学、宗教哲学、瑜伽哲学、印度教和印度文化等多个领域。

在 2013 年 11 月的一次学术交流会上，我有幸与华培教授相识。他博大的文化胸襟以及优雅的君子风范给我留下了深刻印象。他朗读梵文时，那略微低沉的男中音配上优美的韵律，让人感觉梵文是世界上最唯美的语言。于是我暗下决心，将来学习梵文，像华培教授一样能够阅读梵文。当然，若能效法徐梵澄先生将梵文典籍直接译成中文，岂不更妙？怀着对未来美好的憧憬，我向华培教授表达了跟他学习的愿望。他不嫌我对梵文的一无所知，欣然应允。

2016 年 10 月，华培教授的这部著作由李丹阳女士完成初稿的翻译，交由我做进一步的润色。这对我来说并不容易。一则我的英文翻译水平显然不足以应对这么深奥的学术著作。幸好李丹阳女士经验丰富，曾翻译出版多部作品。她的初稿一定程度上成了我的学习指南。我把她的译稿和华培教授的原稿都打印出来，先一字一句地试着自己翻译原稿，然后再和她的译稿两相对照，寻找差距。另外，令人遗憾的是，我没有哲学和宗教学的学科背景，只是出于兴趣，从 1996 年开始，受我爱人耿会武先生的影响，陆续阅读了一些宗教哲学书籍。[③] 2007 年元旦期间我随先生一起到云南西双版纳州景洪市基诺族的村寨作原始宗教研究的田野调查，同年完成了自己的历史学硕士论文《隋唐时期观音信仰中国化研究》。2008 年 9 月，我来到中央民族

---

① 此处引自华培教授正在出版当中的第二部中文译著的序言。该书名拟定为《涉越大川：瑜伽哲学反思与跨文化比较研究》。

② 另有以下单位，如浙江大学基督教与跨文化研究中心、上海大学文学院、深圳大学印度研究中心、深圳理工大学、北京外国语大学亚非学院、中国人民大学佛教与宗教学理论研究所、中国社会科学院梵文研究中心和中国哲学研究室、天津外国语大学比较文学研究所、北京师范大学外国语言文学学院、广东外语外贸大学翻译与跨文化研究中心、清华大学科学技术与社会研究所等等。

③ 当时最喜欢的是四川大学道教与宗教文化研究所陈兵教授的《生与死：佛教轮回说》。呼和浩特：内蒙古人民出版社，1994 年。

大学，师从奇文瑛先生，从事明史的学习和研究。2013 年初，最终完成了二十万字的博士论文《晚明居士群体研究》。在春季的答辩会上，中国社会科学院的定宜庄老师鼓励我说："你下了很大功夫，而且文字功底不错，以后可去出版社做编辑工作。"是的，我喜欢做文字工作。中国的文字真的是太美了，我的理想就是将优美的文字呈给读者。

书中出现的一些专业术语该如何处理和呈现？这是我们思考较多的问题。我们的主要原则是沿用学术界通用的说法。如梵天（*Brahmā*）、毗湿奴（*Viṣṇu*）、湿婆（*Śiva*）、摩耶（*māyā*）这类术语都是学界约定俗成的，我们尽量沿袭旧译。至于巴克提瑜伽（Bhakti Yoga/devotional yoga）的译法，2016 年 11 月 22 日中国社科院世界宗教研究所邀请华培教授去做学术交流，与会学者们曾就此有过讨论。当时的翻译徐达斯先生将其译为"奉爱瑜伽"①，有学者提出，以前一般译为"虔信瑜伽"，这两种译法有何异同？记得关于这个问题会上没有定论。后来我在读书的过程中找到了答案，二者是可以通用的。确切地说，是三者，即巴克提瑜伽、虔信瑜伽、奉爱瑜伽，说的都是一回事。②我同意这一观点，可当我看到中国社科院邱永辉研究员有"虔爱瑜伽"之说，③还是情不自禁地采用了，尽管我认为，虔爱瑜伽是巴克提瑜伽的又一种说法，本质上与虔信瑜伽和奉爱瑜伽没有区别。相应地，巴克提瑜伽的实践者，书中一般称为巴克塔（bhakta）或虔爱者（devotee）。当然，学界也有"奉献者"之说。④

除了英译汉和专业方面功力较弱之外，本书翻译的过程中最大的障碍是梵文。幸好作者一般都会在梵文词后给出英文对应词。同时，有些学者的著作后所附的梵汉译名对照表，成了我们主要的参考资料。⑤可还是会碰到个

① 关于"奉爱瑜伽"的说法，另见李建欣《印度宗教与佛教》，北京：宗教文化出版社，2013 年 8 月，第 316、394 页。又见朱文信《梵·吠檀多·瑜伽：印度宗教思想家维韦卡南达思想研究》，杭州：浙江大学博士论文，2011 年，第 141~155 页。

② 参见王志成《瑜伽的力量》，成都：四川人民出版社，2013 年 1 月，第 63 页。

③ 参见邱永辉《印度教概论》，北京：社会科学文献出版社，2012 年 4 月，第 305~310 页。

④ 李政阳：《身体、符号与益世康修行》，载陈进国主编《宗教人类学》第七辑，北京：社会科学文献出版社，2017 年 8 月，第 256 页。

⑤ 例如，孙晶：《印度六派哲学》，北京：中国社会科学出版社，2015 年 1 月，第 365~408 页，"梵汉译名对照表"；邱永辉：《印度教概论》，北京：社会科学文献出版社，2012 年 4 月，第 384~404 页，"印度教小词典"和"索引"。

别词汇，查了好多资料也找不到一个满意的译法，这时我就会直接求助学术界的师友。如本书第四章第二节 *śilpa-śāstra* 译为《工巧论》，就是出自中国社会科学院孙晶研究员之手。[1]

关于 Krishna 的译法，有意译和音译两种。意译为“黑天”，“黑”表示 Krishna 的肤色；而“天”是传统汉译中加进去的，表示 Krishna 是神。[2] 至于音译，就我所见，如书后词表所列，有克释拿[3]、奎师那等七种之多。本书采用了“克里希纳”这一音译。[4]

关于 Rādhā 的译法，据我所知，有罗陀、拉达等音译。本书采用“茹阿达”[5]这一音译。

此外，Vaiṣṇava（外士那瓦）也是本书贯穿始终的关键词。从词源学上看，它是从 Viṣṇu（毗湿奴）衍生而来的，意思是毗湿奴的崇拜者。根据外士那瓦宗的理论，毗湿奴是薄伽梵（克里希纳）的一个主要名字，故此，Vaiṣṇava 亦指克里希纳的虔爱者。学界一般很少直接音译为“外士那瓦”[6]，而是将音译与意译相结合，译为毗湿奴派。本书在不同语境中，为使行文流畅，兼取这两种译法。所以，读者若遇到外士那瓦或毗湿奴派，当知两者是一码事，均指克里希纳的虔爱者。而高迪亚 – 外士那瓦（Gauḍīya Vaiṣṇava）则特指毗湿奴派中的柴坦尼亚支派或孟加拉支派，主张将神像崇拜仪礼与哈瑞克里希纳曼陀罗的念诵等其他实践相结合，稳定地为克里希纳作奉献服务。根据高迪亚 – 外士那瓦的理论，这样做，便可最终恢复与克里希纳的甜美关

---

① 本书翻译过程中，承蒙孙晶老师通过微信多次指点。还有李剑、王大惟、徐达斯、李政阳、杨培敏等诸位师友的鼎力相助。所以，这本书其实可以说是“集体智慧”的结晶。

② 王靖：《人神之间：论印度教中黑天形象的起源和嬗变》，《世界宗教文化》2017 年第 3 期，第 135 页脚注 3。

③ 参见徐梵澄译的《薄伽梵歌》，文中多处提到克释拿。收录于孙波编著：《徐梵澄文集》第八卷，上海：上海三联书店，华东师范大学出版社，2006 年。

④ 王靖：《人神之间：论印度教中黑天形象的起源和嬗变》，《世界宗教文化》2017 年第 3 期，第 135 页脚注 3。

⑤ 李政阳：《身体、符号与益世康修行》，载陈进国主编《宗教人类学》第七辑，北京：社会科学文献出版社，2017 年 8 月，第 256 页。

⑥ 但年轻一代的学者也在用其音译，参见李政阳的文章。同前注。

系与情感（茹阿萨，*rasa*），从而获得生而为人的真正快乐与圆满成功。[①]

华培教授在过去四十余年的学术生涯中，笔耕不辍，著述等身。本书作于 1998 年，先后以克罗地亚语、西班牙语、英语出版。虽作于二十年前，但今天看来，书中对于巴克提瑜伽理论与实践诸多细节方面的研究还是最前沿的。[②]可以说中文版的问世乃中国大陆学术界之一大幸事，不仅将填补瑜伽哲学、吠檀多哲学、印度教等领域研究的空白，而且将推动相关领域的研究往纵深发展。

本书篇幅虽不长，但从初稿到定稿，历时约三年之久。可以说，呈现在读者面前的每一个文字背后，都浸着作者、译者、编辑、排版人员以及其他所有师友的辛勤汗水和爱心。克罗地亚 Lotos 出版社无偿转让中文翻译版权；捷克摄影师 Param Tomanec 先生提供了书前八张美妙的照片；李丹阳女士为本书做了最基础的翻译工作，并多次请教作者，反复斟酌与完善。作者华培教授嘱我在后记中代他表达对所有朋友的感谢，尤其是云南大学出版社的万斌编辑，是他和同事们的辛勤工作，才有了本书的出版问世。同时，对于李丹阳女士和我在翻译上的尽心尽力，作者坚持要在此表达他深深的感谢。

当然，作为翻译，我们感谢华培教授，也欣赏他所撰写的这本书。我们希望，当读者打开这本书，一页页翻读的时候，同样会对这部作品心生欣赏。是的，随着阅读的深入，你或许会发现自己正由一位有耐心的向导引领着，在巴克提瑜伽的世界里尽情畅游。

我们努力使译文在忠实于原文的基础上，尽量传达原文之美。奈何学力不逮，错漏之处在所难免，还望读者诸君不吝赐教。

李玉伟

2018 年 12 月 19 日于北京

---

① 姜景奎：《再论中世纪印度教帕克蒂运动》，《南亚研究》2004 年第 1 期，第 59 页。

① 2015 年 12 月 9 日，华培教授在中国社会科学院梵文研究中心和中国哲学研究室联合举办的学术交流会上，作了题为“吠檀多：终极的知识”的报告。会后，有学者表示，报告中所论及的茹阿萨理论（rasa-theory）与柴坦尼亚的情感宗教（Caitanya's religion of feeling），这些都是丰富而深奥的领域，目前他的研究中尚未涉猎到。

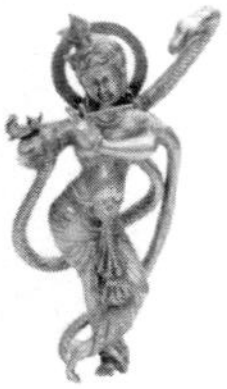

Translators' Afterword

Among the books written by Prof. Valpey, this is the first to be published in Chinese. Two of his academic papers have been previously translated into Chinese and published. One is *The Experience of Authority and the Authority of Experience: the Bhagavad-gītā in dialogue with modern'religious experience'discourse.* [1] The other is *Bodhidharma's"Four Entrances"and the Bhagavad-gītā: An exploration of Chán Buddhism through Vaishnava Hinduism.*[2]

Prof. Valpey likes China very much. It was in 1989 that he came to China for the first time with Mr. Thomas Herzig [3] who studied for his doctor's degree in the Department of Religious Studies, Cambridge University. With an appreciation for Chinese culture, they paid visits to Guang Zhou and Xi'an. From 2007 to 2011, Prof. Valpey was appointed visiting professor in Chinese University of Hong Kong, during which he gave several courses, including " Tradition and Modernity in India " , " Sacred Geography of

---

① Kenneth R. Valpey, " Bodhidharma's ' Four Entrances ' and the Bhagavad-gītā: An exploration of Chán Buddhism through Vaishnava Hinduism " , Zhang Fenglei, ed. , *Religion Studies* 2015 (Autumn) , Beijing: Religion and Culture Publishing House, November 2016, pp. 173-180. Translated by Wang Bo. Revised by Wei Shan.

② Kenneth R. Valpey, " Bodhidharma's ' Four Entrances ' and the Bhagavad-gītā: An exploration of Chán Buddhism through Vaishnava Hinduism " , Zhang Fenglei, ed. , *Religion Studies* 2015 (Autumn) , Beijing: Religion and Culture Publishing House, November 2016, pp. 173-180. Translated by Wang Bo. Revised by Wei Shan.

③ Mr. Thomas Herzig under the pseudonym Gu Daohua (古道华) wrote a novel and published in Chinese later. Gu Daohua, *Yoga for the 21st Century: the story of Li Kuang Shi*, Taiyuan: Beiyue Literature & Art Publishing House, 1994.

India", and "Love in Indian Culture".

The academic exchange between Prof. Valpey and Chinese academic circles began at the end of 2007, when he was teaching in the capacity of the Professorship in Indian Culture and Religion, Chinese University of Hong Kong. Invited by Prof. Lai Pinchao and Prof. Tan Weilun, he participated in a conference in the Department of Philosophy, Peking University, on the subject of "Religious Experience and Interreligious Dialogue." This was a small inter-collegiate conference, in cooperation with the Department of Cultural and Religious Studies, Chinese University of Hong Kong. The paper mentioned previously, *The Experience of Authority and the Authority of Experience: the Bhagavad-gītā in dialogue with modern 'religious experience' discourse* is the presentation he gave at the meeting. Since that time, he has had further opportunities to visit and speak at universities in China. [①] In October, 2012, he gave a lecture series entitled "Indian Religious Thought in Transition" (2 lectures), and a single lecture, "The Comparative Study of Religion," in the Department of Religious Studies, School of Philosophy, Wuhan University. Since then, nearly every year Prof. Valpey has been paying a visit to China, giving lectures at universities and scientific institutes. By March 2018, there have been dozens of schools and institutes inviting him for academic exchange, e.g., Centre for Translation and Interdisciplinary Studies, Tsinghua University; Institute of Global Ethnology and Anthropology, Minzu University of China,

---

① Here I just referenced Prof. Valpey's preface for his second book with a potential title *Advancing Across the Great River: Reflections on Yoga Philosophy and Cross-cultural Comparisons* being published in Chinese at present, in which he said, "Since that time…… I had further opportunities to visit and speak at universities in the People's Republic of China."

and others. [1] The themes of communication have included linguistics, translatology, anthropology, sociology, psychology, animal ethics, philosophy of religion, Yoga philosophy, Hinduism, and Indian culture.

In November 2013, I was fortunate to participate in an academic exchange and first made acquaintance with Prof. Valpey. What impressed me most was his broad cultural vision and manner of gentility. During his lecture, he would read Sanskrit. His slightly low baritone voice with enjoyable rhythm was so attractive that one may think Sanskrit must be the most beautiful language in the world. Thus, I determined to learn Sanskrit in the future so that I could read Sanskrit as he did. Of course, how wonderful it would be if I could follow Mr. Xu Fancheng to translate Sanskrit scriptures into Chinese directly someday! With bright visions of the future, I expressed my desire that I wanted to learn from him. And he gladly agreed despite my being ignorant of the subject.

In October 2016, the first translation draft of this book was finished by Miss Li Danyang and handed over to me for further polishing, which wasn't easy for me. For one thing, it was obvious to me that my English-Chinese translation skill is not good enough for such a profound academic book like this. Happily, Miss Li Danyang is an experienced translator and has published several books before. In this way her draft has, to some extent, become a study guide for me. I had both her translation and Prof. Valpey's

---

[1] Other universities and institutes in which he has lectured include Institute of Christianity And Cross-Cultural Studies, Zhejiang University; College of Liberal Arts, Shanghai University; Center for Hindu Studies, Shenzhen University; Shenzhen Polytechnic; School of Asian and African Studies, Beijing Foreign Studies University; Institute of Studies for Buddhism & Religious Theory, Renmin University of China; Chinese philosophy Research Room & Sanskrit Study Centre of Philosophy Institute, Chinese Academy of Social Sciences; Institute for Comparative Literature, Tianjin Foreign Studies University; School of Foreign Languages and Literature, Beijing Normal University; Translation and Intercultural Studies Center, Guangdong University of Foreign Studies; and Institute of Science, Technology and Society, Tsinghua University, etc.

original printed. First, I tried to translate by myself and then compared with hers, trying to find where the differences were. But my major was neither philosophy nor religion when I was at school. Just for fun, since 1996, I have read some relevant books,[①] influenced by my husband Mr. Geng Huiwu. During the New Year's Day in 2007, I went with him to Jinuo People's village, in Jinghong, Xishuangbanna Dai Autonomous Prefecture, Yunnan, to conduct field research on primitive religion and finished my thesis for master in History entitled *A Study on Chinesization of belief in Guanyin During Sui and Tang Dynasties* in the same year. In September 2008, I went to Minzu University of China for a further study following Prof. Qi Wenying, whose research interest is History of Ming Dynasty. Finally, I completed a 200,000-word dissertation entitled *A Study on the Group of Lay Buddhists in the Late Ming Dynasty*. At the defense meeting, Teacher Ding Yizhuang from Chinese Academy of Social Sciences encouraged me, " It's obvious that you worked very hard and that you have good writing skills, so you could be fit to serve as an editor in a publishing house. " Yes, I like to do literary work. Chinese characters are so beautiful that I think it is my ideal/duty to present them to readers in the best way possible.

So how to present some of the technical terms in this book is a problem about which we thought again and again. One of the main principles is to follow the terms commonly used in the academy. For example, Brahmā, *Viṣṇu*, Śiva, māyā are respectively translated as 梵天，毗湿奴，湿婆，摩耶 which are all conventional terms. Therefore, we didn't change the current translation of such words, but use them directly. As for the translation of Bhakti Yoga (devotional yoga) , it was discussed by scholars present at the academic exchange at World Religions Institute, Chinese Academy of Social Sciences (CASS) when Prof. Valpey was invited to give a visiting lecture on

① At that time my favourite was *Birth and Death*: *Buddhist Idea of Reincarnation* by Prof. Chen Bing from Centre for Studies of Daoism and Religious Culture, Sichuan University. Huhhot: Inner-Mongol People Publishing House, 1994.

November 22nd, 2016. Several scholars asked what's the difference between 虔信瑜伽（devotional yoga）, the general translation in the academic circle, and 奉爱瑜伽（devotional yoga）[1] as translated by Prof. Valpey's interpreter Mr. Xu Dasi. There was no conclusion about this at that time. Later I found the answer to this question during reading, that both are almost interchangeable. In fact, these three, namely 巴克提瑜伽（Bhakti Yoga）, 虔信瑜伽, 奉爱瑜伽, all amount to the same thing-devotional Yoga. [2] I agree with this opinion, however, when I found 虔爱瑜伽（devotional yoga）in the book of Qiu Yonghui, a Research fellow from CASS, [3] I couldn't help adopting it here in this book, although I think it's just another way of saying Bhakti Yoga and there's no difference among 虔信瑜伽, 奉爱瑜伽 and 虔爱瑜伽. Accordingly, the one who practices Bhakti Yoga is here generally called 巴克塔（bhakta）or 虔爱者（devotee）, which is also called 奉献者（devotee）by some scholar. [4]

In addition to my weak English-Chinese translation skill and knowledge of religion and philosophy, the biggest obstacle during translation is Sanskrit. Luckily, the author will generally give the English equivalent just after the Sanskrit word. Also, the comparison tables of translated terms or names in the appendix at the back of some books have become the main reference for me. [5] When I couldn't find a satisfactory translation after reading as

---

① 奉爱瑜伽 is also mentioned by the other scholars. See Li Jianxin: *Religion and Buddhism in India*, Beijing: Religion and Culture Publishing House, 2013, 8, p. 316, p. 394; Zhu Wenxin: *Brahman·Vedānta·Yoag: A Study on Vivekananda's Thoughts of Religion*, Hangzhou: Doctoral Dissertation of Zhejiang University, 2011, pp. 141-155.

② See Wang Zhicheng: *The power of Yoga*, Chengdu: Sichuan Renmin Press, 2013, 1, p. 63.

③ See Qiu Yonghui: *Introduction to Hinduism*, Beijing: Social Sciences Academic Press, 2012, 4, pp.305-310.

④ See Li Zhengyang, "Body, Symbol and ISKCON's Practices", *Anthropology of Religion*, Vol. 7, Beijing: Social Sciences Academic Press, 2017, 8, p. 256.

⑤ E. g. , Sun Jing, *Six Schools of Philosophy in India*, Beijing: China Social Science Press, 2015, 1, pp. 365-408; Qiu Yonghui, Introduction to Hinduism, Beijing: Social Sciences Academic Press, 2014, 4, pp. 384-404.

many materials as I could, I would turn to teachers and friends in academic circles directly. For example, 工巧论（śilpa-śāstra）in Section Ⅳ. 2 is the translation offered by Mr. Sun Jing, research fellow from CASS. ①

Regarding Chinese translation for "Krishna", there're two categories: free translation and transliteration. 黑天 belongs to the first category. 黑（black）means Krishna's complexion; and 天 means Krishna is God. ② As for the transliteration, as far as I can see, there are seven translations, e. g. , 克释拿, ③ 奎师那, etc. , just as is included in the vocabulary at the back of this book. Here in the text we adopted the transliteration 克里希纳. ④

Regarding Chinese translation for "Rādhā", as far as I know, there's only transliteration, e. g. , 罗陀, 拉达, etc. In this book, we adopted 茹阿达. ⑤

In addition, the term "Vaiṣṇava（外士那瓦）" is also a keyword throughout the book, which is etymologically derived from "Viṣṇu（毗湿奴）", a principle name of Bhagavān（Krishna）. "Vaiṣṇava（外士那瓦）" means the worshiper of Viṣṇu and also the devotee of Krishna as well according to Vaiṣṇavism. Generally, in the Chinese academy it is translated as 毗湿奴派（Vaishnava sect）, which is a combination of transliteration and free translation, and is rarely translated as 外士

---

① During the translation process, I am very grateful that Teacher Sun Jing offered guidance to me on Wechat more than once and my friends/teachers such as Li Jian, Wang Dawei, Xu Dasi, Li Zhengyang and Yang Peimin are all very helpful. Thus, this book is actually the crystallization of "collective wisdom".

② Wang Jing, "Between God and Man: on the Origin and Transmutation of Krishna's Image in Hinduism", *The Religious Cultures in the World* No. 3, 2017, footnote 3 on p. 135.

③ See the Chinese version of *Bhagavad-gītā* translated by Xu Fancheng, in Xu Fancheng Anthology, Sun Bo, ed. , Shanghai: Shanghai Joint Publishing Press, East China Normal University Press, 2006.

④ Wang Jing, "Between God and Man: on the Origin and Transmutation of Krishna's Image in Hinduism", *The Religious Cultures in the World* No. 3, 2017, footnote 3 on p. 135.

⑤ See Li Zhengyang, "Body, Symbol and ISKCON's Practices", *Anthropology of Religion*, vol. 7, Beijing: Social Sciences Academic Press, 2017, 8, p. 256.

那瓦，which is a transliteration. [①] Here in this book，in order to keep the writing flow more smooth，we adopted both 外士那瓦 and 毗湿奴派 in accordance with the context. Thus when you read 外士那瓦 or 毗湿奴派 in the text，please keep in mind they are the same in meaning. And Gauḍīya Vaiṣṇava（高迪亚 - 外士那瓦）refers to Bengal Vaiṣṇava or Caitanyite Vaiṣṇava—one who advocates devotional service offered to Krishna through image service（mūrti-sevā）combined with other practices among which chanting Hare Krishna Mantra is of the most importance. According to Caitanyite Vaisnavas，in this way one can finally revive the sweet relationship and bond of affection with Krishna and achieve the true happiness and full success. [②]

During his forty years of academic career，Prof. Valpey has been keeping writing and creating a large number of works. As for this Krishna-Seva book，it was finished in 1998，and translated into several languages and published in Croatian，Spanish，and English. Although it was written twenty years ago，still its research on the details about the theory and practice of Bhakti Yoga is up to date even today. [③] Thus，we may say，the publication of this Chinese version is really a big fortune for the Chinese academic circle，a book which will not only fill a gap in research on Yoga philosophy，Vedānta philosophy and Hinduism，but also push the relevant fields towards greater depth of understanding.

Although not long，this book production took 3 years or so from first draft to finalization. Each and every word presented to the reader is

---

① Yet there is a new generation of young scholars adopting the transliteration. See Li Zhengyang，"Body，Symbol and ISKCON Practice"，*Anthropology of Religion*，vol. 7，Beijing：Social Sciences Academic Press，2017，8，p. 256.

② Jiang Jingkui："On Bhakti Movement of Medieval Hinduism again"，*South Asian Studies*，2004，1，p. 59.

③ On December 9th 2015，Prof. Valpey gave a lecture titled "Vedanta—the 'End of Knowledge'：A Very Brief Overview" at CASS invited by Chinese philosophy Research Room & Sanskrit Study Centre of Philosophy Institute. After the meeting，some scholar said that regarding Rasa-theory and Caitanya's religion of feeling discussed in Prof. Valpey's presentation，he never managed to enter in such deep and rich areas in his study.

impregnated with love and hard sweat of the author, translators, editor, typesetter and all the other teachers and friends who helped in the process of translation and publication. Lotos Publishing House, Croatia, granted the Chinese translation copyright for free; Mr. Param Tomanec, a photographer from Czech Republic, offered eight wonderful photos; Miss Li Danyang did the most basic translation work for the book, consulting the author many times and trying to make it perfect. Prof. Valpey, the author, told me to express his gratitude to all our friends, especially Mr. Wan Bin, for the hard work of him and his colleagues in Yunnan University Press that have brought this book to the light of day. And although it is not for us to say, the author insists that we also register his deep thanks for my dedicated help in translation as well as for Miss Li Danyang's dedicated help.

Of course, we the translators appreciate that Prof. Valpey has written this book, and we anticipate that you, the reader, will also appreciate his writing as you progress through it. Indeed, you may find yourself being welcomed to enter the world of Bhakti Yoga, to enjoy a tour of this world to your heart's content, led by a patient guide.

We tried our best to make the translation faithful to the original and convey the beauty of it. However, due to limitation of knowledge and experience, there might be some mistakes in the translation. We kindly ask for the grant of instruction from all the readers. Thank you so much !

Li Yuwei

December 19th, 2018

Beijing, China